THE
EVERYTHING
VEGAN MEAL PREP
COOKBOOK

Dear Reader,

I can't recall the first time I heard the word *vegan*, but I do remember reading about it. I had been eating a vegetarian diet for years, and I thought a vegan diet was too much. Wasn't giving up meat enough? Why should I give up dairy, cheese, and eggs too?

My body gave me the answer: because I was diagnosed with IBS (Irritable Bowel Syndrome). I had experienced a lifetime of stomach issues, beginning with acid reflux in my childhood and evolving to gallbladder disease in my twenties. The gallbladder disease was easily cured through surgery, but I was flummoxed by IBS.

That's when my real journey into veganism began. I call myself a "secular" vegan because I focus on the passion I feel for delicious vegan food and improved health and well-being, rather than on the rigid rules that some stick to when eating vegan.

Whatever your reasons for learning about veganism, you've come to the right place! This book will provide you with all of the basics of veganism, including what it means, the many health benefits, and tips for delicious vegan meals. You'll find some recipes that are whole-foods based and others that are more on the indulgent side, so enjoy!

Marly McMillen Beelman

Welcome to the EVERYTHING® Series!

These handy, accessible books give you all you need to tackle a difficult project, gain a new hobby, comprehend a fascinating topic, prepare for an exam, or even brush up on something you learned back in school but have since forgotten.

You can choose to read an Everything® book from cover to cover or just pick out the information you want from our four useful boxes: e-questions, e-facts, e-alerts, and e-ssentials.

We give you everything you need to know on the subject, but throw in a lot of fun stuff along the way too.

We now have more than 400 Everything® books in print, spanning such wide-ranging categories as weddings, pregnancy, cooking, music instruction, foreign language, crafts, pets, New Age, and so much more. When you're done reading them all, you can finally say you know Everything®!

QUESTION

Answers to
common questions

FACT

Important snippets
of information

ALERT

Urgent
warnings

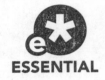

ESSENTIAL

Quick
handy tips

PUBLISHER Karen Cooper

MANAGING EDITOR Lisa Laing

COPY CHIEF Casey Ebert

ASSOCIATE PRODUCTION EDITOR Jo-Anne Duhamel

ACQUISITIONS EDITORS Lisa Laing, Alexander Hatch

DEVELOPMENT EDITOR Sarah Doughty

EVERYTHING® SERIES COVER DESIGNER Erin Alexander

Visit the entire Everything® series at www.everything.com

THE
EVERYTHING®
VEGAN MEAL PREP COOKBOOK

Marly McMillen Beelman

Adams Media

New York London Toronto Sydney New Delhi

For Shawn and Adee, who inspire me to live a healthy, happy, and long life. Also, for those with even a mild curiosity about a vegan diet. May this book inspire your curiosity into action.

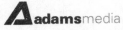

Adams Media
An Imprint of Simon & Schuster, Inc.
57 Littlefield Street
Avon, Massachusetts 02322

An Everything® Series Book.
Everything® and everything.com® are registered trademarks of Simon & Schuster, Inc.

First Adams Media trade paperback edition April 2019

ADAMS MEDIA and colophon are trademarks of Simon & Schuster.

For information about special discounts for bulk purchases, please contact Simon & Schuster Special Sales at 1-866-506-1949 or business@ simonandschuster.com.

The Simon & Schuster Speakers Bureau can bring authors to your live event. For more information or to book an event contact the Simon & Schuster Speakers Bureau at 1-866-248-3049 or visit our website at www.simonspeakers .com.

Interior images by Shawn Beelman

Manufactured in the United States of America

10 9 8 7 6 5 4 3 2 1

Library of Congress Cataloging-in-Publication Data
Names: Beelman, Marly McMillen, author.
Title: The everything® vegan meal prep cookbook / Marly McMillen Beelman.
Description: Avon, Massachusetts: Adams Media, 2019.
Series: Everything®.
Includes bibliographical references and index.
Identifiers: LCCN 2018056082 | ISBN 9781507210178 (pb) | ISBN 9781507210185 (ebook)
Subjects: LCSH: Vegetarian cooking. | Cooking (Natural foods) | LCGFT: Cookbooks.
Classification: LCC TX837 .B393 2019 | DDC 641.5/636--dc23
LC record available at https://lccn.loc .gov/2018056082

ISBN 978-1-5072-1017-8
ISBN 978-1-5072-1018-5 (ebook)

Contents

Introduction

VEGANISM AND MEAL PREPPING are about more than just food, they are about creating an achievable, healthy, and affordable lifestyle. As you may know, veganism offers many health benefits, from boosting weight loss to preventing heart disease, while meal prepping focuses on creating healthy meals that can be stored and enjoyed for days, weeks, or even months. What you may not know, however, is that when veganism and meal prepping join forces, they become quite the dynamic duo. Together, they create easy, delectable, and surprisingly healthy dishes that are ready whenever you need them!

In fact, since store-bought vegan meat replacement products are pre-cooked, the first steps in many meal prepping recipes are eliminated. With meal prepping, you can also make tons of easy recipes to mix and match throughout the week, so you'll never be bored. Plus, prepping vegan recipes can reduce unhealthy temptations. Instead of being enticed to make a last-minute run for takeout, you'll have a refrigerator full of delicious meals and snacks calling your name.

But where do you start? Where do you even buy vegan foods? How do you store meals so they last? Fear not! Whether you are new to the vegan diet, are already vegan and looking for meal prep advice, or are looking for more vegan meal prep recipes to spice up your repertoire, *The Everything® Vegan Meal Prep Cookbook* is here to guide you. In this book, you'll discover everything you need to know about both veganism and prepping meals, from what foods are included in the vegan diet and how to use them to how to store your prepared dishes so they stay fresh longer. You'll also find 300 easy-to-follow recipes, plus a two-week meal prepping plan to get you started. From breakfast scrambles and hearty chilis to savory salads and rich chocolate cake, your new favorite recipes are waiting. Each recipe also provides storage instructions.

With *The Everything® Vegan Meal Prep Cookbook*, preparing flavorful, healthy vegan dishes is a snap! Ready to get started?

CHAPTER 1

Vegan Basics

If you're looking to eat healthier and feel better, veganism is the diet for you. Your next thought is probably: "Veganism is a little too restrictive for me." It's true that there are restrictions with the vegan diet—but there are also a lot of benefits! This chapter will help you navigate the ins and outs of the vegan diet, from what it means exactly to what health benefits it offers and more. Soon you'll forget you ever missed those non-vegan ingredients!

Breaking Down the Vegan Diet

Eating a vegan diet essentially means that you don't consume products made from animals. This includes meat such as beef, pork, poultry, and fish; animal-based dairy; and animal by-products such as gelatin.

FACT

Gelatin is a protein derived from the skin, cartilage, and/or bones of animals. That means any product that uses gelatin, such as marshmallows, is not considered vegan. However, more and more companies are removing gelatin from their products, so check labels as you shop. There are also great plant-based alternatives to gelatin, such as agar-agar, which is derived from red algae.

That's a lot to take in. No ice cream? No scrambled eggs for breakfast? No sausage or pulled pork? No buttery biscuits with creamy gravy? This diet seems like a buzzkill: a boring, restricted lifestyle. However, imagine this scenario: You sit down to a plate with a pulled "pork" barbecue sandwich and sides of French fries, coleslaw, and grilled corn on the cob. Afterward you enjoy a slice of chocolate layered cake with chocolate frosting and a scoop or two of ice cream. Does this sound like deprivation? No! And here's the kicker: it's all vegan.

The "Secular" Vegan

Some people choose to keep their vegan diet at this level: cutting out primarily meat, dairy, and eggs. This is what you may call a "Secular" Vegan. You may even find you want to eat vegan on certain days of the week, or certain times of the day (such as the VB6 schedule, or "vegan before 6 p.m.")—and that's fine too! Your vegan experience is entirely up to you.

If you do eventually choose to take your vegan diet to the next level, you will be cutting out things like honey and refined sugar. That's because honey is made by animals, while some refined sugars are processed using animal bone char. Refined sugar is found in many commercial products, from condiments to breakfast cereals. If you do decide to cut out honey and refined sugar, just be sure to read labels carefully.

Accidental Vegan

As you dive into veganism, you may hear the phrase "accidentally vegan." But what does that even mean? Simply put, accidentally vegan foods are commercially produced foods that weren't created with the intention of being vegan, but as luck would have it, they are! These foods can be less easy to spot than those marked as "Certified Vegan" (products that were intentionally made vegan), so check out the list of accidentally vegan foods and ingredients in Appendix B so you can shop with confidence. You'd be surprised by some of the items, like Oreos, pudding, and cake mixes, that are accidentally vegan!

ESSENTIAL

If you're worried about getting enough protein from a vegan diet, have no fear: There are a number of easy ways to include protein in your vegan meals! Many plant-based ingredients are great sources of protein, from beans and tofu, to quinoa, nuts, and plant-based protein powders. By eating a variety of plant-based foods, you'll have nothing to worry about.

One word of caution: Sometimes the ingredients in a favorite accidentally vegan product will change. It's never a bad idea to double-check a product's ingredients list to make sure the company hasn't recently added a non-vegan ingredient.

The Benefits of the Vegan Diet

Before diving into the how and why of meal planning, it's helpful to know all the benefits of the vegan diet. Of course, being kind to our furry, feathery, and scaly friends is a big one, but there are many other benefits you may not have realized, from helping the planet to improving your health. (And remember, as a secular vegan you can choose how strict or flexible you want to be with the diet, so focus on what feels right for you and your body.)

Reduced Environmental Impact

Did you know that every day you enjoy a vegan diet, you are saving over 1,000 gallons of water and over 30 square feet of forested land? Plants grow naturally with soil and sunshine, but animals require food—and a lot of it. The meat industry uses a lot more resources, like water, grains, and land, to produce less food when compared to the production of plant-based items like rice, beans, and vegetables. The waste emitted from meat production is also one of the largest contributors to global warming. In fact, The UN estimates that about 20 percent of all greenhouse gases comes from the food animal industry. By eliminating meat from your diet, you're reducing your carbon footprint and saving tons of environmental resources!

Weight Loss

The whole- and plant-based foods provided in the vegan diet are a great start toward any weight loss goals! In fact studies have shown that those who followed a vegan diet lost on average 5 pounds more than those who followed a standard omnivore diet. This is primarily because the vegan diet focuses on nutrient-dense ingredients such as greens, vegetables, beans, and nuts that promote weight loss.

Greens and vegetables are loaded with fiber, which improves your gut flora (microorganisms in the digestive tract that control metabolism) and helps you feel full longer. And many greens and vegetables are low in calories! Beans and nuts are also packed with healthy fiber, as well as protein that boosts metabolism and promotes muscle growth. In addition, nuts also contain healthy fats that can prevent belly fat.

ESSENTIAL

A vegan diet can be as healthy or as unhealthy as you make it. Focus on foods that feature filling, nutritious ingredients like beans, vegetables, fruits, and nuts that satisfy your daily nutritional needs. Make these part of your go-to favorite dishes, and then accessorize your meal plan with more indulgent vegan recipes like "pepperoni" pizza and red velvet cookies.

Heart Benefits

The vegan diet is also good for your heart! Studies show that eating a vegan diet can lower your cholesterol and blood pressure levels, and balance your blood sugar levels.

Cholesterol is essential in building strong cells, promoting digestion, and enabling your body to produce vitamin D and certain hormones. Your body produces "good" cholesterol (or HDL) naturally, while the "bad" cholesterol (or "LDL) that contributes to a number of health problems is found in external sources such as meat, dairy, and processed foods. On a vegan diet, you are cutting out those sources of bad cholesterol. Consuming less meat also lowers your blood pressure, as a main cause of high blood pressure is salt, which leads to narrower arteries, causing your blood to exert more force in order to flow through to your vital organs. Finally, your blood sugar can be balanced well on a vegan diet as the leading contributor to unbalanced blood sugar (refined sugar) is cut out or at least consumed in lower quantities.

Your cholesterol, blood pressure, and blood sugar levels are all important factors in heart health, as an imbalance in any of these levels can cause serious issues such as diabetes or heart disease.

FACT

Believe bad genes are out of your hands? The truth is your genes are more closely tied to your diet than you may think! Dr. Dean Ornish, founder of Preventive Medicine Research Institute, discovered in his studies that being on a plant-based diet for just three months changed over 500 genes. Changes included turning on genes that prevent certain diseases and turning off genes that cause breast cancer and prostate cancer.

Reduced Risk of Cancer

Studies have also shown that those who eat a vegan diet also have a reduced risk of certain cancers (including breast, colon, and prostate cancer) than those who regularly eat meat. The main reason for this is that consumption of animal-based proteins such as beef and pork increases a cancer-promoting growth hormone called IGF-1. IGF-1 (Insulin-like Growth Factor 1) is created naturally in the human body and is critical to development. However, when the body contains greater amounts, such as through eating meat, it can lead to the growth of cancerous cells.

In addition, the vegan diet focuses heavily on the consumption of vegetables, which contain a number of cancer-fighting properties such as carotenoids, beta-carotene, and flavones. These organic pigments are what give things like carrots their color. They also act as powerful antioxidants that combat the growth of cancerous cells while promoting the growth of healthy cells. Reducing or eliminating animal-based proteins from your diet, combined with an increased consumption of healthy vegetables and beans, is a prescription for a healthier life!

CHAPTER 2

Meal Prep 101

In a perfect world, you would be able to cook all your meals fresh at home and sit down to eat them at your leisure, but in today's modern society, that's not the case. Most people eat their meals in a variety of places—at home, at work, and even in the car. There are restaurants everywhere and lots of options for takeout, but unfortunately, most of these options don't fall in line with a healthy eating plan, let alone a vegan diet. Because of this, preparing healthy meals in advance—lovingly referred to as meal prepping—is absolutely essential to meeting your goals.

The Science of Meal Prepping

Before jumping into the how of meal prepping, it's helpful to discuss the why. Is there actually a proven benefit to meal prepping? The answer is yes. There are several benefits. Research has found that people who meal prep tend to consume a greater variety of food and have a significantly greater intake of vegetables, salads, and fruits when compared with those who don't meal prep.

In addition, those who spend at least one hour per day (at least seven hours per week) preparing food in advance spend significantly less money on food than those who spend less than an hour each day planning their meals.

Other research found that when you meal prep, you're far more likely to stick to your nutritional guidelines. This is especially helpful when following a vegan diet because there are no surprises. When you know exactly what's in your meals, you know exactly what you're eating and you know that it has no animal products in it.

Aside from the scientific research, there's lots of anecdotal evidence on the benefits of meal prepping. Meal prepping equates to less stress around food since you always know what you're eating and when. Meal prepping also ultimately saves time. You may have to spend a few hours a week preparing your meals for the upcoming days, but you don't have to cook and wash dishes every night after a long day. The trade-off is worth it.

Getting Organized

When it comes to meal prepping, organization is the key to your success. It may seem like a lot of work in the beginning, but the time you take to get yourself organized is time well spent, so don't skip these steps. It's common to prepare meals for three to four days or even the entire week. The number of meals you prepare and the number of days/hours you spend cooking is entirely up to you. No matter what plan you choose, organization is key.

Designing Your Plan

One of the most effective things you can do to get organized is to design your meal plan. You can start on a week-to-week basis, or you can design a schedule for the entire month. Either way, you want to write down exactly what you'll be having for every meal and every snack. You can keep it basic with a notebook and a pen or utilize online meal planners and trackers. There are many free options available. If you're just starting out, it may take a little while to find the system that works best for you, but the more you do this, the easier it will become.

Your schedule may vary, but it's common to set aside an hour or so on a Sunday to sit down, write out your meals, collect the recipes you'll be using, and get your grocery list together. When you start meal planning, it's tempting to go a little overboard looking for fancy recipes or trying to incorporate a lot of variety, but the best thing you can do, at least in the beginning, is keep it simple. Most of the recipes in this book make four or more servings with easy-to-find ingredients, so if you're meal prepping for one, it takes only a handful of recipes to get you through the bulk of the week.

Writing Your Grocery List

Before writing your grocery list, check your pantry and your refrigerator to see what you have on hand. Make a note of what you already have so you don't pick up extra. (One of the goals is to eliminate waste!) If you prefer, you can even take stock of your refrigerator and pantry before writing your meal plan for the week so you can choose recipes that use up most of the items that you already have on hand.

When you write your grocery list, organize the items on your list by where they are found in the grocery store. That way, you don't have to spend time backtracking while you're shopping or constantly rereading your list to make sure you have everything. Put all produce items together, all canned items together, and so on. If there are any specialty items that you need to purchase at separate stores or online, put those items on a separate list and categorize them by store/website.

Ordering in Bulk

When you meal prep, you often use some of the same basic ingredients—like olive oil, almond flour, and coconut milk, for example—repeatedly. You can save yourself time and even money by purchasing these items in larger quantities and stocking up your freezer and pantry. If you don't have one already, purchasing a membership to a wholesale club is a great way to save money and to find these staples in bulk all in one place. Most wholesale clubs are catching on to the growing interest in clean and healthy eating and offering plenty of options for consumers.

ESSENTIAL

Often, stores like T.J. Maxx, Marshalls, and HomeGoods have a food section where you can find specialty food items like coconut oil, coconut flour, avocado oil, nuts, and nut butters for a great price. These stores are constantly changing their inventory, so it's worth a peek to see what they have on a regular basis and stock up on any items that you need or want to try.

Like wholesale clubs, several different websites offer memberships that allow you to purchase healthy food items at a discount. Other websites provide items already discounted and offer periodic discount codes that deepen your savings. Bookmark your favorite websites and check them regularly for sales. When an item that you use regularly goes on sale, purchase a few extra and keep them on hand for when you need them.

Frozen Vegetables

Frozen vegetables are often cheaper than fresh produce, and you can store them longer. As an added bonus, frozen vegetables are often more nutritious because they were picked at peak freshness and frozen immediately, which preserves their nutrients. On the other hand, fresh produce begins losing nutrients as soon as it's picked, and if you purchase it in your local grocery store, sometimes it's been weeks since its picking date. Watch out for sales on frozen vegetables and stock up your freezer when you can.

Storing Your Meals

When meal prepping, proper storage is vital to making sure your food stays fresh and tasty. Proper storage is also helpful if you have to take your meals with you on the go. Spending a little extra time dividing your meals into portions before storing them will save you lots of time when you're ready to eat.

After cooking your meals and sides, divide them into equal portions and put each completed meal in an airtight container. Many of these recipes are designed so that you can pick and choose which items you want to put together. Others are a complete meal on their own.

Once meals are assembled, use a piece of tape to label each meal—Monday breakfast, Monday lunch, Monday dinner, and so on. Many of the meals can also be frozen for later. In addition to taking the time to label food properly, it's important to have the right storage containers. Many companies make airtight stainless steel and glass containers so you can store your food without exposure to plastic. If you choose plastic containers, look for some that are BPA-free and have lids that securely lock in place to keep your food fresh and prevent spills when you're on the go.

Reheating Stored Food

The best way to reheat your stored food to retain moisture and flavor is to warm it through slowly. The easiest way to do this is in a medium skillet on the stovetop or in the oven. If using a skillet, add a little olive oil or vegan butter to the pan and heat on low until food reaches your desired temperature. If using the oven, reheat with the temperature around 250°F and keep a watchful eye on your meal. If you have a toaster oven, you can use that instead of a conventional oven.

Microwaves are quick and easy, but in some cases, you may be sacrificing flavor and texture for convenience. If using a microwave, reheat in thirty-second intervals, making sure to stir your food and check the temperature as you go because microwaves cook—and can overcook—food quickly.

The Importance of Food Quality

The National Academy of Sciences reports that 90 percent of chemicals applied to foods have never been tested for food safety. When there is no information available on how something will affect you long-term, it's best to go by what healthcare professionals call "the precautionary principle"—in other words, when in doubt, leave it out. When following any diet, it's best to choose organic foods that are free of pesticides and as close to their natural state as possible.

When choosing vegetables, buy organic whenever possible. If purchasing all organic isn't in your budget, consider what the Environmental Working Group calls the Dirty Dozen Plus. The list includes:

- Strawberries
- Spinach
- Nectarines
- Apples
- Grapes
- Peaches
- Cherries
- Pears
- Tomatoes
- Celery
- Potatoes
- Bell peppers
- Hot peppers

These are the fruits and vegetables most likely to contain high levels of pesticides. Prioritize purchasing organic versions of these whenever possible.

Once you get into the groove of meal prepping for a vegan diet, you're going to wonder why you didn't start sooner. You'll experience lower levels of stress, you'll save money, you'll consume a wider variety of nutrients, and you'll be lowering your risk of diabetes and heart disease. That's a combination that can't be beat.

CHAPTER 3

Breakfast

Blueberry Overnight Oats

Overnight oats are a perfect way to start your meal prepping journey. Combine the ingredients to this simple recipe on a Sunday night and enjoy a tasty, healthy, and easy breakfast on Monday and Tuesday. Repeat throughout the week!

INGREDIENTS | SERVES 2

1 cup rolled oats, divided

1 tablespoon chia seeds

2 tablespoons almonds

1½ cups water

2 teaspoons stevia

1 teaspoon vanilla extract

½ cup fresh blueberries, divided

1 tablespoon granola

1. Add 1 tablespoon oats, chia seeds, almonds, water, stevia, and vanilla to a blender. Blend until smooth to create a "milk" base. Add ¼ cup blueberries to "milk" and pulse until smooth.

2. Add remaining oats to a large bowl. Pour "milk" mixture over oats. Stir to combine. Pour oats into two medium sealed containers. Refrigerate at least 2 hours, up to 5 days.

3. Serve hot or cold, topped with granola and remaining fresh blueberries.

PER SERVING Calories: 303 | Fat: 9.5 g | Protein: 10.23 g | Sodium: 6 mg | Fiber: 9.0 g | Carbohydrates: 43.8 g | Sugar: 6.0 g

Peanut Butter Overnight Oats

Peanut butter makes for a delicious and healthy addition to this overnight oats recipe. It's the perfect filling breakfast, but you can also enjoy it as a snack or even dessert.

INGREDIENTS | SERVES 2

1 cup rolled oats

2 tablespoons chia seeds

2 tablespoons peanut butter powder

2 teaspoons stevia

1½ cups unsweetened almond milk

2 tablespoons dairy-free chocolate chips, chopped

2 tablespoons granola

½ cup fresh banana slices

1. Add rolled oats, chia seeds, peanut butter powder, and stevia to a large bowl. Stir to combine. Add milk to mixture. Stir to combine.

2. Pour into two medium sealed containers. Refrigerate at least 2 hours, up to 5 days.

3. Serve warm or cold, topped with chocolate chips, granola, and banana slices.

PER SERVING Calories: 417 | Fat: 14.8 g | Protein: 13.7 g | Sodium: 198 mg | Fiber: 12.2 g | Carbohydrates: 60.5 g | Sugar: 14.2 g

German Chocolate Overnight Oats

Make breakfast an indulgence with these German Chocolate Overnight Oats. The simple process in this recipe makes it an easy addition in your everyday life.

INGREDIENTS | SERVES 2

1 cup rolled oats

4 tablespoons chocolate vegan protein powder

2 tablespoons cocoa powder

2 tablespoons chia seeds

2 teaspoons stevia

1½ cups unsweetened vanilla almond milk

1 teaspoon coconut oil, divided

2 tablespoons unsweetened coconut flakes, divided

2 tablespoons slivered almonds, divided

3 teaspoons dairy-free chocolate chips, divided

Plant-Based Milks

Almond milk is just one of the many plant-based milks out there! Others include soy, coconut, cashew, oatmeal, and hemp. You can make your own to avoid last-minute trips to the grocery store when you run out. Check out the recipe in Chapter 7 for Easy Homemade Oat Milk!

1. Add rolled oats, protein powder, cocoa powder, chia seeds, and stevia to a large bowl. Stir to combine.

2. Pour almond milk over oatmeal mixture. Stir to combine.

3. Pour equal amounts mixture into two medium lidded containers. Refrigerate at least 2 hours, up to 5 days.

4. For a single serving, place ½ coconut oil in a medium skillet over medium heat. Add ½ coconut flakes and ½ slivered almonds. Cook approximately 3 minutes, stirring occasionally, until coconut flakes and almonds are toasted.

5. Top one container overnight oats with toasted coconut flakes, almonds, and ½ chocolate chips. Repeat topping instructions for second batch.

PER SERVING Calories: 421 | Fat: 20.4 g | Protein: 15.0 g | Sodium: 169 mg | Fiber: 13.6 g | Carbohydrates: 48.6 g | Sugar: 5.9 g

Peanut Butter Pecan Granola

Granola is an essential in a vegan kitchen because of its versatility as either a nutritious, filling breakfast, or a delicious topping on things like smoothies and desserts. Make this granola and store it in your cupboard for an easy breakfast served with almond milk or over dairy-free yogurt, or even served plain as a snack.

INGREDIENTS | SERVES 12

6 cups rolled oats
1 cup pecans, roughly chopped
1 cup almonds
½ cup pumpkin seeds
½ cup maple syrup
½ cup creamy peanut butter
2 tablespoons coconut oil
1 cup raisins

Nuts and Seeds for Weight Loss

A 2010 study in *Nutrients* confirmed that including nuts and seeds in your diet is important for your health. Some people avoid nuts because they believe nuts contribute to weight gain. However, studies show that nuts are nutrient-dense foods full of fiber and other bioactive compounds, and that regular consumption may even help with weight loss.

1. Preheat oven to 300°F. Line two large baking sheets with parchment paper.

2. Add oats, pecans, almonds, and seeds to a large bowl. Stir to combine.

3. In a small microwave-safe bowl add syrup, peanut butter, and coconut oil. Stir to combine. Heat mixture in microwave for 11-second increments until smooth enough to pour. Pour over oat mixture and stir, ensuring oats and nuts are coated.

4. Pour granola mixture onto prepared pans, distributing equally across each pan. Place pans in oven and bake 10 minutes.

5. Remove pans from oven and stir mixture. Return to oven and bake another 8 minutes until granola is golden brown.

6. Remove pans from oven and add raisins. Stir and then set aside to cool 15 minutes.

7. Store granola in a large airtight container at room temperature up to 14 days, in refrigerator up to 1 month, or freezer up to 2 months.

PER SERVING Calories: 492 | Fat: 23.3 g | Protein: 13.7 g | Sodium: 5 mg | Fiber: 8.9 g | Carbohydrates: 59.3 g | Sugar: 19.1 g

Easy Vegan Tofu Scramble

If you love the flavor and texture of scrambled eggs, this tofu scramble is a perfect substitution for you. It's a savory dish that you can serve with toast for a simple, hearty breakfast any morning. This recipe is a staple that you'll return to time and time again.

INGREDIENTS | SERVES 4

1 (15-ounce) package extra-firm tofu
1 teaspoon olive oil
½ cup water
¼ cup nutritional yeast flakes
½ teaspoon ground turmeric
½ teaspoon paprika
1 teaspoon garlic powder
1 teaspoon mild miso paste
1 tablespoon ground flaxseed

Understanding Tofu

There are a variety of tofu types. The most common is extra-firm or firm, found in the produce section of many grocery stores. Some recipes use silken tofu, which is sold in a hermetically sealed container and can be found in the health food section of your grocery store.

1. Wrap tofu in paper towels. Stand over sink and press tofu gently to remove excess liquid.

2. Place olive oil in a medium skillet over medium-high heat. Add pressed tofu, breaking it up into smaller pieces. Cook about 5 minutes, stirring occasionally.

3. In a small bowl combine water, yeast, turmeric, paprika, garlic powder, miso, and flaxseed.

4. Pour mixture over tofu and stir to coat. Reduce heat to medium and cook until sauce is absorbed by tofu, about 5 minutes.

5. Let cool 10 minutes, then store tofu scramble in a large lidded container in refrigerator up to 5 days. To serve, cook in microwave in 30-second intervals until heated through.

PER SERVING Calories: 137 | Fat: 7.8 g | Protein: 13.2 g | Sodium: 74 mg | Fiber: 2.0 g | Carbohydrates: 5.2 g | Sugar: 0.8 g

Breakfast Biscuit Casserole

This indulgent vegan breakfast casserole boasts layers of biscuit, vegan sausage crumbles, scrambled tofu, and melted cheese. Make it on the weekend and refrigerate or freeze individual servings to enjoy later.

INGREDIENTS | SERVES 10

2 cups all-purpose flour

4 teaspoons baking powder

¼ teaspoon baking soda

1 teaspoon salt

⅓ cup dairy-free margarine, sliced

⅔ cup plain soy milk

2 teaspoons apple cider vinegar

2 cups vegan sausage crumbles

1 batch Easy Vegan Tofu Scramble (see this chapter for recipe)

1 cup vegan Cheddar shreds

1. Preheat oven to 400°F. Spray a 9" × 13" baking dish with vegetable spray.

2. Place flour, baking powder, baking soda, and salt in a food processor. Pulse 4 seconds to combine. Add margarine, soy milk, and vinegar. Pulse again 3 seconds until combined. Press mixture evenly across bottom of prepared pan.

3. Spread vegan sausage crumbles evenly over top of biscuit layer. Spread scrambled tofu over sausage crumbles. Top with shredded vegan cheese. Cover pan with aluminum foil.

4. Place pan in oven. Bake 30 minutes.

5. Remove from oven. Let cool completely, about 20 minutes, before covering with foil or plastic wrap. Store in refrigerator up to 7 days. Alternatively cut into individual slices and freeze up to 2 months.

6. To serve, heat individual slices in microwave in 30-second intervals until heated through.

PER SERVING Calories: 236 | Fat: 9.4 g | Protein: 11.7 g | Sodium: 772 mg | Fiber: 2.7 g | Carbohydrates: 26.2 g | Sugar: 0.7 g

Cheesy Vegan Breakfast Burritos

Make these flavorful vegan breakfast burritos with savory scrambled tofu, hash brown potatoes, and vegan cheese. Freeze individual burritos and reheat for a quick and satisfying weekday breakfast.

INGREDIENTS | SERVES 6

1 tablespoon vegetable oil

1 (14-ounce) bag frozen hash brown potatoes, thawed

½ teaspoon salt

⅛ teaspoon ground black pepper

6 (10") flour tortillas

1 cup vegan Cheddar shreds

1 batch Easy Vegan Tofu Scramble (see this chapter for recipe)

Freezing Individual Servings

There are multiple ways of freezing individual servings. You can store each serving in a freezer-safe container. Alternatively, you can wrap each serving in plastic wrap or aluminum foil. Finally, you can place individual servings on a tray and place the tray in the freezer. Once the servings on the tray are frozen, transfer them to a freezer bag and place the bag in the freezer.

1. Add oil to a medium skillet over medium-high heat. Add hash brown potatoes. Cook until potatoes are browned on both sides, about 10 minutes total. Sprinkle with salt and pepper.

2. Assemble burritos by distributing hash browns evenly in center of each tortilla. Top with equal amounts cheese and tofu scramble. Turn up tortilla ends, then fold bottom half over top and roll tightly.

3. Let cool 10 minutes, then freeze burritos by wrapping each in foil. Place in a freezer bag and freeze up to 2 months. To reheat, remove foil and place burrito on a plate in microwave. Heat 3 minutes on high.

PER SERVING Calories: 362 | Fat: 15.0 g | Protein: 14.1 g | Sodium: 784 mg | Fiber: 4.2 g | Carbohydrates: 44.3 g | Sugar: 2.2 g

Vegan Bacon and Cheese Breakfast Sandwiches

Breakfast doesn't have to be complicated, and these hearty breakfast sandwiches are a perfect example. Vegan bacon takes the stage, topped with grilled onion, tofu scramble, and vegan Cheddar cheese.

INGREDIENTS | SERVES 6

6 vegan English muffins, sliced in half

1 teaspoon vegetable oil

¼ medium red onion, peeled and thinly sliced

12 slices vegan bacon

1 batch Easy Vegan Tofu Scramble (see this chapter for recipe)

6 slices vegan Cheddar cheese

Where Do I Find Vegan Bread Products?

You can find vegan bread products at a variety of stores, including your local grocery store. Simply read the ingredients and look for things like milk, casein, and eggs. Oftentimes, dairy will be listed as an allergen if it's included in the ingredients.

1. Toast English muffins in toaster oven 4 minutes until golden brown.

2. Add oil to a medium skillet over medium-high heat. Add onion. Stir and cook 5 minutes until onion is tender. Remove from skillet.

3. Add vegan bacon to skillet and cook 4 minutes on each side. Let cool 5 minutes, then slice in half.

4. Distribute tofu scramble equally onto English muffin bottoms. Top with vegan cheese slices, followed by cooked onions. Distribute bacon pieces over onions. Place tops of English muffins on bacon pieces.

5. Wrap each sandwich in aluminum foil. Place in a freezer bag and freeze up to 2 months. To serve, remove foil, place sandwich on plate, and microwave on high 4 minutes until thawed and cheese is melted.

PER SERVING Calories: 319 | Fat: 13.1 g | Protein: 16.9 g | Sodium: 675 mg | Fiber: 4.2 g | Carbohydrates: 36.4 g | Sugar: 2.9 g

Sweet Potato Biscuit Sandwiches

Sweet potatoes bring a touch of sweetness to this savory recipe. Biscuits are transformed into slider-sized sandwiches with layers of smoky potato, tofu scramble, and melted vegan cheese.

INGREDIENTS | SERVES 8

1 medium sweet potato, perforated with a fork

2 tablespoons liquid smoke sauce, divided

2 tablespoons agave nectar

½ teaspoon salt

1 batch Homemade Vegan Biscuits (see Chapter 4 for recipe)

1 batch Easy Vegan Tofu Scramble (see this chapter for recipe)

8 slices vegan Cheddar cheese

What Is Parchment Paper?

Parchment paper is a specially treated paper made for use in the oven. It makes cleanup much easier. Use it on baking sheets, in cake pans, and even in the bottom of cupcake tins. You can buy parchment paper in rolls or even precut sheets in most grocery stores.

1. Preheat oven to 400°F. Cover a large baking pan with parchment paper.

2. Place potato in microwave and cook on high heat 2 minutes until tender. Remove and set aside to cool slightly 3 minutes.

3. Add olive oil and 1 tablespoon liquid smoke to a large skillet over medium heat. Peel cooled potato, then cut into 8 slices. Place slices in skillet. Pour remaining liquid smoke and agave nectar over slices. Cook 4 minutes until bottom is golden, then flip and cook other side another 4 minutes. Sprinkle with salt and set aside to cool.

4. Slice biscuits in half. Place bottom half of each biscuit back on baking sheet. Top with sweet potato slice, followed by tofu scramble. Add one slice vegan cheese to each. Place pan back in oven 6 minutes to allow cheese to melt.

5. Remove from oven and place top half of biscuit on each sandwich. Let cool about 5 minutes before transferring to a large lidded container. Refrigerate 10 days, or freeze up to 2 months.

6. To serve, place biscuit sandwiches in a toaster oven and cook until heated through, about 5 minutes.

PER SERVING Calories: 388 | Fat: 13.0 g | Protein: 13.8 g | Sodium: 953 mg | Fiber: 3.7 g | Carbohydrates: 55.2 g | Sugar: 4.4 g

Easy Vegan Biscuits and Gravy

Here's a simple way to enjoy vegan biscuits and gravy—complete with vegan sausage.
Make this on the weekends and enjoy a hearty breakfast any day of the week.

INGREDIENTS | SERVES 8

1 (16-ounce) can refrigerated vegan biscuits
1 teaspoon olive oil
1 (14-ounce) package vegan sausage
¼ cup all-purpose flour
3½ cups plain soy milk
2 teaspoons nutritional yeast flakes
1 teaspoon salt
½ teaspoon ground black pepper

Finding Specific Vegan Ingredients

Most of the ingredients in this cookbook are chosen specifically because of their availability. However, some specific ingredients, such as the vegan bacon and vegan sausage, can be purchased at health food stores or even online.

1. Bake biscuits according to package directions. Store in a large sealed container in refrigerator up to 7 days.

2. Add oil to a large skillet over medium heat. Add vegan sausage to skillet and break into pieces. Cook until sausage is crispy around the edges, about 10 minutes. Transfer to a paper towel.

3. In the same skillet, add in flour. Gradually add soy milk, stirring continuously. Simmer 3 minutes, until gravy forms. Add yeast, salt, and pepper, stirring to combine. Mix in sausage crumbles, then remove from heat.

4. Let cool 10 minutes, then pour sausage gravy into a large sealed container and store in refrigerator up to 7 days.

5. When ready to serve, heat one biscuit about 4 minutes in toaster oven. Heat ⅛ gravy in microwave about 30 seconds. Place biscuit on a medium plate and drizzle with warmed gravy.

PER SERVING Calories: 292 | Fat: 10.1 g | Protein: 12.4 g | Sodium: 1,053 mg | Fiber: 2.9 g | Carbohydrates: 34.8 g | Sugar: 5.4 g

Avocado Toast

Healthy recipes don't get much easier than this Avocado Toast. Use this basic recipe to create a delicious breakfast. Once you get the hang of it, be sure to experiment with toppings, like sliced tomatoes, chopped walnuts, mushrooms, and more.

INGREDIENTS | SERVES 4

4 slices whole-wheat bread
1 clove garlic, halved
2 medium avocados, halved and pitted
1 tablespoon nutritional yeast flakes
½ teaspoon salt
¼ teaspoon ground black pepper
1 teaspoon lemon juice
½ teaspoon dried chives

1. Toast bread in toaster oven 4 minutes.

2. While toast is still warm, rub cut side of halved garlic clove across one side of each toast slice. Transfer toast to a small sealed container and refrigerate up to 3 days.

3. Spoon avocado flesh into a large lidded bowl. Add remaining ingredients, using a fork to mash avocado and combine all ingredients. Place lid on container and refrigerate up to 3 days until ready to serve.

4. When ready to serve, remove one slice of toast per serving, and warm in a toaster oven 1 minute. Top with a generous portion of avocado spread.

PER SERVING Calories: 199 | Fat: 10.3 g | Protein: 5.9 g | Sodium: 442 | Fiber: 6.8 g | Carbohydrates: 20.3 g | Sugar: 1.6 g

Egg-Free Pancakes

You can make delicious, fluffy pancakes without eggs with this simple recipe.
Serve it for breakfast on a Sunday morning, and then freeze the leftovers
so you can heat them up for breakfast Monday through Friday.

INGREDIENTS | SERVES 8

2 tablespoons vegan butter

1 tablespoon chia seeds

1¼ cup vanilla almond milk

¼ cup unsweetened applesauce

2 tablespoons agave nectar

1 teaspoon vanilla extract

1¼ cups whole-wheat flour

2 teaspoons baking powder

½ teaspoon baking soda

¼ teaspoon salt

½ cup maple syrup

Cooking Without Eggs

Nervous about cooking without eggs? Don't be. Ingredients like ground flaxseed and chia seeds substitute well. An added bonus is that cooking without eggs reduces the amount of cholesterol in your finished dishes!

1. Place vegan butter in a medium microwave-safe bowl. Heat 30 seconds. Add chia seeds, almond milk, applesauce, agave, and vanilla. Stir to combine. Set aside.

2. In a separate large bowl combine flour, baking powder, baking soda, and salt.

3. Heat a large skillet greased with vegetable cooking spray over medium-high heat 30 seconds.

4. Pour almond milk mixture into dry ingredients and stir to combine. Some lumps are fine.

5. Once skillet is hot, pour in ¼ cup pancake batter. Cook about 4 minutes until bubbles form. Use a spatula to flip pancakes and cook other side another 3 minutes until golden brown. Set finished pancakes aside and repeat with remaining batter.

6. Place pancakes in a large sealed container and refrigerate up to 7 days. Alternatively, freeze up to 2 months.

7. To serve, heat pancakes in toaster oven 1 minute, then drizzle with maple syrup.

PER SERVING Calories: 162 | Fat: 2.2 g | Protein: 2.9 g | Sodium: 320 mg | Fiber: 2.7 g | Carbohydrates: 33.6 g | Sugar: 17.4 g

Banana Pancakes

These fluffy vegan Banana Pancakes are so moist, thanks to the bananas in the batter. You'll love them for your weekend breakfasts and brunches and also your weekday mornings.

INGREDIENTS | SERVES 12

6 tablespoons vegan butter, divided

2½ cups unsweetened almond milk

1 tablespoon apple cider vinegar

2 tablespoons chia seeds

2 teaspoons vanilla extract

1 cup peeled mashed bananas (about 2 medium)

2½ cups whole-wheat flour

1 tablespoon coconut sugar

1 tablespoon baking powder

½ teaspoon baking soda

¼ teaspoon salt

2 teaspoons vegetable oil, divided

½ cup maple syrup

1. In a large microwave-safe bowl add 3 tablespoons vegan butter. Microwave 30 seconds until melted. Add almond milk, vinegar, chia seeds, and vanilla to bowl. Stir to combine. Add mashed bananas and stir to combine.

2. In a medium bowl combine flour, sugar, baking powder, baking soda, and salt. Pour into banana mixture and stir until just combined.

3. Add 1 teaspoon vegetable oil to a large skillet over medium heat. Once surface is hot, about 30 seconds, add ¼ cup batter in skillet. Use back of measuring cup to flatten batter. Cook 4 minutes until bubbles form, then flip and cook another 2 minutes. Transfer to a large plate to cool and repeat steps with remaining oil and batter.

4. Place pancakes in a large sealed container and refrigerate up to 7 days. Alternatively, freeze up to 2 months.

5. To serve, heat pancakes in toaster oven 1 minute, top with remaining butter, then drizzle with maple syrup.

PER SERVING Calories: 187 | Fat: 4.7 g | Protein: 4.0 g | Sodium: 303 mg | Fiber: 4.0 g | Carbohydrates: 33.8 g | Sugar: 11.5 g

Whole-Wheat Vegan Waffles

Use a fork to cut through the crispy shell of these whole-wheat waffles and discover the tender, delicious center. These waffles are full of fiber but still remain light and fluffy. They can be served any time of day—just be sure to drizzle them with maple syrup!

INGREDIENTS | SERVES 12

1¾ cups whole-wheat pastry flour
2 tablespoons coconut sugar
1 teaspoon baking powder
½ teaspoon baking soda
1 tablespoon ground flaxseed
1½ cups unsweetened almond milk
1 tablespoon apple cider vinegar
2 tablespoons vegetable oil
1 teaspoon vanilla extract
½ cup maple syrup

Cooking with Whole-Wheat Pastry Flour

Whole-wheat pastry flour is milled from a softer wheat, resulting in a low-protein whole wheat. If whole wheat makes you think of thick, dense baked goods, you'll be pleasantly surprised by whole-wheat pastry flours. Look for it in the health food section of most grocery stores.

1. Turn on waffle iron and grease with vegetable cooking spray.

2. In a large bowl combine flour, sugar, baking powder, baking soda, and flaxseed.

3. In a separate large bowl combine almond milk, vinegar, oil, and vanilla. Pour into flour mixture and stir until just combined.

4. Dispense ¼ cup batter onto waffle iron. Use the back of measuring cup to spread the batter to edges of iron. Close lid and cook waffle 7 minutes until golden and crispy. Set waffle aside and repeat with remaining batter.

5. Place waffles in a large sealed container and refrigerate up to 7 days. Alternatively, freeze up to 2 months.

6. To serve, heat waffles in toaster oven 1 minute, then drizzle with maple syrup.

PER SERVING Calories: 134 | Fat: 2.8 g | Protein: 2.0 g | Sodium: 117 mg | Fiber: 2.6 g | Carbohydrates: 24.8 g | Sugar: 10.0 g

Vegan Chocolate Waffles

Crispy on the outside, tender on the inside, these Vegan Chocolate Waffles are served with chocolate-infused maple syrup. This recipe will make breakfast memorable!

INGREDIENTS | SERVES 5

For Waffles

2 tablespoons coconut oil, melted
2 tablespoons agave nectar
1¼ cup unsweetened vanilla almond milk
1 teaspoon vanilla extract
1¼ cups whole-wheat pastry flour
2 teaspoons baking soda
¼ cup cocoa powder
¼ teaspoon ground nutmeg
¼ teaspoon salt

For Chocolate Maple Syrup

¼ cup dairy-free chocolate chips
½ cup maple syrup

1. Turn on waffle iron and grease with vegetable cooking spray.

2. **To make Waffles:** in a large bowl combine coconut oil, agave nectar, almond milk, and vanilla.

3. In a separate large bowl combine flour, baking soda, cocoa powder, nutmeg, and salt. Pour milk mixture into flour mixture and stir until just combined.

4. Dispense ¼ cup batter onto waffle iron. Use the back of measuring cup to spread the batter to edges of iron. Close lid and cook waffle 7 minutes until golden and crispy. Set waffle aside and repeat with remaining batter.

5. **To make Chocolate Maple Syrup:** combine chocolate chips and maple syrup in a medium microwave-safe bowl and microwave 30 seconds. Stir until chocolate melts. Store in a lidded container in refrigerator until ready to use (up to 7 days).

6. Place waffles in a large sealed container and refrigerate 7 days. Alternatively, freeze up to 2 months.

7. To serve, heat waffles in toaster oven 1 minute. Heat chocolate maple syrup in microwave 30 seconds and stir, then drizzle over waffles.

PER SERVING Calories: 339 | Fat: 10.5 g | Protein: 4.4 g | Sodium: 669 mg | Fiber: 6.7 g | Carbohydrates: 57.9 g | Sugar: 27.9 g

Coffee Cake

This Coffee Cake is a perfect example of how vegan recipes can taste just as good as their dairy- and egg-laden counterparts. This recipe boasts a soft cake in the center, with a crumbly topping dotted with pumpkin seeds. It's the best way to start the day.

INGREDIENTS | SERVES 9

For Crumble Topping

½ cup packed light brown sugar
1 teaspoon ground cinnamon
⅛ teaspoon salt
½ cup vegan butter, softened
1½ cups all-purpose flour

For Coffee Cake

¾ cup vegan butter
1 cup granulated sugar
1 cup unsweetened almond milk
1 tablespoon ground flaxseed
1 tablespoon cornstarch
1 teaspoon apple cider vinegar
1½ cups all-purpose flour
2 teaspoons baking powder
½ teaspoon baking soda
½ teaspoon salt

1. Preheat oven to 350°F. Spray a 9" × 9" pan with vegetable cooking spray.

2. **To make Crumble Topping:** combine brown sugar, cinnamon, salt, vegan butter, and flour in a medium bowl. Stir until combined. Set aside.

3. **To make Coffee Cake:** in a large bowl cream together vegan butter and sugar. Add almond milk, flaxseed, cornstarch, and vinegar. Stir to combine.

4. In a medium bowl combine flour, baking powder, baking soda, and salt. Add flour mixture to milk mixture. Stir until just combined.

5. Pour batter into prepared baking dish. Evenly distribute crumble topping across top of batter. Bake for about 30 minutes until a toothpick inserted in the middle of the cake comes out clean. Crumble topping should be golden brown.

6. When done, remove from oven and let cool 15 minutes. Cover with a lid or plastic wrap and refrigerate up to 7 days. Alternatively, slice and freeze individual pieces up to 2 months.

7. To serve, heat in microwave in 30-second intervals until heated through.

PER SERVING Calories: 303 | Fat: 11.2 g | Protein: 3.1 g | Sodium: 432 mg | Fiber: 1.2 g | Carbohydrates: 45.5 g | Sugar: 22.3 g

Vegan French Toast

It may be hard to imagine an egg- and dairy-free French toast recipe, but this one will show you it's possible. It's an easy-to-make dish that yields six servings of deliciousness!

INGREDIENTS | SERVES 6

1½ cups vanilla soy milk

1 tablespoon all-purpose flour

1 tablespoon ground flaxseed

1 tablespoon + ½ cup maple syrup, divided

1 tablespoon nutritional yeast flakes

¼ teaspoon ground cinnamon

1 tablespoon coconut oil, divided

6 slices whole-wheat bread

1. Preheat oven to 350°F. Spray a large baking sheet with vegetable cooking spray.

2. Mix together milk, flour, flaxseed, 1 tablespoon maple syrup, nutritional yeast flakes, and cinnamon in a large bowl.

3. Add ½ coconut oil to a large skillet over medium-high heat. Dredge 3 bread slices in milk mixture, ensuring both sides are coated. Place soaked slices in skillet and cook until golden brown on bottom, about 5 minutes. Use a spatula to flip pieces and cook another 5 minutes. When done, remove from skillet and place on prepared baking sheet. Repeat process with remaining oil and slices of bread.

4. Bake finished French toast 10 minutes.

5. Remove from oven and let cool 10 minutes. Transfer to a large sealed container and refrigerate up to 7 days or freeze up to 2 months.

6. When ready to serve, cook in toaster oven 1 minute. Serve with maple syrup.

PER SERVING Calories: 210 | Fat: 4.5 g | Protein: 6.4 g | Sodium: 172 mg | Fiber: 2.8 g | Carbohydrates: 36.2 g | Sugar: 19.6 g

Baked Blackberry Donuts with Berry Glaze

Make this batch of vegan blackberry donuts in your oven and enjoy a dairy-free, egg-free breakfast treat in less than 30 minutes! Freeze the rest and reheat for a quick and satisfying treat for the rest of the week.

INGREDIENTS | SERVES 6

For Donuts
1 tablespoon ground flaxseed
3 tablespoons water
½ cup granulated sugar
1 cup vanilla almond milk
2 teaspoons apple cider vinegar
¼ cup vegan butter, melted
1½ cups all-purpose flour
1 teaspoon baking powder
¼ teaspoon baking soda
½ teaspoon ground nutmeg
½ cup fresh blackberries, chopped

For Berry Glaze
¾ cup powdered sugar
1 teaspoon coconut oil
4 fresh blackberries, finely chopped
2 teaspoons vanilla almond milk

Perfect Baked Donuts
There are two tricks to making perfect baked donuts. First, you'll need a donut pan, found in the bakeware section of many department stores. Second, adding a small amount of ground nutmeg gives baked donuts a distinctive donut taste.

1. Preheat oven to 350°F. Spray donut pan with vegetable cooking spray.

2. **To make Donuts:** in a large bowl combine flaxseed and water. Add sugar, 1 cup milk, vinegar, and butter. Stir to combine.

3. In a separate large bowl add flour, baking powder, baking soda, and nutmeg. Stir to combine. Gently pour chopped blackberries into flour mixture. Stir to combine. Pour in milk mixture and gently stir until just combined.

4. Pour batter into donut pan. Use a spoon to evenly distribute batter in each compartment, filling to the top. Bake 15 minutes until donuts are slightly golden on top. Remove from the oven and let cool 5 minutes.

5. **To make the Berry Glaze:** combine powdered sugar and coconut oil in a medium bowl. Add blackberries (along with juice) to mixture. Stir to combine. Add almond milk, one teaspoon at a time, until desired consistency is reached. Coat each donut with glaze and let icing set, about 10 minutes.

6. Store donuts in a large sealed container at room temperature up to 3 days, or in refrigerator up to 10 days. Alternatively, you can freeze them up to 2 months. Place donuts on a tray and place in freezer. Once donuts are frozen, about 30 minutes, transfer to a large freezer bag.

7. To serve, heat in microwave until thawed, about 1 minute.

PER SERVING Calories: 179 | Fat: 4.7 g | Protein: 0.6 g | Sodium: 80 mg | Fiber: 1.3 g | Carbohydrates: 33.9 g | Sugar: 32.2 g

Pumpkin Cinnamon Sugar Donuts

Enjoy these fluffy vegan Pumpkin Cinnamon Sugar Donuts that are baked, not fried, and coated with cinnamon and pumpkin-spiced sugar. They're sure to please!

INGREDIENTS | SERVES 6

For Donuts

1¼ cups all-purpose flour
½ cup packed light brown sugar
1 teaspoon pumpkin pie spice
½ teaspoon ground cinnamon
½ teaspoon salt
1 teaspoon baking powder
3 tablespoons vegan butter, melted
¼ cup canned pumpkin purée
¾ cup unsweetened almond milk

For Cinnamon Sugar Topping

3 tablespoons vegan butter, melted
⅓ cup granulated sugar
½ teaspoon pumpkin pie spice
½ teaspoon ground cinnamon

1. Preheat oven to 350°F. Spray a donut pan with vegetable cooking spray.

2. **To make Donuts:** in a large bowl combine flour, brown sugar, pumpkin pie spice, cinnamon, salt, and baking powder.

3. In a medium bowl combine vegan butter, pumpkin purée, and almond milk. Pour pumpkin mixture into flour mixture. Stir until just combined.

4. Pour donut batter into donut pan and use a spoon to spread evenly into donut compartments. Bake 15 minutes until donuts are slightly golden on bottom.

5. **To make Cinnamon Sugar Topping:** place melted vegan butter in a small bowl. In a medium bowl combine sugar, pumpkin pie spice, and cinnamon.

6. Once donuts are done, remove from oven and let cool 2 minutes. Once cool enough to handle, dip top of each donut in melted vegan butter, then dip in cinnamon sugar mixture. Repeat with each donut.

7. Store donuts in a large sealed container at room temperature up to 3 days, or in refrigerator up to 10 days. Alternatively, you can freeze them up to 2 months. Place donuts on a tray and place in freezer. Once donuts are frozen, about 30 minutes, transfer to a large freezer bag.

8. To serve, heat in microwave until thawed, about 1 minute.

PER SERVING Calories: 249 | Fat: 3.7 g | Protein: 3.0 g | Sodium: 357 mg | Fiber: 1.4 g | Carbohydrates: 51.1 g | Sugar: 29.5 g

Chocolate Glazed Baked Donuts

These vegan Chocolate Glazed Baked Donuts are decorated with sprinkles to make for a fun and colorful start to your day. Make a double batch and take them to the office to share with others. See how many people can tell these delicious donuts are vegan!

INGREDIENTS | SERVES 6

For Donuts

1¼ cups all-purpose flour
1 teaspoon baking powder
½ teaspoon baking soda
¼ teaspoon ground nutmeg
1 tablespoon ground flaxseed
7 tablespoons water
⅓ cup packed light brown sugar
1 (5.3-ounce) container vanilla soy yogurt
2 tablespoons vegan butter, softened
¼ cup sprinkles

For Chocolate Glaze

½ cup dairy-free semisweet chocolate chips
2 tablespoons coconut oil
1 tablespoon light corn syrup

1. Preheat oven to 350°F. Coat one donut pan with vegetable cooking spray.

2. **To make Donuts:** in a large bowl combine flour, baking powder, baking soda, and nutmeg. Set aside.

3. In a medium bowl combine flaxseed and water. Add brown sugar, yogurt, and vegan butter. Stir to combine.

4. Pour yogurt mixture into flour mixture and stir to combine. Spoon batter into prepared donut pan and bake 15 minutes until donuts are golden brown.

5. **To make Chocolate Glaze:** combine all ingredients in a small microwave-safe bowl. Microwave 30 seconds. Stir until smooth and creamy.

6. Dip cooled donuts in chocolate glaze. Top with sprinkles.

7. Store donuts in a large sealed container at room temperature up to 3 days, or in refrigerator up to 10 days. Alternatively, you can freeze them up to 2 months. Place donuts on a tray and place in freezer. Once donuts are frozen, about 30 minutes, transfer to a large freezer bag.

8. To serve, heat in microwave until thawed, about 1 minute.

PER SERVING Calories: 386 | Fat: 15.7 g | Protein: 4.2 g | Sodium: 222 mg | Fiber: 2.5 g | Carbohydrates: 61.7 g | Sugar: 37.4 g

Toasted Coconut Donuts

These Toasted Coconut Donuts are reminiscent of the mini donuts found in packs of six. Of course, the store-bought donuts are not vegan, so this recipe is a great substitution. Freeze the ones you don't eat right away, then reheat and enjoy a tasty breakfast any day of the week.

INGREDIENTS | SERVES 6

For Donuts

1 teaspoon coconut oil
½ cup unsweetened coconut flakes
1¼ cups all-purpose flour
½ cup packed light brown sugar
¼ teaspoon ground nutmeg
½ teaspoon salt
½ teaspoon baking soda
1 teaspoon baking powder
3 tablespoons vegan butter, melted
1 tablespoon ground flaxseed
3 tablespoons water
¾ cup unsweetened vanilla almond milk

For Topping

1 cup powdered sugar
1 tablespoon unsweetened vanilla almond milk

1. Preheat oven to 350°F. Spray donut pan with vegetable cooking spray.

2. **To make Donuts:** place coconut oil in a large skillet over medium heat. Add coconut flakes and stir until coconut is coated. Cook 5 minutes, stirring frequently, until coconut is golden. Set aside.

3. In a large bowl combine flour, brown sugar, nutmeg, salt, baking soda, and baking powder.

4. In a small bowl combine vegan butter, flaxseed, water, and almond milk. Pour wet mixture into flour mixture. Add 2 tablespoons toasted coconut flakes and stir until just combined.

5. Pour batter into donut compartments, filling each generously. Bake 15 minutes until donuts are slightly golden on bottom.

6. **To make Topping:** combine powdered sugar and almond milk in a medium bowl.

7. Once donuts are done, remove from oven and let cool 3 minutes. Once cool, remove from pan, dip top part of each donut in topping, and sprinkle with leftover toasted coconut flakes. Repeat with remaining donuts.

8. Store donuts in a large sealed container at room temperature up to 3 days, or in refrigerator up to 10 days. Alternatively, you can freeze them up to 2 months. Place donuts on a tray and place in freezer. Once donuts are frozen, about 30 minutes, transfer to a large freezer bag.

9. To serve, heat in microwave until thawed, about 1 minute.

PER SERVING Calories: 314 | Fat: 8.1 g | Protein: 3.5 g | Sodium: 450 mg | Fiber: 2.5 g | Carbohydrates: 57.3 g | Sugar: 34.7 g

Cinnamon Crunch Scones

Enjoy a luxurious, relaxed start to your day with these delicious vegan Cinnamon Crunch Scones. These scones are easy to freeze and reheat for a breakfast treat any day of the week.

INGREDIENTS | SERVES 16

For Cinnamon Crunch Topping
¾ cup packed light brown sugar
1 teaspoon ground cinnamon
1 tablespoon plain soy milk

For Scones
3 cups all-purpose flour
⅓ cup granulated sugar
4 teaspoons baking powder
1 teaspoon baking soda
½ teaspoon salt
½ teaspoon ground cinnamon
1 cup dairy-free margarine, cold, sliced
¾ cup plain soy milk
1 teaspoon apple cider vinegar
1 tablespoon ground flaxseed
1 tablespoon cornstarch
4 tablespoons water
1 teaspoon vanilla extract

Health Benefits of Cinnamon

Spices are a great way to increase the healthiness of your everyday dishes. For example, cinnamon contains antioxidants that can reduce inflammation. Cinnamon can also lower blood pressure, and can also lower blood sugar levels after a meal.

1. Preheat oven to 350°F. Line two baking sheets with parchment paper.

2. **To make Cinnamon Crunch Topping:** combine ingredients in a small bowl. Set aside.

3. **To make Scones:** in a large bowl combine flour, sugar, baking powder, baking soda, salt, and cinnamon. Add sliced margarine and use a pastry knife or two butter knives used in a scissor motion to cut margarine into flour until mixture resembles coarse crumbs.

4. In a medium bowl combine soy milk, vinegar, ground flaxseed, cornstarch, water, and vanilla. Pour soy milk mixture over flour mixture. Stir dough gently until just combined.

5. Prepare a work surface by lightly flouring it. Place dough on surface and shape into a large flat circle. Sprinkle cinnamon crunch topping over top, lightly pressing into dough.

6. Cut dough into 16 wedges. Transfer wedges onto prepared baking sheets and bake 25 minutes until golden around edges.

7. Let cool 10 minutes, then store scones in a large sealed container at room temperature up to 3 days, or in refrigerator up to 7 days. Alternatively, you can freeze them up to 2 months. Place cooled scones on a large tray and place in freezer. Once scones are frozen, about 30 minutes, transfer to a large freezer bag.

8. To serve, heat in microwave until thawed, about 1 minute.

PER SERVING Calories: 197 | Fat: 5.2 g | Protein: 2.9 g | Sodium: 362 mg | Fiber: 1.0 g | Carbohydrates: 33.8 g | Sugar: 14.3 g

Chocolate Biscotti

Chocolate chips in the batter add bits of tenderness to these crispy double-chocolate biscotti cookies. Dunk one in a cup of hot coffee or tea and discover the appeal of biscotti cookies.

INGREDIENTS | SERVES 20

½ cup dairy-free margarine

1 cup + 2 teaspoons granulated sugar, divided

2 teaspoons baking powder

½ teaspoon baking soda

2 tablespoons ground flaxseed

2 tablespoons cornstarch

½ cup plain soy milk

1 teaspoon apple cider vinegar

2½ cups all-purpose flour

¼ cup cocoa powder

½ cup dairy-free chocolate chips

1. Preheat oven to 375°F. Line two baking sheets with parchment paper.

2. In a large bowl beat together margarine, 1 cup sugar, baking powder, and baking soda on high until light and creamy, about 1 minute.

3. Move margarine mixture to one side of bowl. In other side, pour in flaxseed, cornstarch, soy milk, and vinegar. Stir to combine. Use mixer to combine flaxseed mixture with batter.

4. Add flour, ½-cup at a time, and use mixer to combine. Add cocoa powder and continue mixing until combined. Stir in chocolate chips.

5. Divide dough in half and create two balls, placing one on each prepared pan. Use your hands to shape each one into a rectangle measuring approximately 11" × 4". Sprinkle each with 1 teaspoon sugar.

6. Place pans in oven and bake 20 minutes. Remove from oven and let cool about 10 minutes.

7. Reduce oven temperature to 300°F and slice loaves into ½" slices. Bake 10 minutes, then turn slices over and bake another 10 minutes.

8. Place on a wire rack to cool completely, about 15 minutes. Place in a large air-tight container and store at room temperature up to 14 days, refrigerator up to 1 month, or freezer up to 2 months.

PER SERVING Calories: 159 | Fat: 4.5 g | Protein: 2.3 g | Sodium: 115 mg | Fiber: 1.5 g | Carbohydrates: 27.4 g | Sugar: 12.9 g

Raspberry Chocolate Croissants

These croissants are a delicacy, with a flaky crust filled with melted dark chocolate and raspberries. Believe it or not, they are ready in less than 30 minutes, and you can store them in the refrigerator and enjoy them throughout the week.

INGREDIENTS | SERVES 12

1 sheet Pepperidge Farm Puff Pastry Sheets, thawed

¼ cup unsweetened almond milk

1 teaspoon vegan butter, melted

4 ounces dairy-free bittersweet baking chocolate, broken into pieces

12 fresh raspberries

1. Preheat oven to 375°F. Line a baking sheet with parchment paper.

2. Unroll puff pastry sheet and use a knife to cut along lines where pastry was folded in packaging. Then turn sheet and create three cuts on long side of sheet. This will create 12 squares of pastry dough.

3. In a medium bowl combine almond milk and vegan butter. Brush mixture over top of 1 pastry square. Place 1 chocolate piece at one corner of square. Place 1 raspberry on top chocolate and roll pastry dough diagonally over chocolate and raspberry. Place pastry seam-side down on baking sheet. Repeat with remaining pastry squares.

4. Brush top of each pastry with more milk mixture. Bake 20 minutes until golden on top.

5. Let cool 3 minutes. Transfer to a large sealed container and store in refrigerator up to 5 days or freezer up to 2 months. To serve, heat in toaster oven 1 minute.

PER SERVING Calories: 78 | Fat: 5.0 g | Protein: 0.6 g | Sodium: 15 mg | Fiber: 0.9 g | Carbohydrates: 7.4 g | Sugar: 4.2 g

CHAPTER 4

Breads, Biscuits, and Muffins

Easy Vegan Dinner Rolls

Soft and buttery, these Easy Vegan Dinner Rolls are a perfect recipe to add something extra to your next family dinner.

INGREDIENTS | SERVES 12

1 tablespoon vegetable oil

½ cup water

½ cup plain soy milk

1 tablespoon packed light brown sugar

7 tablespoons vegan butter, melted, divided

2½ cups all-purpose flour, divided

2½ teaspoons rapid-rise instant yeast

1 teaspoon salt

Whole-Wheat Flour and Breads

Whole-wheat flour requires different amounts of moisture than white flour, and the bran and germ present can inhibit the dough from rising properly. This can result in a flatter, denser finished product. Only use whole-wheat flour when specifically called for in a recipe for the best results.

1. Grease a 9" × 9" baking dish with vegetable oil.

2. Combine water, milk, brown sugar, and 3 tablespoons melted butter in a large bowl. Set aside.

3. In a separate large bowl combine 2 cups all-purpose flour, yeast, and salt. Create a well in middle of flour with two fingers and pour milk mixture into well.

4. Use your hands to knead dough 2 minutes. Add up to ½ cup additional all-purpose flour as needed until dough pulls away slightly from sides of bowl. It will be sticky.

5. Pinch off golf ball–sized sections of dough. Dip each section in oil from prepared pan and gently work into a ball. Place dough balls 1" apart in pan. Spray a sheet of plastic wrap with vegetable cooking spray and cover pan. Let sit 35 minutes until balls have doubled in size.

6. When ready to bake, preheat oven to 350°F. Remove plastic wrap from pan and bake 25 minutes until golden brown on top. Remove rolls from oven and immediately coat with remaining melted butter.

7. Let rolls cool 10 minutes, then store in a large sealed container in refrigerator up to 5 days or freezer up to 2 months. If frozen, let sit on counter 10 minutes to defrost before serving. To serve, preheat oven to 300°F and reheat rolls 12 minutes on an ungreased baking pan.

PER SERVING Calories: 142 | Fat: 4.2 g | Protein: 3.3 g | Sodium: 245 mg | Fiber: 1.0 g | Carbohydrates: 21.7 g | Sugar: 1.2 g

Easy Corn Bread

This lightly sweet vegan Easy Corn Bread is made with just a few ingredients. It's easy to make at home and results in a perfect side dish for soups, chilis, and stews. Because it's not overly sweet, you can use this corn bread for your stuffing recipes too! Top warmed slices with some vegan butter before serving.

INGREDIENTS | SERVES 12

1 cup whole-wheat pastry flour

1 cup cornmeal

½ teaspoon baking soda

1 teaspoon baking powder

½ teaspoon salt

1 cup canned corn kernels, drained

½ cup vegan butter

⅓ cup agave nectar

1 cup unsweetened almond milk

1 tablespoon apple cider vinegar

1. Preheat oven to 375°F. Spray an 8" × 8" baking dish with vegetable cooking spray.

2. Combine flour, cornmeal, baking soda, baking powder, and salt in a large bowl. Add corn and stir until corn is coated.

3. In a medium microwave-safe bowl add vegan butter. Microwave 20 seconds until melted, then add agave nectar, milk, and vinegar. Stir to combine. Pour into bowl with corn mixture and stir until just combined.

4. Pour batter into prepared pan and bake 30 minutes until corn bread is golden on top.

5. Remove from oven and let cool about 15 minutes. Place in a large sealed container and refrigerate up to 5 days, or freeze up to 1 month. To serve, reheat in microwave or toaster oven in 30-second intervals until heated through.

PER SERVING Calories: 137 | Fat: 3.8 g | Protein: 2.3 g | Sodium: 264 mg | Fiber: 2.4 g | Carbohydrates: 22.9 g | Sugar: 5.0 g

Homemade Vegan Biscuits

These Homemade Vegan Biscuits are light and airy, with a crispy crust—just like the traditional biscuits you know and love. The buttery flavor infused in these biscuits will make them a favorite for breakfast, dinner, and everything in between!

INGREDIENTS | SERVES 10

2 cups all-purpose flour
1 tablespoon baking powder
½ teaspoon baking soda
¾ teaspoon salt
½ cup vegan butter, cut into 1" slices
¾ cup unsweetened almond milk
1 teaspoon apple cider vinegar

1. Preheat oven to 400°F.

2. In a food processor combine flour, baking powder, baking soda, and salt. Add vegan butter. Pulse in several short bursts until coarse crumbs form.

3. In a small bowl combine milk and vinegar. Pour into food processor with flour mixture and pulse again, until just combined.

4. Use a large spoon to drop biscuit dough onto an ungreased baking sheet. Bake 18 minutes until golden on top.

5. Let biscuits cool 10 minutes, then store in a large sealed container in refrigerator up to 7 days or freezer up to 2 months. To serve, cook in microwave in 30-second intervals until heated through. For crispier biscuits, turn your oven or toaster oven to 300°F and bake 10 minutes.

PER SERVING Calories: 131 | Fat: 4.1 g | Protein: 2.7 g | Sodium: 462 mg | Fiber: 0.8 g | Carbohydrates: 19.8 g | Sugar: 0.1 g

Sweet Potato Dinner Rolls

Soft, tender, homemade Sweet Potato Dinner Rolls are a favorite to serve with any meal, including holiday dinners. Make them year-round and freeze for homemade heat-and-serve dinner rolls!

INGREDIENTS | SERVES 15

1 tablespoon vegetable oil
1 medium sweet potato, perforated with a fork
½ cup water
¾ cup unsweetened almond milk
1 tablespoon packed light brown sugar

2½ teaspoons rapid-rise instant yeast
3½ cups all-purpose flour, divided
1 teaspoon salt
1 tablespoon ground flaxseed
5 tablespoons vegan butter, melted, divided
2 cups whole-wheat pastry flour

1. Grease a 9" × 13" baking dish with vegetable oil.

2. Microwave sweet potato 2 minutes. Remove with oven mitts and cut into large chunks.

3. In a food processor add sweet potato, water, milk, and brown sugar. Pulse until creamy. Transfer to a large bowl and let mixture cool slightly about 5 minutes. (It should be same temperature as your finger when you dip it into mix).

4. In a separate large bowl whisk together yeast, 3 cups all-purpose flour, salt, and flaxseed. Create a well in middle of flour with a spatula and scoop sweet potato mixture and 3 tablespoons melted vegan butter into well. Knead dough in bowl 5 minutes. Add up to ½ cup remaining all-purpose flour as needed until dough pulls slightly away from sides of bowl. It will still be sticky.

5. Pinch off golf ball–sized pieces of dough. Dip each piece in oil from prepared pan and gently work dough into a ball. Place dough balls 1" apart in prepared pan.

6. Spray a sheet of plastic wrap with vegetable cooking spray and cover pan. Let dough balls rise 40 minutes until doubled in size.

7. When ready to bake, preheat oven to 350°F. Remove plastic wrap from pan and bake 25 minutes until golden brown on top. Remove rolls from oven and immediately coat with remaining melted vegan butter.

8. Let rolls cool 10 minutes, then store rolls in a large sealed container in refrigerator up to 5 days or freezer up to 2 months. If frozen, let sit on counter 10 minutes to defrost before serving. To serve, preheat oven to 300°F and bake rolls 15 minutes until heated through.

PER SERVING Calories: 205 | Fat: 3.0 g | Protein: 5.2 g | Sodium: 197 mg | Fiber: 3.5 g | Carbohydrates: 37.8 g | Sugar: 1.4 g

Working with Yeast

There are different types of yeast available. Active dry yeast requires yeast proofing (dissolving it in warm water with sugar) before proceeding with the recipe. Alternatively, rapid-rise yeast has been processed into smaller pieces and includes additives that help it rise faster. As a result, recipes with rapid-rise yeast do not require yeast proofing.

Coffee Cake Muffins

*Picture the very best vegan coffee cake recipe—transformed into muffins.
That's what these deliciously sweet Coffee Cake Muffins deliver. You'll love
this recipe for breakfast, brunch, snack time, and even dessert!*

INGREDIENTS | SERVES 12

For Topping
¼ cup coconut sugar
2 teaspoons ground cinnamon
¼ cup creamy peanut butter
2 teaspoons molasses
½ cup instant oats

For Muffins
½ cup vegan butter
½ cup agave nectar
¼ cup coconut sugar
½ cup unsweetened applesauce
1 cup unsweetened almond milk
1 tablespoon ground flaxseed
1 tablespoon cornstarch
1 teaspoon apple cider vinegar
1½ cups whole-wheat pastry flour
2 teaspoons baking powder
½ teaspoon baking soda
½ teaspoon salt

1. **To make Topping:** combine coconut sugar, cinnamon, peanut butter, and molasses in a bowl. Add instant oatmeal and stir until combined. Set aside.

2. **To make Muffins:** preheat oven to 350°F. Line muffin tins with parchment paper or grease with vegetable cooking spray.

3. In a large bowl cream together vegan butter, agave nectar, and coconut sugar. Add applesauce, milk, flaxseed, cornstarch, and vinegar. Stir to combine.

4. In a medium bowl combine flour, baking powder, baking soda, and salt. Add flour mixture to milk mixture and stir until just combined.

5. Pour batter into prepared muffin tins. Evenly distribute topping across muffins. Bake 22 minutes until a toothpick inserted in middle of muffins comes out clean. Topping should be golden brown.

6. When done, remove from oven and let cool about 15 minutes. Store in a large sealed container in refrigerator up to 7 days or freezer up to 2 months. To serve, cook in microwave in 30-second intervals until heated through, or cook in an oven or toaster oven set at 300°F for 8 minutes.

PER SERVING Calories: 206 | Fat: 6.4 g | Protein: 3.4 g | Sodium: 301 mg | Fiber: 3.2 g | Carbohydrates: 33.7 g | Sugar: 16.7 g

Garlic Breadsticks

These homemade Garlic Breadsticks are perfect to make ahead of time, freeze, and then pop in a toaster oven to have with your favorite meals. They have a crispy crust infused with garlic, yielding to a tender middle.

INGREDIENTS | SERVES 20

1½ cups water
2¼ teaspoons active dry yeast
1 tablespoon packed light brown sugar
½ cup whole-wheat flour
4 cups + 1 tablespoon all-purpose flour, divided

3 teaspoons salt, divided
5 tablespoons vegan butter, melted, divided
1 teaspoon garlic powder
1 tablespoon nutritional yeast flakes
1 teaspoon dried oregano

1. Preheat oven to 200°F. Line a 18" × 13" sheet pan with parchment paper.

2. Place water in a medium microwave-safe bowl and heat 11 seconds. Water should be about the same temperature as your finger. Add yeast and sugar. Stir gently and set aside.

3. In a large bowl add whole-wheat flour, 4 cups all-purpose flour, and 1½ teaspoons salt. Stir to combine. Pour yeast mixture and 2 tablespoons melted vegan butter over flour mixture and stir to combine.

4. Place dough on a floured surface and knead 3 minutes. Tear off pieces of dough about the size of your palm and roll into long pieces. Place dough on prepared pan, allowing 3" between each piece.

5. Cover pan with a dish towel. Turn off oven and place pan in oven. Allow dough to rise about 40 minutes.

6. Prepare garlic topping by combing remaining 3 tablespoons vegan butter, garlic powder, remaining salt, and nutritional yeast in a small bowl.

7. When breadsticks have doubled in size, remove pan from oven. Preheat oven to 375°F. Gently spread ½ garlic topping across each breadstick and sprinkle with dried oregano. Place pan back in oven and bake 15 minutes until breadsticks are golden brown. Remove from oven and coat with remaining topping mixture.

8. Let breadsticks cool 10 minutes, then store in a large sealed container in refrigerator up to 7 days or freezer up to 2 months. If frozen, let sit on counter 10 minutes to defrost before serving. To serve, preheat oven to 300°F and bake 10 minutes on an ungreased baking pan.

PER SERVING Calories: 119 | Fat: 1.4 g | Protein: 3.3 g | Sodium: 370 mg | Fiber: 1.2 g | Carbohydrates: 22.7 g | Sugar: 0.8 g

Growing Your Own Herbs

It's easy to grow herbs at home. Begin by growing them in small pots indoors, especially if your location experiences colder climates. Some of the best herbs to begin with include basil, oregano, sage, and parsley. You can find all the information you need for successful home-grown herbs online! Add a reminder on your phone to water them regularly, and you'll be well on your way to a green thumb.

Vegan Irish Soda Bread

If you love a crispy artisanal bread, then try this Vegan Irish Soda Bread with raisins and hints of orange. Sure, it's great for St. Patrick's Day, but it's also a perfect go-to bread all year long!

INGREDIENTS | SERVES 10

1¾ cups plain soy milk

1 tablespoon apple cider vinegar

3 cups whole-wheat flour

1¼ cups all-purpose flour

1 tablespoon packed light brown sugar

1 teaspoon salt

1 teaspoon baking soda

4 tablespoons vegan butter

1 cup raisins

1 teaspoon orange zest

1 tablespoon ground flaxseed

1 tablespoon cornstarch

Why Do Vegans Use So Much Flaxseed?

Flaxseeds are loaded with omega-3s, which make them an important food to include in a vegan diet. In addition, ground flaxseed, when combined with water or milk, creates a gel similar to eggs. This gel is the perfect egg replacement in vegan baked goods.

1. Preheat oven to 400°F. Line a 18" × 13" sheet pan with parchment paper.

2. In a small bowl combine soy milk and vinegar. Set aside.

3. Add whole-wheat flour, 1 cup all-purpose flour, sugar, salt, and baking soda to a food processor. Pulse 3 seconds to combine. Add vegan butter and pulse until it resembles a coarse meal, about 10 seconds. Add raisins, orange zest, flaxseed, and cornstarch. Pulse to combine.

4. Pour mixture from food processor into a large bowl. Create a well in middle with a spatula. Pour soy milk mixture into well and stir from center outward, incorporating flour as you mix.

5. Knead dough in bowl and sprinkle with remaining ¼ all-purpose flour until a dough ball forms. Place dough ball on prepared pan. Use a knife to cut a shallow "X" into top of dough.

6. Bake 45 minutes. When you tap loaf, it should have a hollow sound. When done, remove from oven and let cool 15 minutes.

7. Store whole bread or slices in a large sealed container in refrigerator up to 7 days or freezer up to 2 months. If frozen, let sit on counter 10 minutes to defrost before serving. When serving, preheat oven to 300°F and bake 15 minutes until heated through.

PER SERVING Calories: 285 | Fat: 3.6 g | Protein: 8.6 g | Sodium: 409 mg | Fiber: 5.4 g | Carbohydrates: 56.5 g | Sugar: 11.5 g

Oven-Baked Naan Bread

Pillow-soft, Oven-Baked Naan Bread is easy to make and delicious to eat with soups, stews, salads, curries, and more! Make a batch to freeze and reheat with any meal.

INGREDIENTS | SERVES 8

1 teaspoon active dry yeast
¾ cup warm water
2 teaspoons packed light brown sugar
2 cups all-purpose flour
1 teaspoon salt
¼ teaspoon baking powder
¼ teaspoon baking soda
3 tablespoons vegan sour cream
2 tablespoons olive oil

1. In a small bowl gently combine yeast, water, and brown sugar. Allow mixture to sit until it becomes frothy about 5 minutes.

2. In a large bowl combine flour, salt, baking powder, and baking soda. Set aside.

3. Add vegan sour cream and oil to yeast mixture. Stir to combine. Pour sour cream mixture into flour mixture and stir. Cover with a kitchen towel and place in a warm area. Let dough rise about 45 minutes.

4. Grease a 18" × 13" baking sheet with vegetable cooking spray. Punch down dough, then tear and shape in 10 golf ball–sized balls. Place on baking sheet and set aside to rise another 30 minutes.

5. When dough is ready, preheat oven to 350°F and grease a 9" × 13" baking pan with vegetable cooking spray. Flatten dough balls into small discs, about 6" in diameter. Return to prepared pan. Bake 5 minutes each side.

6. Let naan cool 10 minutes, then store in a large sealed container in refrigerator up to 7 days or freezer up to 2 months. If frozen, let sit on counter 10 minutes to defrost before serving. When serving, preheat oven to 300°F and bake 10 minutes on an ungreased baking sheet.

PER SERVING Calories: 158 | Fat: 4.5 g | Protein: 3.4 g | Sodium: 350 mg | Fiber: 1.4 g | Carbohydrates: 25.8 g | Sugar: 1.2 g

Savory Zucchini Bread

This Savory Zucchini Bread is made with fresh zucchini, basil, tomatoes, and other delicious summertime ingredients.

INGREDIENTS | SERVES 10

1 cup whole-wheat flour

2 cups all-purpose flour

1 tablespoon baking powder

1 teaspoon baking soda

1 teaspoon salt

1 medium zucchini, ends removed, roughly chopped

1 medium tomato, roughly chopped

½ cup fresh basil leaves, chopped

½ cup chopped scallions

1 cup water

1 tablespoon apple cider vinegar

3 tablespoons vegetable oil

3 thin slices fresh tomato

1. Preheat oven to 350°F. Spray a 9" × 5" loaf pan lightly with vegetable cooking spray.

2. In a large bowl combine both flours, baking powder, baking soda, and salt. Set aside.

3. Add zucchini to a food processor. Pulse 3 seconds. Add tomato, basil, and scallions to food processor and pulse another 3 seconds. Use a spatula to push any pieces in side of bowl down. Pulse again until shredded. Add water, vinegar, and vegetable oil. Pulse again to combine.

4. Pour contents from food processor into bowl with flour. Stir until just combined. Pour batter into prepared loaf pan. Top with tomato slices.

5. Bake 70 minutes until a toothpick inserted in middle of loaf comes out clean. Top of loaf should be a golden brown.

6. Let cool 10 minutes, then store in a large sealed container in refrigerator up to 5 days or freezer up to 2 months. If frozen, let sit on counter for 10 minutes to defrost before serving. To serve, preheat oven to 300°F and bake 10 minutes on an ungreased baking sheet.

PER SERVING Calories: 177 | Fat: 4.3 g | Protein: 4.7 g | Sodium: 508 mg | Fiber: 2.5 g | Carbohydrates: 29.8 g | Sugar: 1.2 g

"Cheesy" Pull-Apart Bread

Go crazy for this vegan "Cheesy" Pull-Apart Bread. Why? Because it requires only a few ingredients and takes just minutes to make. Make it on the weekend and reheat and serve as an appetizer or a side to your favorite meals throughout the week.

INGREDIENTS | SERVES 10

1 (16-ounce) store-bought round loaf white bread
½ cup vegan butter
2 cloves garlic, peeled and finely chopped
½ teaspoon salt
12 ounces vegan mozzarella shreds
½ cup sliced green onion

How Is Vegan Cheese Made?

Vegan cheese has gone through several changes over the years. It used to lack flavor and wouldn't melt when heated. Today's vegan cheeses are typically oil-based and bound together with starch to create a stretchy, melty cheese. Some vegan cheeses are also made with nuts.

1. Preheat oven to 350°F. Line a baking sheet with aluminum foil.

2. Use a serrated knife to make vertical and horizontal cuts in round loaf, cutting to bottom of crust, but not through crust.

3. In a small bowl combine butter, garlic, and salt. Use a butter knife to spread mixture through each cut in bread.

4. Insert cheese shreds in bread cuts, leaving some on top of loaf for a melted cheese crust. Sprinkle top with onion slices.

5. Place loaf on prepared baking sheet and cover with a piece of foil. Bake 15 minutes.

6. Remove pan from oven and carefully remove top piece of foil. Return pan to oven and bake another 10 minutes until bread has toasted edges and cheese has melted.

7. Let cool 20 minutes, then store entire loaf or sections of loaf in a large sealed container in refrigerator up to 7 days or freezer up to 2 months. If frozen, let sit on counter 10 minutes to defrost before serving. To serve, preheat oven to 300°F and bake 10 minutes on an ungreased baking sheet.

PER SERVING Calories: 270 | Fat: 12.4 g | Protein: 5.4 g | Sodium: 744 mg | Fiber: 2.6 g | Carbohydrates: 31.7 g | Sugar: 2.7 g

Whole-Wheat Harvest Bread

You'll want to make this recipe for crusty, lightly sweet Whole-Wheat Harvest Bread again and again to add a special touch to a typical dinner.

INGREDIENTS | SERVES 12

3 cups whole-wheat flour
1 cup all-purpose flour
1 teaspoon salt
2¼ teaspoons instant yeast
1½ cups lukewarm water

1. In a large bowl mix together whole-wheat flour, all-purpose flour, salt, and yeast.

2. Add water. Stir to incorporate. Dough will be sticky. Cover bowl with a dish towel. Set aside at least 8 hours or overnight.

3. Spray a baking sheet with vegetable cooking spray. Pour dough onto a lightly floured surface and mold it into a round loaf. Place on prepared baking sheet. Cover with plastic wrap sprayed with a light coating of vegetable cooking spray. Set aside 2 hours to let dough rise.

4. Preheat oven to 400°F and bake 50 minutes until top is golden brown.

5. Let cool 20 minutes, then store entire loaf or slices in a large sealed container in refrigerator up to 7 days or freezer up to 2 months. If frozen, let sit on counter 10 minutes to defrost before serving. To serve, preheat oven to 300°F and bake 10 minutes on an ungreased baking sheet.

PER SERVING Calories: 142 | Fat: 0.7 g | Protein: 5.3 g | Sodium: 194 mg | Fiber: 3.7 g | Carbohydrates: 29.9 g | Sugar: 0.2 g

Cinnamon Swirl Bread

Nothing compares to homemade bread, especially when there's cinnamon involved. Enjoy every slice of this homemade vegan cinnamon bread with swirls of gooey, sweet cinnamon.

INGREDIENTS | SERVES 12

¾ cup plain soy milk

1 tablespoon apple cider vinegar

¾ cup vegan butter, softened and divided

¼ cup + 2 tablespoons water

3¼ cups all-purpose flour, divided

2¼ teaspoons instant yeast

¼ cup granulated sugar

½ teaspoon salt

1 cup packed light brown sugar

1 tablespoon ground cinnamon

1. Combine soy milk and vinegar in a small saucepan. Place over medium heat until simmering, about 2 minutes. Remove from heat. Add ¼ cup vegan butter and stir until melted, about 30 seconds. Let cool about 10 minutes until lukewarm, then add water and stir. Set aside.

2. In a large bowl combine 2¼ cups flour, yeast, granulated sugar, and salt. Add soy milk mixture to flour mixture. Stir to combine. Mixture should be sticky.

3. Add remaining flour, ½ cup at a time, stirring well after each addition. Once dough starts to form into a ball, knead mixture in bowl about 5 minutes. Spray top of dough ball with vegetable cooking spray and cover with a damp cloth. Place in a warm place to rise 1 hour.

4. Combine brown sugar, cinnamon, and remaining ½ cup vegan butter in a small bowl.

5. Spray a 9" × 5" loaf pan with vegetable cooking spray. Roll out dough into a rectangle. Once rolled out, spread cinnamon sugar mixture on top. Starting at far end, roll dough toward you and pinch seam. Place in prepared pan. Cover with a damp cloth and let rise 30 minutes.

6. Preheat oven to 350°F. Once loaf has risen, bake 40 minutes until browned. Remove from oven and set aside to cool about 15 minutes.

7. Store entire loaf or slices in a large sealed container in refrigerator up to 7 days or freezer up to 2 months. If frozen, let sit on counter 10 minutes to defrost before serving. To serve, preheat oven to 300°F and bake 10 minutes on an ungreased baking sheet.

PER SERVING Calories: 265 | Fat: 5.2 g | Protein: 4.3 g | Sodium: 189 mg | Fiber: 1.5 g | Carbohydrates: 49.4 g | Sugar: 22.1 g

Chai Tea Muffins with Pumpkin Seeds

Wake up to vegan Chai Tea Muffins with Pumpkin Seeds to start your day in a healthy and tasty way! Of course, these muffins are good any time of the day!

INGREDIENTS | MAKES 12 MUFFINS

1 bag chai tea

½ cup hot water

¾ cup vanilla almond milk

⅓ cup vegetable oil

2 tablespoons ground flaxseed

2 tablespoons cornstarch

6 tablespoons water

1 teaspoon apple cider vinegar

¾ cup light packed brown sugar

1½ cups all-purpose flour

½ cup whole-wheat flour

2 teaspoons baking powder

1 teaspoon baking soda

½ teaspoon salt

1 teaspoon ground cinnamon

½ teaspoon ground cloves

½ teaspoon ground nutmeg

2 tablespoons pumpkin seeds

1. Preheat oven to 350°F and line a muffin pan with muffin papers.

2. Place tea bag in hot water and allow to steep 2 minutes.

3. In meantime, add milk, oil, flaxseed, cornstarch, water, vinegar, and brown sugar to a small bowl. Remove tea bag from hot water and pour tea into milk mixture. Stir to combine.

4. In a medium bowl combine flours, baking powder, baking soda, salt, cinnamon, cloves, and nutmeg. Add milk mixture and stir to combine.

5. Use a measuring cup or a cookie dough dispenser to equally distribute batter among muffin papers. Spread a few pumpkin seeds on top of each muffin.

6. Place in oven and bake 25 minutes until a toothpick inserted in center of muffin comes out clean When muffins are ready, remove from oven and let cool 5 minutes before serving.

7. Store in a large sealed container in refrigerator up to 7 days. Alternatively, you can freeze muffins up to 2 months. To serve, cook in microwave or toaster oven in 30-second intervals until heated through.

PER SERVING (1 muffin) Calories: 235 | Fat: 6.9 g | Protein: 4.0 g | Sodium: 297 mg | Fiber: 2.7 g | Carbohydrates: 39.6 g | Sugar: 14.4 g

Carrot Cake Muffins

Enjoy carrot cake for breakfast with these spicy, whole-grain vegan Carrot Cake Muffins. They're lightly sweetened and topped with a delicate cream cheese drizzle.

INGREDIENTS | MAKES 12 MUFFINS

For Muffins

1½ cups whole-wheat pastry flour
1 teaspoon baking soda
1½ teaspoons ground cinnamon
¼ teaspoon ground nutmeg
¼ teaspoon salt
1 cup chopped peeled carrots
½ cup coconut sugar
1 tablespoon vegetable oil
¼ cup unsweetened applesauce
1 tablespoon chia seeds
1 teaspoon vanilla extract
½ cup unsweetened almond milk
1 tablespoon apple cider vinegar

For Drizzle

¼ cup vegan cream cheese, softened
2 tablespoons maple syrup
½ teaspoon vanilla extract
1 tablespoon peanut butter powder

Is Sugar Vegan?

Some granulated sugars are processed with bone char to make the sugar white. As a result, some vegans won't eat granulated sugar. However, every person who takes on a vegan diet has to make decisions on what works best for their way of life. You can look online to find brands that aren't processed with bone char.

1. Preheat oven to 350°F. Spray a muffin pan with vegetable cooking spray.

2. **To make Muffins:** add flour, baking soda, cinnamon, nutmeg, and salt to a medium bowl. Stir to combine. Set aside.

3. In a food processor add carrots. Pulse until broken down into large pieces. Add coconut sugar, vegetable oil, applesauce, chia seeds, vanilla, milk, and vinegar. Pulse again until carrots are broken down into a grated texture.

4. Pour carrot mixture into flour mixture. Stir until just combined (be careful not to overmix). Divide batter evenly among muffin pan compartments.

5. Bake 22 minutes. A toothpick inserted in middle of one muffin should come out clean. When done, remove from oven and cool 7 minutes before transferring to a rack to cool an additional 5 minutes.

6. **To make Drizzle:** place vegan cream cheese and maple syrup in a small microwave-safe bowl. Microwave 30 seconds. Stir, then add vanilla and peanut butter powder and stir until a spreadable consistency is achieved. Drizzle over top of each muffin after baking.

7. Store muffins in a large airtight container in refrigerator up to 7 days. Alternatively, you can freeze muffins up to 2 months. To serve, cook in microwave in 30-second intervals until heated through.

PER SERVING (1 muffin) Calories: 135 | Fat: 2.9 g | Protein: 2.2 g | Sodium: 211 mg | Fiber: 2.9 g | Carbohydrates: 25.1 g | Sugar: 11.2 g

Heavenly Banana Nut Bread

This supermoist Heavenly Banana Nut Bread is a vegan dream. Each delicious slice is filled with ripe bananas and walnuts.

INGREDIENTS | SERVES 9

½ cup walnut halves

3 medium bananas (1 cup, mashed)

½ cup vegan butter, room temperature

1 cup packed light brown sugar

1 teaspoon vanilla extract

½ cup vanilla almond milk

1 tablespoon ground flaxseed

1 tablespoon cornstarch

1¾ cups all-purpose flour

1 teaspoon baking soda

½ teaspoon baking powder

¼ teaspoon salt

1. Preheat oven to 350°F. Spray a 9" × 5" loaf pan with vegetable cooking spray.

2. Place walnuts on a baking sheet and place in oven. Bake 5 minutes until walnuts are toasted. Remove from oven and let cool about 5 minutes and then chop.

3. In a food processor add bananas, vegan butter, sugar, vanilla, almond milk, ground flaxseed, and cornstarch. Pulse until smooth and creamy. Set aside.

4. In a large bowl combine flour, baking soda, baking powder, and salt. Fold in toasted nuts. Add wet ingredients and stir until just combined.

5. Pour batter into prepared pan and bake 60 minutes until crust is golden brown and a toothpick inserted in center comes out clean.

6. Let bread cool 20 minutes, then store in a large airtight container in refrigerator up to 7 days. Alternatively, you can freeze loaf up to 2 months. To serve, cook slices in microwave or toaster oven in 30-second intervals until heated through.

PER SERVING Calories: 315 | Fat: 9.0 g | Protein: 4.2 g | Sodium: 319 mg | Fiber: 2.4 g | Carbohydrates: 54.7 g | Sugar: 26.7 g

Peanut Butter Pumpkin Muffins

Peanut Butter Pumpkin Muffins bring together the flavors of oatmeal, pumpkin, and peanut butter in each delicious bite. It's a perfect start to any day.

INGREDIENTS | MAKES 16 MUFFINS

For Topping
¼ cup rolled oats
¼ cup chopped pecans
1 tablespoon coconut sugar
1 tablespoon coconut oil
1 teaspoon ground cinnamon, divided

For Muffins
1 cup all-purpose flour
½ cup whole-wheat flour
1 cup rolled oats
1 teaspoon baking powder
1 teaspoon baking soda
½ teaspoon salt
1 teaspoon ground cinnamon
1 cup canned pumpkin
1 tablespoon ground flaxseed
2 tablespoons cornstarch
¾ cup unsweetened almond milk
¾ cup coconut sugar
¼ cup creamy peanut butter
2 tablespoons vegetable oil
1 teaspoon vanilla extract

Pumpkin for the Win!

Pumpkin is loaded with healthy nutrients, like fiber, potassium, and beta-carotene. You'll also find important minerals in pumpkin, like calcium and magnesium. And pumpkin adds moisture and flavor to your baked goods so add it to your favorite recipes!

1. Preheat oven to 350°F. Line two muffin pans with sixteen muffin papers.

2. **To make Topping:** mix together oatmeal, pecans, coconut sugar, coconut oil, and cinnamon in a small bowl. Set aside.

3. **To make Muffins:** mix together flours, 1 cup oatmeal, baking powder, baking soda, salt, and cinnamon in a medium bowl. Set aside.

4. In a separate medium bowl mix together pumpkin, flaxseed, cornstarch, milk, coconut sugar, peanut butter, vegetable oil, and vanilla.

5. Pour flour mixture into pumpkin mixture and stir until just combined. Drop batter into lined muffin tins so each muffin cup is about ¾ of the way full. Top each with 1 teaspoon Topping.

6. Bake 25 minutes until lightly golden on top. Remove from oven and let cool about 10 minutes.

7. Store muffins in a large airtight container in refrigerator up to 7 days. Alternatively, you can freeze muffins up to 2 months. To serve, cook in microwave in 30-second intervals until heated through.

PER SERVING (1 muffin) Calories: 173 | Fat: 6.4 g | Protein: 3.5 g | Sodium: 192 mg | Fiber: 2.4 g | Carbohydrates: 26.6 g | Sugar: 10.9 g

Cinnamon Sugar Monkey Bread

These homemade bread bites are infused with sticky sweet cinnamon. Make this recipe on the weekend and enjoy the delicious bites as snacks throughout the week.

INGREDIENTS | SERVES 16

For Bread

4½ teaspoons active dry yeast
½ cup packed light brown sugar
2 cups warm water
½ cup olive oil, divided
5 cups all-purpose flour

1½ teaspoons salt
1 cup whole-wheat flour
1 cup granulated sugar
1½ tablespoons ground cinnamon, divided

For Glaze

1 cup powdered sugar
3 tablespoons vanilla soy milk

1. **To make Bread:** combine yeast, brown sugar, and water in a small bowl. Let sit 3 minutes until frothy. Add ¼ cup olive oil and stir slightly.

2. In a large bowl stir together all-purpose flour and salt. Pour yeast mixture into flour mixture and stir well. Dough should be slightly sticky.

3. Turn dough onto a clean, well-floured surface and knead in whole- wheat flour, about 5 minutes until dough is no longer sticky.

4. Place dough in a large well-oiled bowl and cover with a cloth. Let dough rise in a warm place 1 hour until doubled in size.

5. Preheat oven to 350°F. Prepare a 12-cup Bundt pan by pouring remaining ¼ cup oil in bottom and using your fingers to run it up the sides and in pan crevices.

6. Place granulated sugar on a large plate. Punch down dough and tear off in small pieces, shaping into balls. Roll balls in sugar and then drop into Bundt pan. Repeat until there's a layer of dough at bottom of pan. Sprinkle with ½ tablespoon cinnamon. Repeat dough and cinnamon layers until ¾ of pan is full.

7. Bake 50 minutes until golden on top. Once done, set aside to cool about 10 minutes. Use oven mitts to invert pan onto a large serving dish.

8. **To make Glaze:** combine powdered sugar with milk. Drizzle glaze over top of monkey bread.

9. Store entire loaf or broken-up sections in large sealed containers in refrigerator up to 7 days or freezer up to 2 months. If frozen, let sit on counter 10 minutes to defrost before serving. To serve, preheat oven to 300°F and bake 10 minutes on an ungreased baking sheet.

PER SERVING Calories: 362 | Fat: 10.3 g | Protein: 5.6 g | Sodium: 222 mg | Fiber: 2.6 g | Carbohydrates: 61.9 g | Sugar: 25.5 g

Orange Poppy Seed Muffins

If you love muffins for breakfast, you'll want to make these delicious vegan Orange Poppy Seed Muffins. Full of flavor and topped with an orange-infused glaze, they are perfect for breakfast any day of the week.

INGREDIENTS | MAKES 12 MUFFINS

For Muffins

½ cup vegan butter
¾ cup granulated sugar
½ cup soy buttermilk
1 cup vegan sour cream
Zest of 1 orange
1 teaspoon vanilla extract
2 cups all-purpose flour
1½ tablespoons poppy seeds
½ teaspoon salt
2 teaspoons baking powder
½ teaspoon baking soda

For Glaze

½ cup powdered sugar
2 tablespoons freshly squeezed orange juice

Homemade Soy Buttermilk

Soy buttermilk is simple to make at home! Just combine 1 cup soy milk with 2 teaspoons apple cider vinegar.

1. Preheat oven to 350°F and line a muffin pan with paper muffin cups.

2. **To make Muffins:** in a medium bowl cream vegan butter and sugar with an electric mixer. Add soy buttermilk, vegan sour cream, orange zest, and vanilla and mix again until light and creamy.

3. In a small bowl stir together dry ingredients. Add to wet ingredients and stir until just combined (don't overmix).

4. Drop batter into prepared muffin cups and bake approximately 20 minutes until tops are golden brown and a toothpick inserted in center comes out clean. Remove from oven and cool on a wire rack about 10 minutes.

5. **To make Glaze:** combine powdered sugar and orange juice. Drizzle glaze over muffins.

6. Store muffins in a large airtight container in refrigerator up to 7 days. Alternatively, you can freeze muffins up to 2 months. To serve, cook in microwave in 30-second intervals until heated through.

PER SERVING (1 muffin) Calories: 217 | Fat: 7.2 g | Protein: 2.7 g | Sodium: 305 mg | Fiber: 2.3 g | Carbohydrates: 36.0 g | Sugar: 16.9 g

CHAPTER 5

Smoothies

Chocolate Peanut Butter Protein Smoothie

Enjoy this Chocolate Peanut Butter Protein Smoothie, made with just six simple ingredients. You'll have lots of energy to fuel your day!

INGREDIENTS | SERVES 2

1 large banana, peeled and sliced

2 teaspoons cocoa powder

¾ cup unsweetened almond milk

2 tablespoons vegan chocolate protein powder

1 tablespoon all-natural unsweetened peanut butter

1 cup ice

1. Add banana, cocoa powder, almond milk, and protein powder to a blender. Pulse until smooth. Add peanut butter and pulse again until smooth. Add ice and pulse until smooth.

2. Pour smoothie into two medium lidded containers. Seal and refrigerate immediately, up to 3 days.

3. When ready to serve, shake or stir smoothie and enjoy.

PER SERVING Calories: 163 | Fat: 5.8 g | Protein: 9.5 g | Sodium: 149 mg | Fiber: 3.2 g | Carbohydrates: 21.4 g | Sugar: 11.6 g

Green Tea Banana Smoothie

Add some healthiness to your day with this Green Tea Banana Smoothie. This rich and creamy smoothie includes a little pick-me-up from green tea. It's as delicious as it is healthy and easy to make!

INGREDIENTS | SERVES 2

1 cup water, room temperature

1 green tea bag

1 cup unsweetened almond milk

2 large bananas, peeled and sliced

2 cups fresh spinach

1 cup ice

1. Pour water into a medium cup and add green tea bag. Allow tea to steep 5 minutes, then discard tea bag.

2. Pour almond milk, bananas, and spinach in a blender. Pour in seeped tea. Pulse until smooth. Add ice and pulse until smooth.

3. Pour into two medium lidded containers. Refrigerate immediately, up to 3 days. When ready to serve, shake or stir smoothie and enjoy.

PER SERVING Calories: 143 | Fat: 1.9 g | Protein: 2.8 g | Sodium: 114 mg | Fiber: 4.7 g | Carbohydrates: 33.5 g | Sugar: 17.0 g

Very Berry Smoothie

The flavors from strawberries, raspberries, and blackberries combine into this naturally sweetened, creamy smoothie. Serve for breakfast, lunch, or even as a refreshing, light dessert.

INGREDIENTS | SERVES 2

1 cup chopped fresh strawberries
½ cup fresh raspberries
¼ cup fresh blackberries
1 large banana, peeled and sliced
1 cup unsweetened almond milk
1 cup crushed ice

Freezing Bananas

If you've ever found yourself with the dilemma of a bunch of bananas on the verge of going brown, you can freeze them. Peel bananas, chop them onto a tray, and place the tray in the freezer. Once the bananas freeze, transfer to a freezer bag. Add frozen banana slices to smoothies and shakes.

1. Combine all ingredients in a blender. Blend until well combined.

2. Pour into two medium lidded containers. Refrigerate immediately, up to 3 days. When ready to serve, shake or stir smoothie and enjoy.

PER SERVING Calories: 122 | Fat: 2.0 g | Protein: 2.4 g | Sodium: 91 mg | Fiber: 6.7 g | Carbohydrates: 27.8 g | Sugar: 14.5 g

Piña Colada Green Smoothie

This Piña Colada Green Smoothie can be a simple way to get your vegetables with the added benefit of actually liking them. Pineapples add delicious flavor and, combined with coconut, make this healthy smoothie taste like a tropical vacation.

INGREDIENTS | SERVES 2

¼ cup unsweetened coconut flakes
1 cup coconut water
2 cups fresh spinach
1 large banana, peeled and sliced
1 cup diced fresh pineapple
1 cup crushed ice

1. Place coconut flakes and coconut water in a blender. Pulse until smooth. Add spinach, banana, and pineapple and pulse until smooth. Add ice and pulse until smooth.

2. Pour into two medium lidded containers. Refrigerate immediately, up to 3 days. When ready to serve, shake or stir smoothie and enjoy.

PER SERVING Calories: 174 | Fat: 6.3 g | Protein: 2.7 g | Sodium: 24 mg | Fiber: 5.6 g | Carbohydrates: 30.1 g | Sugar: 17.2 g

Basic Green Smoothie

This Basic Green Smoothie is full of healthy greens, fruits, and vegetables. Use this recipe as is or to build from by adding other favorite ingredients.

INGREDIENTS | SERVES 2

2 cups fresh spinach

1 large banana, peeled and sliced

1 medium red apple, cored and quartered

1 cup chopped peeled carrots

1 cup unsweetened almond milk

1 tablespoon ground flaxseed

1 cup ice

1. Place spinach, banana, apple, carrots, milk, and flaxseed in a blender. Pulse until smooth. Add ice and blend until incorporated.

2. Pour into two medium lidded containers. Refrigerate immediately, up to 3 days. When ready to serve, shake or stir smoothie and enjoy.

PER SERVING Calories: 173 | Fat: 3.3 g | Protein: 3.6 g | Sodium: 159 mg | Fiber: 7.9 g | Carbohydrates: 37.3 g | Sugar: 21.2 g

Vegan Shamrock Shake Smoothie

Delight in the luck o' the Irish with the fresh, minty flavor of this Vegan Shamrock Shake Smoothie. This green treat is made healthy with nutritious ingredients like bananas, spinach, and fresh mint leaves. And the avocados make it rich and creamy! Get ready to dance a jig!

INGREDIENTS | SERVES 2

1 cup fresh spinach

1 cup banana slices

¼ cup avocado, peeled and chopped

1 cup unsweetened vanilla almond milk

6 fresh mint leaves

1 cup ice

1. Add spinach, bananas, avocados, almond milk, and mint leaves to a blender. Pulse until smooth. Add ice and pulse until a thick, creamy consistency develops.

2. Pour into two medium lidded containers. Refrigerate immediately, up to 3 days. When ready to serve, shake or stir smoothie and enjoy.

PER SERVING Calories: 132 | Fat: 5.6 g | Protein: 2.3 g | Sodium: 104 mg | Fiber: 4.8 g | Carbohydrates: 21.2 g | Sugar: 9.5 g

Using Blenders

Using a high-powered blender is important for making smoothies, especially when using greens like spinach or kale. A high-quality blender definitely pays in creating smoothies, shakes, soups, nondairy ice creams, and more.

Creamy Chocolate Banana Smoothie

This smoothie is taking on a flair of indulgence with its creamy texture and rich chocolate flavor. Bananas contribute to the creaminess of this recipe, and they also add sweetness.

INGREDIENTS | SERVES 2

1 tablespoon chocolate vegan protein powder

2 cups banana slices

2 medjool dates, pitted

1½ cups unsweetened vanilla almond milk

1 cup ice

1. Add all ingredients to a blender. Blend until smooth.

2. Pour into two medium lidded containers. Freeze immediately, up to 3 days. When ready to serve, remove from freezer and allow to sit 15 minutes before drinking.

PER SERVING Calories: 195 | Fat: 2.3 g | Protein: 5.6 g | Sodium: 175 mg | Fiber: 5.2 g | Carbohydrates: 42.2 g | Sugar: 24.2 g

Working with Medjool Dates

Medjool dates are one of the world's oldest cultivated fruits. They have a rich, caramel flavor, making them a perfect and healthy way to sweeten smoothies. To soften before use, simply soak in water for 10 minutes.

Blueberry Smoothie

Colorful blueberries add lots of antioxidants to this smoothie. Combined with a vanilla protein powder and bananas for sweetness, this recipe will keep you coming back for more.

INGREDIENTS | SERVES 2

2 tablespoons vanilla vegan protein powder

1½ cups unsweetened vanilla almond milk

2 cups banana slices

1 cup fresh blueberries

3 cups ice

1. Add protein powder and almond milk to a medium jar. Screw on lid and shake vigorously to blend. Place jar in refrigerator to keep cool up to 3 days until ready to make your smoothie.

2. Immediately prior to serving smoothie, pour ½ almond milk mixture into blender. Add ½ banana slices, ½ blueberries, and ½ ice and blend until smooth.

PER SERVING Calories: 237 | Fat: 3.1 g | Protein: 9.0 g | Sodium: 215 mg | Fiber: 6.4 g | Carbohydrates: 48.7 g | Sugar: 28.2 g

Vegan Key Lime Pie Smoothie

The flavors of key lime pie are brought to life in this lime-infused smoothie. Skip the high-calorie pie and have this creamy refreshment instead. Enjoy for breakfast, lunch, or even dessert.

INGREDIENTS | SERVES 2

2 tablespoons vanilla vegan protein powder

1½ cups unsweetened vanilla almond milk

¾ cup lime juice

2 teaspoons lime zest

1 cup fresh spinach, divided

3 cups ice, divided

1 graham cracker, crushed and divided

1. Add protein powder, almond milk, lime juice, and lime zest to a medium jar. Screw on lid and shake vigorously to blend.

2. Place jar in refrigerator up to 3 days until ready to make your smoothie.

3. Immediately prior to serving a smoothie, pour ½ lime juice mixture into blender. Add ½ spinach and ½ ice and blend until smooth. Top with ½ graham cracker crumbs and enjoy.

PER SERVING Calories: 117 | Fat: 3.4 g | Protein: 8.2 g | Sodium: 258 mg | Fiber: 1.9 g | Carbohydrates: 17.6 g | Sugar: 5.9 g

Vanilla Strawberry Lime Smoothie

This smoothie is like a strawberry limeade but better. Imagine an infusion of sweet vanilla, strawberries, and lime juice, made creamy with almond milk. It's a delicious, nutritious drink!

INGREDIENTS | SERVES 2

1½ cups unsweetened vanilla almond milk

2 tablespoons vanilla vegan protein powder

¼ cup lime juice

1 teaspoon lime zest

1 cup chopped fresh strawberries, divided

2 cups ice, divided

1. Add almond milk, protein powder, lime juice, and lime zest to a medium jar. Screw on lid and shake vigorously to blend.

2. Place jar in refrigerator to keep cool up to 3 days until ready to make your smoothie.

3. Immediately prior to serving, pour ½ lime juice mixture into blender. Add ½ strawberries and ½ ice and blend until smooth. Serve cold.

PER SERVING Calories: 93 | Fat: 2.8 g | Protein: 7.5 g | Sodium: 213 mg | Fiber: 2.5 g | Carbohydrates: 12.3 g | Sugar: 6.7 g

CHAPTER 6

Salads

Vegan Cobb Salad

The Vegan Cobb Salad sports layers of favorite ingredients, like avocados, vegan chicken strips, bacon-flavored almond slivers, and more. It is the quintessential American salad—deliciously veganized!

INGREDIENTS | SERVES 2

2 teaspoons olive oil, divided

1 cup Gardein Seven Grain Crispy Tenders, thawed

6 strips vegan bacon

5 cups spring mix salad blend

1 cup Easy Vegan Tofu Scramble (see Chapter 3 for recipe)

1 cup cherry tomatoes, chopped

½ avocado, peeled and chopped

1 cup vegan Cheddar shreds

½ cup Vegan Ranch Dressing (see Chapter 7 for recipe)

Making Bacon

If you don't have store-bought vegan bacon available, make your own. Combine 1 cup almond slivers with 1 tablespoon each of liquid smoke, maple syrup, and soy sauce. Then add 1 teaspoon paprika and ½ teaspoon ground turmeric. Stir and bake at 325°F on a parchment-lined baking sheet 5 minutes. Voilà: vegan "bacon."

1. Place a large skillet over medium heat. Add 1 teaspoon oil and crispy tenders. Cook 7 minutes on each side until golden brown. Use tongs to remove tenders to a cutting board and cut into bite-sized pieces.

2. Add remaining oil to skillet then add vegan bacon. Cook 3 minutes, then flip and cook 3 minutes on other side. Transfer to a small plate and let cool 5 minutes, then break into small pieces.

3. Refrigerate all ingredients in separate medium containers up to 7 days.

4. Immediately before serving, place ½ salad mix in a large bowl. Top with rows of vegan bacon, crispy tender pieces, tofu scramble, tomatoes, avocado, and shredded cheese. Drizzle with Vegan Ranch Dressing.

PER SERVING Calories: 898 | Fat: 58.7 g | Protein: 50.3 g | Sodium: 1,937 mg | Fiber: 14.9 g | Carbohydrates: 52.4 g | Sugar: 5.0 g

Vegan Potato Salad

Imagine Mom's best recipe for potato salad—veganized! This is a slightly sweet, creamy, mustard-based potato salad with an extra dose of summertime flavor for everyone, vegan or not! Add a pop of summer color by topping the salad with fresh cherry tomatoes.

INGREDIENTS | SERVES 12

6 small red potatoes with skins, cut into ½" cubes

5 cups water

½ cup finely chopped peeled red onion

1 cup Vegan Mayonnaise (see Chapter 7 for recipe)

3 tablespoons yellow mustard

2 tablespoons apple cider vinegar

3 tablespoons chopped sweet pickles

4 tablespoons agave nectar

1 teaspoon celery seed

1 batch Easy Vegan Tofu Scramble (see Chapter 3 for recipe)

1. Place potatoes in a large pan over high heat. Pour in water and bring to a boil. Cook until potatoes are just tender, about 10 minutes.

2. Place onion in a large lidded container. When potatoes are done, strain to remove excess liquid. Pour immediately over onions and seal container.

3. In a small bowl stir together mayonnaise, mustard, vinegar, pickles, agave nectar, and celery seed.

4. Pour mayonnaise mixture and tofu scramble over potatoes and onions and stir gently until combined. Refrigerate at least 1 hour before serving. Salad will last up to 6 days in refrigerator.

PER SERVING Calories: 163 | Fat: 5.6 g | Protein: 7.9 g | Sodium: 280 mg | Fiber: 2.7 g | Carbohydrates: 21.2 g | Sugar: 5.7 g

Seven-Layer Salad

This is a classic Midwestern potluck dish, but it is also perfect for holiday dinners. Seven-Layer Salad has all the layers you love, like vegan bacon, tofu scramble, peas, and more. No one will miss the meat or dairy!

INGREDIENTS | SERVES 12

For Salad

1 teaspoon olive oil

1 (15-ounce) block extra-firm tofu, pressed

1 teaspoon Garlic & Herb seasoning

⅛ teaspoon ground turmeric

2 tablespoons nutritional yeast flakes

½ teaspoon salt

5 cups mixed greens, torn into small pieces

7 green onions, sliced

1 (10-ounce) bag frozen peas

½ cup vegan bacon bits

1½ cups vegan Cheddar shreds

For Vegan Mayonnaise Dressing

2 cups Vegan Mayonnaise (see Chapter 7 for recipe)

½ cup plain dairy-free yogurt

2 teaspoons garlic powder

1 teaspoon onion powder

2 tablespoons agave nectar

½ teaspoon salt

⅛ teaspoon ground black pepper

Pressing Tofu

Because tofu is packed in water, many recipes require pressing it to remove the water. This also helps the tofu better absorb the flavors it's cooked in. To press tofu, remove it from its packaging, wrap it in paper towels, and gently press it while standing over a sink. Alternatively, you can set the wrapped tofu on a plate and place something heavy on top, like an iron skillet, for several minutes until excess water is drained.

1. **To make Salad:** add olive oil to a large skillet over medium heat. Place tofu in skillet and use a spatula to break it into small pieces. Cook about 1 minute. Add seasoning, turmeric, nutritional yeast, and salt and stir until tofu is coated. Cook additional 10 minutes, occasionally stirring to prevent tofu from browning.

2. Remove from heat and let cool 10 minutes before placing in a medium lidded bowl. Place in refrigerator while preparing remaining ingredients.

3. Fill a large serving dish with mixed greens. Spread green onions evenly over greens. Spread frozen peas on top of green onions.

4. Evenly spread tofu pieces on top of frozen peas. Sprinkle vegan bacon bits on top, followed with shredded vegan cheese. Cover and refrigerate up to 5 days.

5. **To make Vegan Mayonnaise Dressing:** add mayonnaise, dairy-free yogurt, garlic powder, onion powder, agave nectar, salt, and pepper to a small bowl and stir until well combined. Cover and refrigerate up to 5 days.

6. Immediately before serving, layer dressing over salad. Serve.

PER SERVING Calories: 187 | Fat: 12.4 g | Protein: 9.0 g | Sodium: 796 mg | Fiber: 2.1 g | Carbohydrates: 10.8 g | Sugar: 3.3 g

Vegan Harvest Salad

This is the perfect vegan salad: made just like the kind everyone knows and loves, but veganized! And it's just as good—and more heart-friendly too!

INGREDIENTS | SERVES 6

2 tablespoons liquid smoke

2 tablespoons maple syrup, divided

2 teaspoons olive oil, divided

1 tablespoon low-sodium soy sauce

1 (15-ounce) can chickpeas, drained

½ cup chopped sweet potatoes

2 tablespoons nutritional yeast flakes

½ teaspoon salt

⅛ teaspoon ground black pepper

6 cups romaine lettuce, torn into small pieces

½ cup cored and diced red apple

½ cup pecan halves

2 tablespoons roasted pumpkin seeds

1 batch Vegan Ranch Dressing (see Chapter 7 for recipe)

1. Preheat oven to 350°F. Line a baking sheet with parchment paper.

2. In a medium bowl combine liquid smoke, 2 tablespoons maple syrup, 1 teaspoon olive oil, and soy sauce. Add chickpeas and stir until thoroughly coated.

3. Pour over prepared baking sheet and bake 40 minutes, stirring occasionally throughout bake. Once done, set aside to cool 10 minutes, then transfer to a medium lidded container and refrigerate up to 10 days.

4. Place a skillet over medium heat. Add 1 teaspoon olive oil. Add potatoes and stir until coated with olive oil. Sprinkle with nutritional yeast and stir until coated. Cook until tender, about 7 minutes.

5. Sprinkle with salt and pepper, then set aside to cool 5 minutes. Transfer to a medium lidded container and refrigerate up to 7 days.

6. To serve, place lettuce in a serving bowl. Add chickpeas and sweet potatoes, apples, pecans, and pumpkin seeds. Toss to combine. Drizzle with Vegan Ranch Dressing.

PER SERVING Calories: 233 | Fat: 11.3 g | Protein: 7.7 g | Sodium: 622 mg | Fiber: 6.2 g | Carbohydrates: 26.2 g | Sugar: 10.9 g

Easy Pasta Salad

Italian flavors are infused in this easy recipe. It's the perfect light, convenient salad to take along with lunches, potlucks, or backyard barbeques, or it can be a side dish you can eat throughout the week. This crowd-pleasing recipe will inspire you to make it again and again!

INGREDIENTS | SERVES 8

3 cups water

2 cups uncooked multicolored rotini pasta

1 cup broccoli florets

1 cup cauliflower florets

¼ cup chopped green onion

¼ cup sliced black olives

½ cup dairy-free Italian dressing, divided

1. In a large pot, bring water to a boil over high heat. Add pasta and boil 8 minutes.

2. Place broccoli, cauliflower, green onions, and olives in a large lidded bowl.

3. When pasta is done, strain, then rinse in cold water. Pour pasta over broccoli mixture. Add ½ Italian dressing and gently stir to combine. Set aside to cool 10 minutes. Cover and refrigerate up to 4 days.

4. To serve, add remaining dressing. Serve cold.

PER SERVING Calories: 103 | Fat: 3.8 g | Protein: 2.5 g | Sodium: 197 mg | Fiber: 1.1 g | Carbohydrates: 14.4 g | Sugar: 2.5 g

Brussels Sprouts Slaw

Just like cabbage, Brussels sprouts make a delicious slaw when shredded and mixed with a lime-infused cilantro dressing. This simple but flavorful Brussels Sprouts Slaw will be the hit of your summer picnics. Serve it as a salad or even as a condiment on sandwiches or tacos.

INGREDIENTS | SERVES 6

2 cups Brussels sprouts, roughly chopped

¼ cup roughly chopped green onion

¼ cup roughly chopped seeded red bell pepper

1 jalapeño, seeded and chopped

¼ cup cilantro leaves, chopped

2 tablespoons lime juice

1 tablespoon agave nectar

1 tablespoon sesame seed oil

3 tablespoons Vegan Mayonnaise (see Chapter 7 for recipe)

1 tablespoon sesame seeds

1. Add Brussels sprouts to a food processor along with green onion, bell pepper, jalapeño, and cilantro. Pulse until ingredients are shredded into small pieces similar to slaw.

2. Transfer to a large lidded bowl and add lime juice, agave nectar, sesame seed oil, and mayonnaise. Stir until combined. Cover and refrigerate up to 7 days.

3. To serve, top with sesame seeds.

PER SERVING Calories: 66 | Fat: 4.0 g | Protein: 2.1 g | Sodium: 77 mg | Fiber: 1.7 g | Carbohydrates: 6.4 g | Sugar: 2.9 g

Broccoli Salad

Increase your consumption of high-energy foods with this crispy and healthy Broccoli Salad. Enjoy the flavors of broccoli, infused with a slightly sweet mayonnaise, vegan bacon, pumpkin seeds, raisins, and more.

INGREDIENTS | SERVES 10

For Salad

6 cups broccoli florets

¼ cup chopped green onion

1 cup frozen peas, thawed

¼ cup pumpkin seeds

¼ cup raisins

For Dressing

¾ cup Vegan Mayonnaise (see Chapter 7 for recipe)

2 tablespoons apple cider vinegar

2 tablespoons agave nectar

1 tablespoon chia seeds

4 slices vegan bacon

1. Place a steamer insert into a medium saucepan and add enough water so that it's just below the level of the basket. Bring water to a boil over high heat, then add broccoli florets. Steam until florets are tender but still crunchy, about 5 minutes. Remove from heat, strain, and run under cold water.

2. Place onion in a large lidded bowl. Pour broccoli over onion. Stir in peas, pumpkin seeds, and raisins.

3. In a small bowl combine Vegan Mayonnaise, vinegar, agave nectar, and chia seeds. Pour over broccoli mixture and stir to combine. Cover and refrigerate up to 7 days.

4. Place a medium skillet over medium heat and add vegan bacon strips. Cook 5 minutes on each side. Set aside to let cool 5 minutes before breaking into pieces. Place in a small sealed container and refrigerate up to 10 days.

5. To serve, sprinkle vegan bacon crumbles over salad. Serve cold.

PER SERVING Calories: 105 | Fat: 4.0 g | Protein: 4.8 g | Sodium: 247 mg | Fiber: 3.3 g | Carbohydrates: 13.6 g | Sugar: 6.4 g

Spring Wedge Salad

The crispy, refreshing wedge salad is a classic American dish. Here, this retro salad is veganized and easy to make at home. It uses simple ingredients, like crunchy iceberg lettuce, with other favorite toppings.

INGREDIENTS | SERVES 4

4 slices vegan bacon

¾ cup Vegan Mayonnaise (see Chapter 7 for recipe)

2 tablespoons plain soy milk

1 tablespoon apple cider vinegar

½ teaspoon garlic powder

½ teaspoon salt

⅛ teaspoon ground black pepper

1 head iceberg lettuce, cored and quartered

½ cup chopped green onion

½ cup chopped seeded yellow pepper

8 cherry tomatoes, halved

1. Place a medium skillet over medium heat and add vegan bacon. Cook 5 minutes on each side. Set aside to cool 5 minutes before breaking into pieces. Place in a small sealed container and refrigerate up to 10 days.

2. In a small lidded bowl stir together mayonnaise, soy milk, vinegar, garlic powder, salt, and pepper. Cover and refrigerate up to 5 days.

3. Place lettuce in a medium lidded container and refrigerate up to 5 days.

4. To serve, arrange iceberg wedges on plates, drizzle with the vegan ranch dressing made in step 2, and top each wedge with bacon crumbles, onions, bell peppers, and tomato halves.

PER SERVING Calories: 146 | Fat: 8.6 g | Protein: 7.0 g | Sodium: 844 mg | Fiber: 3.7 g | Carbohydrates: 11.5 g | Sugar: 5.0 g

Vegan Miso Slaw

This coleslaw is smothered with a miso-infused sauce. It's a sweet but tangy flavor that can be served alone, as a side dish, or even as a condiment. If you haven't tried adding slaw over nachos, you're missing out!

INGREDIENTS | SERVES 6

½ cup Vegan Mayonnaise (see Chapter 7 for recipe)

2 tablespoons apple cider vinegar

2 tablespoons mild miso paste

2 tablespoons agave nectar

⅛ teaspoon celery seed

⅓ teaspoon ground turmeric

¼ teaspoon salt

2 tablespoons chia seeds

3 cups shredded cabbage mixed with slivered carrots

1. Combine everything except cabbage mix in a small bowl. Set aside.

2. Place cabbage mix in a medium lidded bowl. Pour in coleslaw sauce. Stir to combine. Cover and refrigerate up to 7 days.

PER SERVING Calories: 86 | Fat: 4.0 g | Protein: 3.2 g | Sodium: 524 mg | Fiber: 2.6 g | Carbohydrates: 9.3 g | Sugar: 5.5 g

Vegan Taco Salad

This Vegan Taco Salad recipe is an easy meal full of your favorite taco ingredients. Meal prepping instructions make it easy to prep on the weekend and serve within minutes on weekdays.

INGREDIENTS | SERVES 4

3 cups vegan crumbles

4 tablespoons taco seasoning

1 (15-ounce) can chili beans, drained

4 cups field greens

1 (14-ounce) package tortilla chips

½ cup chopped green onion

2 cups vegan Cheddar shreds

1 cup mild chunky salsa

1 cup vegan sour cream

1 cup chopped cherry tomatoes

½ cup black olives

½ cup Catalina light salad dressing

1. In a medium microwave-safe bowl combine vegan crumbles, taco seasoning, and chili beans. Microwave in 30-second increments until heated through.

2. Store field greens by placing paper towels in bottom of a large container. Put greens in the container and place paper towels on top. Greens will stay fresh up to 7 days in refrigerator.

3. Place remaining ingredients in separate containers. They will last in refrigerator up to 7 days. Vegan crumble mixture will also last up to 7 days in refrigerator, or can be frozen up to 1 month.

4. To serve, recook vegan crumble mixture in microwave until heated through, about 2 minutes. Remove enough chips for one serving and break into pieces in a medium bowl. Top chips with ¼ vegan crumble mixture, followed by ¼ of each topping. Drizzle with Catalina dressing.

PER SERVING Calories: 1,128 | Fat: 53.2 g | Protein: 28.5 g | Sodium: 2,891 mg | Fiber: 24.1 g | Carbohydrates: 131.6 g | Sugar: 13.9 g

Vegan Caesar Salad

This amazing Vegan Caesar Salad is set apart from others because of the great dressing. A standard Caesar salad requires raw eggs and anchovies. That doesn't sound too appealing to many people, so this vegan version will be your go-to recipe moving forward!

INGREDIENTS | SERVES 6

¼ cup olive oil

3 cloves garlic, peeled

1 baguette, sliced into 1" pieces

2 tablespoons lemon juice

1 tablespoon Dijon mustard

½ cup Vegan Mayonnaise (see Chapter 7 for recipe)

1 tablespoon nutritional yeast flakes

1 teaspoon agave nectar

1 tablespoon apple cider vinegar

3 heads romaine lettuce hearts, torn into small pieces

2 tablespoons shredded vegan Parmesan

Flavor with Lemons

Having fresh lemons around is a great way to add flavor to your dishes. Sprinkle lemon zest from the peel over salads and pasta dishes, and even add to baked goods like lemon bars. In addition, lemon juice combined with a little salt and pepper makes a perfect sauce for salads, steamed vegetables, and more.

1. Preheat oven to 375°F. Line a baking sheet with parchment paper.

2. In a medium bowl stir together olive oil and garlic. Set aside 10 minutes.

3. Place baguette pieces on prepared pan. Drizzle garlic olive oil over baguette pieces, using a spatula or your hands to toss pieces until well covered. Bake 10 minutes until golden, tossing occasionally. Let cool and then store at room temperature in a large airtight container up to 7 days.

4. In the same bowl with remaining olive oil add lemon juice, mustard, mayonnaise, nutritional yeast flakes, agave nectar, and vinegar. Stir to combine. Transfer to a medium sealed container and refrigerate up to 7 days.

5. When ready to serve, place lettuce in a large salad bowl. Drizzle with dressing. Toss until the lettuce is coated with dressing. Sprinkle with croutons and vegan Parmesan.

PER SERVING Calories: 306 | Fat: 13.6 g | Protein: 10.6 g | Sodium: 572 mg | Fiber: 7.9 g | Carbohydrates: 36.0 g | Sugar: 7.1 g

Five-Bean Salad

This colorful Five-Bean Salad features lots of beans, fresh vegetables, and a slightly sweet sauce that ties it all together. Take it to a potluck and share with others!

INGREDIENTS | SERVES 10

2 tablespoons apple cider vinegar

⅓ cup olive oil

2 tablespoons maple syrup

2 tablespoons tamari

1 teaspoon dried oregano

1 teaspoon dried basil

¼ cup chopped fresh flat-leaf parsley

1 green onion, finely chopped

1 (15-ounce) can cannellini beans, drained and rinsed

1 (15-ounce) can light red kidney beans, drained and rinsed

1 (15-ounce) can pinto beans, drained and rinsed

1 (15-ounce) can chickpeas, drained and rinsed

1 (15-ounce) can black beans, drained and rinsed

1 large zucchini, ends removed, quartered and sliced

¼ cup sliced red radishes

½ cup chopped peeled red onion

1 medium red bell pepper, seeded and diced

1. Combine vinegar, olive oil, maple syrup, tamari, oregano, basil, parsley, and green onion in a small lidded bowl. Cover and refrigerate up to 7 days.

2. Add all beans to a large lidded bowl. Add all vegetables and combine. Drizzle ¾ dressing over bean mixture. Stir to combine. Cover and refrigerate 4 hours, up to 7 days.

3. To serve, drain any extra juices that may have accumulated in bottom of dish, then drizzle with remaining dressing.

4. To freeze, make entire salad except for zucchini, radishes, and bell peppers. Transfer to a large freezer bag and freeze up to 3 months. When ready to serve, remove from freezer and allow to sit at room temperature until thawed, about 1 hour. Add chopped zucchini, radishes, and bell peppers.

PER SERVING Calories: 300 | Fat: 11.3 g | Protein: 11.9 g | Sodium: 541 mg | Fiber: 7.7 g | Carbohydrates: 37.0 g | Sugar: 5.5 g

What Is Tamari?

Tamari is a gluten-free and oftentimes lower-sodium version of soy sauce. It has a similar flavor to soy sauce and can be used in place of it in most recipes. You can find tamari in the international section of most grocery stores.

Chinese Salad

An Asian-style salad, this vegan Chinese Salad is served with shredded cabbage, edamame, and crunchy chow mein noodles and is topped with a delicious dressing infused with sesame and ginger flavors.

INGREDIENTS | SERVES 6

For Salad
2 tablespoons tamari
1 teaspoon sesame oil
2 tablespoons agave nectar, divided
¼ teaspoon ground black pepper
1 (15-ounce) container extra-firm tofu, pressed and cut into ½" cubes
4 cups chopped romaine lettuce
1 cup shredded red cabbage
¼ cup grated peeled carrots
¼ cup shelled edamame beans
1 green onion, thinly sliced
¼ cup chow mein noodles
2 tablespoons sesame seeds

For Vinaigrette
2 tablespoons rice vinegar
½ teaspoon garlic powder
2 teaspoons sesame oil
1 teaspoon ground ginger
1 teaspoon tamari

1. Preheat oven to 350°F.

2. **To make Salad:** in an 8" × 8" square baking dish, stir together tamari, 1 teaspoon sesame oil, 1 tablespoon agave nectar, and pepper. Add tofu and marinate 10 minutes, stirring occasionally. Transfer to oven and bake 15 minutes.

3. Remove from oven and let cool about 5 minutes. Transfer to a large lidded container and refrigerate up to 7 days.

4. **To make Vinaigrette:** whisk together vinegar, garlic powder, remaining sesame oil, remaining agave nectar, ginger, and tamari. Transfer to a small lidded container. Refrigerate up to 7 days.

5. When ready to serve, place romaine lettuce in large bowl. Top with cabbage, carrots, edamame, green onions, and baked tofu. Add chow mein noodles and sesame seeds. Drizzle with vinaigrette. Toss to coat.

PER SERVING Calories: 150 | Fat: 7.9 g | Protein: 9.7 g | Sodium: 434 mg | Fiber: 2.2 g | Carbohydrates: 11.2 g | Sugar: 5.0 g

CHAPTER 7

Sauces and Dressings

Vegan Velvet Cheese Sauce

This kid-friendly Vegan Velvet Cheese Sauce is so creamy it will redefine your idea of vegan cheese. Serve this versatile sauce over baked potatoes or steamed broccoli or even on sandwiches. Add some salsa to create a delicious nacho cheese sauce.

INGREDIENTS | SERVES 12

¼ cup vegan butter

¼ cup all-purpose flour

1 cup hot water

1 tablespoon soy sauce

¼ teaspoon ground turmeric

½ teaspoon garlic powder

¼ cup nutritional yeast flakes

1 (15-ounce) can pumpkin purée

1 (15-ounce) can chickpeas, including liquid

2 cups vegan Cheddar shreds

1. In a small saucepan melt vegan butter over low heat about 2 minutes. Turn heat up to medium and whisk in flour until mixture is smooth and bubbly. Whisk in water, soy sauce, turmeric, and garlic powder and nutritional yeast. Remove from heat.

2. In a food processor add pumpkin and chickpeas (including liquid). Pulse 1 minute or until mixture is very smooth. Add mixture from saucepan and vegan cheese. Pulse 1 minute.

3. Transfer mixture back to saucepan over medium heat. Cover and cook 5 minutes until cheese has melted and sauce is smooth.

4. Let cool 10 minutes before transferring to a small lidded container. Cover and store in the refrigerator up to 7 days.

5. To serve, cook in microwave until heated through, about 1 minute.

PER SERVING (2 tbsp) Calories: 129 | Fat: 6.8 g | Protein: 2.9 g | Sodium: 330 mg | Fiber: 3.3 g | Carbohydrates: 14.7 g | Sugar: 2.4 g

Sun-Dried Tomato Aioli

This creamy Sun-Dried Tomato Aioli is a great condiment to add to your favorite recipes, like veggie burgers or French fries. With a simple, two-step process it will be ready in just minutes and adds rich flavor to any dish.

INGREDIENTS | MAKES ¾ CUP

¼ cup sun-dried tomatoes

½ cup Vegan Mayonnaise (see this chapter for recipe)

1 teaspoon garlic powder

1 tablespoon olive oil

1. Soak tomatoes in hot water 10 minutes. Once soaked, place in a food processor, along with mayonnaise, garlic powder, and olive oil. Pulse 3 seconds, then use a spatula to push ingredients down and pulse again.

2. Transfer to a small lidded container and refrigerate up to 7 days.

PER SERVING (¾ cup) Calories: 375 | Fat: 29.8 g | Protein: 12.4 g | Sodium: 1,146 mg | Fiber: 3.5 g | Carbohydrates: 15.4 g | Sugar: 8.0 g

Date-Sweetened Barbecue Sauce

Avoid processed sugar by making your own naturally sweetened barbecue sauce. This Date-Sweetened Barbecue Sauce is a perfect condiment for veggie burgers, and it will make your summer grilling even healthier than before!

INGREDIENTS | SERVES 16

1 (15-ounce) can tomato sauce

1 cup pitted medjool dates (approximately 8 dates), softened

2 tablespoons tomato paste

2 tablespoons vegan Worcestershire sauce

1 tablespoon apple cider vinegar

1 tablespoon liquid smoke

1 tablespoon ground flaxseed

1 teaspoon paprika

1 teaspoon garlic powder

1 teaspoon dehydrated onions

1. Place all ingredients in a food processor and pulse 3 seconds. Use a spatula to press down any ingredients that may have moved to the top of the container and pulse again until desired saucy consistency.

2. Transfer to a small lidded container, cover, and refrigerate up to 10 days.

PER SERVING (2 tbsp) Calories: 39 | Fat: 0.3 g | Protein: 0.8 g | Sodium: 148 mg | Fiber: 1.4 g | Carbohydrates: 9.5 g | Sugar: 7.3 g

Vegan White Barbecue Sauce

*Use this savory, sweet Vegan White Barbecue Sauce as a dipping sauce,
or drizzle it over veggie burgers, French fries, and more.*

INGREDIENTS | SERVES 6

1 cup Vegan Mayonnaise (see this chapter for recipe)
1 teaspoon Dijon mustard
½ teaspoon garlic powder
½ teaspoon dehydrated onions
½ teaspoon ground black pepper
¼ cup apple cider vinegar
¼ teaspoon salt
½ teaspoon smoked paprika

1. Stir all ingredients together in a small bowl.

2. Transfer to a small lidded container, cover, and refrigerate up to 10 days.

PER SERVING (2 tbsp) Calories: 76 | Fat: 5.6 g | Protein: 3.5 g | Sodium: 488 mg | Fiber: 0.7 g | Carbohydrates: 2.5 g | Sugar: 1.0 g

Date-Sweetened Ketchup

This date-sweetened ketchup recipe is made with just a few simple ingredients that combine to create the perfect naturally sweetened ketchup—with no preservatives! Use this wholesome ketchup in place of regular ketchup in all your favorite recipes.

INGREDIENTS | SERVES 16

¼ cup medjool dates, pitted and chopped
1 (6-ounce) can tomato paste
1 (8-ounce) can tomato sauce
1 tablespoon apple cider vinegar
1 tablespoon tamari
1 teaspoon garlic powder
1 teaspoon onion powder
½ teaspoon paprika
½ teaspoon salt

1. Place dates in a small microwave-safe bowl. Heat for 15 seconds until tender.

2. Add all ingredients to a food processor and pulse 3 seconds. Use a spatula to press down any ingredients that may have moved to the top of the container and pulse again until desired saucy consistency is reached.

3. Transfer to a small lidded container, cover, and refrigerate up to 10 days.

PER SERVING (2 tbsp) Calories: 20 | Fat: 0.1 g | Protein: 0.7 g | Sodium: 167 mg | Fiber: 0.9 g | Carbohydrates: 5.0 g | Sugar: 3.3 g

Vegan Ranch Dressing

This Vegan Ranch Dressing is popular for a very good reason: it's creamy with just the right balance of herbs, sweetness, and subtle garlic flavor! You'll love this dairy-free version, made with vegan mayonnaise, fresh garlic, and fresh herbs.

INGREDIENTS | SERVES 8

½ cup Vegan Mayonnaise (see this chapter for recipe)

½ cup unsweetened almond milk

1 tablespoon apple cider vinegar

½ teaspoon garlic powder

1 tablespoon finely chopped green onion

⅛ teaspoon salt

¼ teaspoon dry mustard

1 tablespoon chopped fresh chives

2 teaspoons dried parsley

¼ teaspoon dried dill weed

1. In a small bowl whisk together Vegan Mayonnaise, almond milk, and vinegar.

2. Add garlic powder and green onion to milk mixture, along with salt and dry mustard. Stir to combine, then stir in chives, parsley, and dill.

3. Store in a small airtight container in refrigerator up to 7 days.

PER SERVING (2 tbsp) Calories: 30 | Fat: 2.3 g | Protein: 1.4 g | Sodium: 187 mg | Fiber: 0.4 g | Carbohydrates: 1.1 g | Sugar: 0.4 g

Vegan Pumpkin Ranch Dressing

This Vegan Pumpkin Ranch Dressing is everyone's favorite—but veganized and served with a fall flair! It has just a touch of pumpkin and is delicious over salads or served as a dip with chopped vegetables.

INGREDIENTS | SERVES 6

1 cup plain dairy-free yogurt

2 tablespoons Vegan Mayonnaise (see this chapter for recipe)

1 tablespoon apple cider vinegar

1 tablespoon nutritional yeast flakes

1 tablespoon maple syrup

2 tablespoons pumpkin purée

½ teaspoon garlic powder

½ teaspoon salt

¼ teaspoon dried thyme

¼ teaspoon dried sage

1. Add all ingredients together in a small bowl and stir to combine.

2. Transfer to a small lidded container and refrigerate up to 10 days.

PER SERVING (2 tbsp) Calories: 48 | Fat: 0.8 g | Protein: 1.8 g | Sodium: 246 mg | Fiber: 0.5 g | Carbohydrates: 7.0 g | Sugar: 4.4 g

Ginger Peanut Butter Dipping Sauce

This slightly sweet Ginger Peanut Butter Dipping Sauce transforms peanut butter into a creamy sauce perfect over your favorite dishes, such as veggie burgers, kebabs, fried tofu, and vegan wraps.

INGREDIENTS | SERVES 4

¼ cup all-natural peanut butter

1 tablespoon sesame oil

1 teaspoon soy sauce

1 tablespoon hoisin sauce

1 tablespoon sriracha

½ teaspoon garlic powder

½ teaspoon ground ginger

½ cup water

1. Combine peanut butter, sesame oil, soy sauce, hoisin sauce, sriracha, garlic powder, and ginger in a medium bowl. Add water and stir to combine.

2. Transfer to a small lidded container and refrigerate up to 21 days.

PER SERVING (2 tbsp) Calories: 141 | Fat: 11.3 g | Protein: 3.9 g | Sodium: 214 mg | Fiber: 1.0 g | Carbohydrates: 6.6 g | Sugar: 3.6 g

Vegan Mayonnaise

Make this homemade Vegan Mayonnaise from simple ingredients and enjoy it on veggie burgers, mixed into salads, spread on sandwiches, and more!

INGREDIENTS | SERVES 17

1 (15-ounce) package firm tofu, pressed

4 tablespoons rice vinegar

4 tablespoons vegetable oil

2 teaspoons agave nectar

2 teaspoons salt

½ teaspoon dried mustard

4 tablespoons nutritional yeast flakes

1. Combine all ingredients in a food processor and pulse until smooth. Use a spatula to press down any ingredients at the top of the bowl and pulse again 3 seconds.

2. Spoon mayonnaise into a small lidded container and refrigerate up to 10 days.

PER SERVING (2 tbsp) Calories: 53 | Fat: 4.1 g | Protein: 2.5 g | Sodium: 278 mg | Fiber: 0.4 g | Carbohydrates: 1.4 g | Sugar: 0.7 g

Blackberry Hoisin Sauce

This Blackberry Hoisin Sauce takes just five minutes to make and will transform your vegan Asian dishes! The slightly sweet sauce can be used as a condiment on veggie burgers, sandwiches, salads, and more.

INGREDIENTS | SERVES 4

2 tablespoons blackberry jam

1 tablespoon soy sauce

1 teaspoon garlic powder

1 teaspoon ginger powder

1 teaspoon rice vinegar

Stir all ingredients together in a medium lidded bowl. Cover and refrigerate up to 10 days.

PER SERVING (2 tbsp) Calories: 34 | Fat: 0.0 g | Protein: 0.5 g | Sodium: 222 mg | Fiber: 0.3 g | Carbohydrates: 8.0 g | Sugar: 4.9 g

Red Bell Pepper Aioli

This creamy, zesty red pepper aioli is a delicious condiment to add on veggie burgers or hot dogs or even alongside French fries. It's also great as a dip with vegetables or chips.

INGREDIENTS | SERVES 4

1 cup chopped seeded red bell pepper

4 tablespoons Vegan Mayonnaise (see this chapter for recipe)

1 teaspoon garlic powder

2 teaspoons agave nectar

1 tablespoon ground flaxseed

1. Combine all ingredients in a food processor and pulse until smooth. It will be runny at first, but flaxseed will thicken sauce within 3 minutes.

2. Transfer to a medium lidded container and refrigerate up to 10 days.

PER SERVING (2 tbsp) Calories: 60 | Fat: 2.8 g | Protein: 2.1 g | Sodium: 141 mg | Fiber: 1.5 g | Carbohydrates: 6.7 g | Sugar: 4.3 g

Smoky Chipotle Hummus

Make this Smoky Chipotle Hummus and use it as a dip, or as a condiment on your favorite sandwiches. This tasty recipe will give you a great boost of fiber, while adding a little protein to your diet as well.

INGREDIENTS | SERVES 6

2 tablespoons olive oil

½ cup chopped peeled yellow onion

2 cloves garlic, peeled and roughly chopped

1 (15-ounce) can chickpeas, rinsed and drained

¼ cup tahini

¼ cup lemon juice

1 tablespoon soy sauce

1 tablespoon Tabasco Chipotle Pepper Sauce

1 teaspoon smoked paprika

2 tablespoons sesame seeds

1. Place olive oil in a medium skillet over medium heat. Add chopped onions and cook until translucent, about 5 minutes. Add garlic and turn heat off.

2. Place chickpeas, tahini, lemon juice, and soy sauce in a blender or food processor. Pulse until chickpeas are mostly smooth. Remove lid and push down any ingredients on the side of the bowl and pulse again. Add cooked onions and garlic (including oil from skillet), Tabasco, and paprika. Pulse until smooth.

3. Transfer to a medium lidded container and refrigerate up to 10 days. To serve, top with sesame seeds.

PER SERVING (2 tbsp) Calories: 186 | Fat: 11.2 g | Protein: 6.0 g | Sodium: 263 mg | Fiber: 4.5 g | Carbohydrates: 16.1 g | Sugar: 2.7 g

What Is Tahini?

Tahini is essentially sesame seeds that have been toasted and ground to a creamy paste. You can also use tahini to make salad dressings and sauces. Look for it in the international section of your grocery store. It will last up to 4 months if stored in the refrigerator.

Green Monster Hummus

Enjoy this delicious Green Monster Hummus, made with spinach for added nutrition and color. Serve with pita chips or crackers, or even as a condiment on sandwiches.

INGREDIENTS | SERVES 6

1 (15-ounce) can chickpeas, rinsed and drained

¼ cup tahini

1 teaspoon garlic powder

1 tablespoon lemon juice

1 tablespoon soy sauce

2 tablespoons water

¼ cup olive oil

1 teaspoon salt

1 teaspoon dried oregano

1 teaspoon dried basil

2 cups fresh spinach

1. Pour all ingredients into a food processor and pulse until well combined. Scrape down sides of food processor bowl and process again until hummus is a fine consistency.

2. Transfer to a medium lidded bowl and refrigerate up to 10 days.

PER SERVING (2 tbsp) Calories: 203 | Fat: 14.1 g | Protein: 5.5 g | Sodium: 643 mg | Fiber: 4.1 g | Carbohydrates: 14.0 g | Sugar: 1.9 g

Vegan Special Sauce

Don't give up your dream of the perfect burger: Simply make this delicious special sauce recipe at home and smear it on your favorite veggie patties. This is a restaurant-quality sauce that's so good, you can even use it as a dip for French fries.

INGREDIENTS | SERVES 4

½ cup Vegan Mayonnaise (see this chapter for recipe)

2 tablespoons French dressing

3 teaspoons sweet relish

2 green onions, only white parts, finely chopped

1 teaspoon white vinegar

1 teaspoon granulated sugar

1. Combine all ingredients in a small bowl.

2. Transfer to a small lidded container and refrigerate up to 21 days.

PER SERVING (2 tbsp) Calories: 100 | Fat: 6.9 g | Protein: 2.7 g | Sodium: 376 mg | Fiber: 0.6 g | Carbohydrates: 5.6 g | Sugar: 4.3 g

Sweet Mustard Dipping Sauce

This homemade Sweet Mustard Dipping Sauce is perfect for dipping, but also for drizzling over veggie burgers, salads, and more. This is a supereasy, tangy-sweet sauce you can make in minutes!

INGREDIENTS | SERVES 4

¾ cup Vegan Mayonnaise (see this chapter for recipe)
2 tablespoons agave nectar
2 tablespoons yellow mustard
1 tablespoon apple cider vinegar
½ teaspoon garlic powder

1. Combine all ingredients in a small bowl.

2. Transfer to a small sealable container and refrigerate up to 5 days.

PER SERVING (2 tbsp) Calories: 107 | Fat: 6.4 g | Protein: 4.1 g | Sodium: 503 mg | Fiber: 1.0 g | Carbohydrates: 8.1 g | Sugar: 5.8 g

Easy Vegan Parmesan

Cashews, combined with a perfect mixture of herbs and other tasty ingredients, create the perfect nondairy vegan Parmesan. This recipe can be served over pasta, popcorn, and even chips.

INGREDIENTS | SERVES 20

1 cup cashews
3 tablespoons nutritional yeast flakes
1 tablespoon mild miso paste
1 tablespoon ground flaxseed
½ teaspoon ground turmeric
1 teaspoon paprika
½ teaspoon garlic powder
½ teaspoon salt

1. Place cashews and nutritional yeast in a food processor. Pulse 3 seconds until nuts are broken down into smaller, crumbly pieces. Add remaining ingredients and pulse until mixture becomes a coarse meal.

2. Transfer to a medium lidded container and refrigerate up to 10 days. Mixture can also be frozen up to 1 month.

PER SERVING (2 tbsp) Calories: 45 | Fat: 3.3 g | Protein: 1.5 g | Sodium: 95 mg | Fiber: 0.5 g | Carbohydrates: 2.9 g | Sugar: 0.5 g

Asian Awesome Sauce

This tangy-sweet Asian Awesome Sauce is perfect over cauliflower fried rice or air-fried tofu, or even as a condiment for dishes like veggie burgers.

INGREDIENTS | SERVES 4

¼ cup rice wine vinegar

2 tablespoons agave nectar

½ cup orange juice

1 clove garlic, peeled and roughly chopped

1 teaspoon chili garlic sauce

1 tablespoon cornstarch

¼ cup water

¼ cup fresh cilantro leaves

1. Place vinegar, agave nectar, juice, garlic, and garlic sauce in a food processor. Pulse 2 seconds until garlic is minced.

2. Combine cornstarch with water in a small microwave-safe bowl. Microwave 15 seconds and stir. Repeat heating until mixture thickens. Once thickened, let cool 1 minute, then add to food processor and pulse until well incorporated.

3. Add cilantro and pulse 3 seconds until roughly chopped, leaving plenty of bits of leaves throughout.

4. Transfer to a small sealed container and refrigerate up to 10 days. To serve, allow to sit 3 minutes at room temperature, or heat 3 seconds in microwave.

PER SERVING (2 tbsp) Calories: 46 | Fat: 0.0 g | Protein: 0.3 g | Sodium: 29 mg | Fiber: 0.1 g | Carbohydrates: 10.6 g | Sugar: 7.3 g

Easy Homemade Oat Milk

This Easy Homemade Oat Milk can save you those last-minute trips to the store when you realize you're out of soy or almond milk. It's easy to make, creamy, and full of flavor.

INGREDIENTS | SERVES 6

⅔ cup rolled oats

2 cups water

½ teaspoon vanilla extract

1. Combine oats and water in a medium bowl and soak 20 minutes. Once soaked, transfer to a blender and blend 2 minutes until completely smooth.

2. To use this milk in a recipe, use as is. To use for drinking, stir in vanilla, then strain through a nut-milk bag. Place nut-milk bag over a large bowl. Pour oat milk into bag to strain thicker oat bits. Squeeze bag to get all milk out. Transfer milk back to blender and blend until smooth. Then transfer to a lidded container and refrigerate up to 4 days.

PER SERVING (2 tbsp) Calories: 43 | Fat: 0.8 g | Protein: 1.6 g | Sodium: 0 mg | Fiber: 1.1 g | Carbohydrates: 7.2 g | Sugar: 0.3 g

Sweet Potato Nacho "Cheese" Sauce

This Sweet Potato Nacho "Cheese" Sauce is everything you want from a creamy, spicy cheese sauce. You might even forget that it's plant-based. Serve with tortilla chips or drizzled over your favorite veggie burgers. For a crunchy kick, sprinkle with chopped red bell pepper.

INGREDIENTS | SERVES 4

1 tablespoon cornstarch

1 cup water

3 cups diced sweet potato

½ cup nutritional yeast flakes

1 teaspoon lemon juice

½ teaspoon salt

¼ teaspoon onion powder

¼ teaspoon garlic powder

¼ teaspoon paprika

1 (4.5-ounce) can diced tomatoes and green chilies

1. Combine cornstarch and water in a medium pot. Add sweet potatoes and place over medium heat. Bring to a boil, then reduce heat to a simmer and cook 10 minutes until potatoes are tender. Drain water, conserving ½ cup.

2. Pour sweet potato mixture into a blender with nutritional yeast flakes, lemon juice, salt, onion powder, garlic powder, paprika, and reserved water. Blend until smooth. Add tomatoes with chilies including liquid, and pulse 3 seconds to combine.

3. Let cool 10 minutes, then transfer to a large sealed container and refrigerate up to 10 days.

4. To serve, cook in microwave until heated through—about 1 minute.

PER SERVING (2 tbsp) Calories: 131 | Fat: 0.3 g | Protein: 5.8 g | Sodium: 454 mg | Fiber: 4.9 g | Carbohydrates: 26.1 g | Sugar: 5.0 g

CHAPTER 8

Sides

Fresh Corn Salsa

This quick and easy Fresh Corn Salsa is delicious on homemade burrito bowls, tacos, salads, and more. It's a simple way to add farm-fresh flavor to your everyday meals.

INGREDIENTS | SERVES 8

3 ears fresh corn, still in husk

2 teaspoons finely chopped seeded jalapeños

¼ cup minced peeled red onion

¼ cup fresh cilantro leaves, chopped

Juice from 1 lime

½ teaspoon salt

1. Place corn, still in husk, in microwave and cook 12 minutes. Wearing gloves, place hot ears of corn on a cutting board. Chop off bottoms of corn, then use gloved hands to press corn out of husk from other end. Allow to sit on cutting board to cool about 5 minutes.

2. Hold 1 cooled corncob upright with base resting on bottom of cutting board and use a serrated knife to cut downward to remove corn from cob. Repeat with remaining corncobs.

3. Place corn in a large sealable container and add jalapeños, red onion, and cilantro. Squeeze juice from lime over corn, then add salt and stir until well combined.

4. Place in a medium lidded container and refrigerate up to 7 days, or freeze up to 2 months.

PER SERVING Calories: 35 | Fat: 0.5 g | Protein: 1.3 g | Sodium: 151 mg | Fiber: 0.9 g | Carbohydrates: 7.8 g | Sugar: 2.7 g

Air Fryer French Fries

*Do crispy French fries conjure up images of an unhealthy, greasy side dish,
leaving you with a heavy feeling? These fries are made with minimal oil and will
make your veggie burger nights take on a healthier new meaning!*

INGREDIENTS | SERVES 2

2 medium russet potatoes, cut into ¼"
strips
1 teaspoon olive oil
½ teaspoon salt
⅛ teaspoon ground black pepper

What's an Air Fryer?

An air fryer works like a convection oven to
cook food with hot air. Use it to create
browned and crispy foods without all the
oil necessary in cooking fried foods the traditional way.

1. Heat your air fryer to 400°F.

2. Place potato slices in a large bowl and drizzle oil over top. Use fingers or a spoon to ensure each potato slice is coated in oil.

3. Transfer potato slices to air fryer basket. Cook 20 minutes, removing basket and stirring potatoes halfway through.

4. Remove from air fryer and transfer to a large lidded container and refrigerate up to 5 days. To serve, heat in toaster oven 1 minute until heated through and season with salt and pepper.

PER SERVING Calories: 187 | Fat: 2.3 g | Protein: 4.6 g |
Sodium: 605 mg | Fiber: 4.0 g | Carbohydrates: 37.2 g |
Sugar: 1.9 g

Vegan Garlic Mashed Potatoes

Savory potatoes, garlic, and olive oil are the main ingredients in these delicious Vegan Garlic Mashed Potatoes. It's an easy recipe with minimal ingredients and big flavor!

INGREDIENTS | SERVES 4

6 medium red potatoes, chopped
2 cloves garlic, peeled and chopped
4 tablespoons olive oil
¾ cup unsweetened almond milk
1 teaspoon salt
¼ teaspoon ground black pepper

Are Potatoes Healthy?

Potatoes are indeed full of healthy nutrients your body needs! In fact, they're a fairly low-calorie food option, depending on the added ingredients and the way they're prepared. Over half of the fiber found in a potato is in the skin.

1. Place chopped potatoes in a large pot and fill with water so it comes to about 2" above potatoes. Place over medium-high heat and bring to a boil. Reduce heat to a simmer and cook about 10 minutes until potatoes are fork-tender. Sprinkle garlic over top and remove from heat. Let cool about 5 minutes.

2. Strain potatoes, then place in a large sealable container. Add olive oil and use a fork or potato masher to mash potatoes. Add milk and continue to mash until well mixed. Add salt and pepper and stir.

3. Store in refrigerator up to 7 days. To serve, cook in microwave in 30-second intervals until heated through.

PER SERVING Calories: 357 | Fat: 13.9 g | Protein: 6.3 g | Sodium: 646 mg | Fiber: 4.9 g | Carbohydrates: 51.8 g | Sugar: 3.8 g

Easy Vegan Stuffing

This Easy Vegan Stuffing is quick and savory. It's simple to make for a meal, but it also makes a special and delicious side for your holiday dinner table.

INGREDIENTS | SERVES 8

¼ cup vegan butter

1 cup chopped celery

1 cup chopped peeled yellow onion

2½ cups vegetable broth

1 (14-ounce) package herb-seasoned corn-bread stuffing

1. Preheat oven to 375°F. Spray bottom and sides of a 9" × 13" baking pan or casserole dish.

2. Heat vegan butter in a large saucepan over medium heat until melted. Add celery and onion. Cook until tender, about 7 minutes.

3. Pour in vegetable broth and stir. Cook until just boiling, then pour in stuffing and stir to combine. Remove from heat.

4. Pour stuffing into prepared baking dish. Bake 20 minutes until stuffing is golden and crusty on top. Remove from oven and let cool about 15 minutes.

5. Once cooled, cover dish and refrigerate up to 5 days. To serve, either heat in microwave in 30-second intervals until heated through, or place in oven preheated to 250°F and cook 10 minutes.

PER SERVING Calories: 231 | Fat: 4.2 g | Protein: 5.3 g | Sodium: 856 mg | Fiber: 8.0 g | Carbohydrates: 41.4 g | Sugar: 3.7 g

Vegan Cheesy Corn Casserole

This easy corn casserole is a cheesy, corn bread–like dish that is sure to please any dinner crowd! Make it ahead of time and reheat for meals throughout the week.

INGREDIENTS | SERVES 8

1 (15-ounce) can whole kernel corn, drained

1 (15-ounce) can cream-style corn

1 (8-ounce) package vegan corn muffin mix

1 cup vegan sour cream

4 tablespoons vegan butter, melted

1 cup vegan Cheddar shreds

Is Store-Bought Corn Bread Vegan?

In years past, most store-bought corn-bread mixes were not vegan. That's because they were made with lard, which is animal fat. Some mixes also included eggs and dairy. However, times have changed, and now there are several store-bought corn-bread mixes made without lard, eggs, or dairy.

1. Preheat oven to 350°F. Spray a 9" × 9" baking dish with vegetable cooking spray.

2. Combine whole and creamed corn, muffin mix, sour cream, and melted butter in a large bowl. Pour into prepared baking dish and bake 45 minutes until golden brown.

3. Remove from oven and turn heat up to 375°F. Top dish with Cheddar shreds and cover with aluminum foil. Return to oven and bake another 10 minutes until cheese is melted.

4. Remove and let cool 10 minutes before covering and refrigerating up to 7 days. To serve, remove cover, place in microwave and cook in 30-second intervals until heated through.

PER SERVING Calories: 288 | Fat: 14.5 g | Protein: 3.5 g | Sodium: 619 mg | Fiber: 5.6 g | Carbohydrates: 39.5 g | Sugar: 8.1 g

Cauliflower Gratin

Cauliflower Gratin is the perfect side dish. It's delicious and healthy, which makes it perfect for a Tuesday night dinner or a dish you can take to dinner gatherings.

INGREDIENTS | SERVES 6

1 large head cauliflower, cut into florets

1 small yellow onion, peeled and chopped

1 tablespoon olive oil

1 cup plain soy milk

1 cup vegan Cheddar shreds, divided

½ teaspoon salt

½ teaspoon garlic powder

2 tablespoons nutritional yeast flakes

¼ cup bread crumbs

1. Preheat oven to 350°F. Spray a 9" × 9" baking dish with vegetable cooking spray.

2. Place a steamer insert into a medium saucepan and add enough water so that it is just below bottom of basket. Bring water to a boil over high heat, then add cauliflower florets and steam covered until tender, about 5 minutes. Remove from heat.

3. Add onion, olive oil, milk, ½ cheese shreds, salt, garlic powder, and nutritional yeast flakes to a food processor and pulse until smooth. Pour mixture into a medium microwave-safe bowl and microwave 1 minute. Stir and repeat cooking until sauce thickens.

4. Pour steamed cauliflower into prepared baking dish. Pour cheese sauce over cauliflower. Top with remaining shredded cheese and bread crumbs.

5. Cover with aluminum foil and bake 15 minutes until cheese is melted. Remove foil with tongs and bake uncovered another 10 minutes to brown bread crumbs.

6. Remove from oven and let cool about 15 minutes. Cover and refrigerate up to 7 days. To serve, heat individual servings in microwave in 1-minute intervals until heated through.

PER SERVING Calories: 152 | Fat: 8.0 g | Protein: 5.4 g | Sodium: 465 mg | Fiber: 4.5 g | Carbohydrates: 17.2 g | Sugar: 3.9 g

Balsamic Glazed Steamed Green Beans

*Start with fresh steamed green beans, and add the most delicious
glaze to transform dinner into something very special!*

INGREDIENTS | SERVES 6

1 pound fresh green beans, stem ends removed

1 tablespoon Vegan Mayonnaise (see Chapter 7 for recipe)

1 teaspoon balsamic vinegar

1 teaspoon agave nectar

⅛ teaspoon salt

Cooking with Vegan Mayonnaise

Vegan mayonnaise has been around for a while, but it was once only available in health food stores. These days you can find vegan mayonnaise, which is made with vegetable oil instead of eggs, at most grocery stores. For creamy vegan mayonnaise, try Hellmann's or Just Mayo. For a tangier mayonnaise, try Vegenaise.

1. Insert a steamer basket in a large saucepan and fill pan with water until it comes to just below bottom of steamer basket. Bring water to a boil over high heat, then add green beans. Cover and steam until tender, about 8 minutes. Set aside.

2. In a small bowl combine mayonnaise, balsamic vinegar, agave nectar, and salt. Set aside.

3. Use tongs to remove green beans from steamer basket. Transfer to a large lidded container (or individual serving containers). Drizzle with balsamic glaze and use tongs to toss beans in sauce.

4. Store in refrigerator up to 5 days. To serve, cook individual servings in microwave in 30-second intervals until heated through.

PER SERVING Calories: 31 | Fat: 0.5 g | Protein: 1.6 g | Sodium: 76 mg | Fiber: 2.0 g | Carbohydrates: 6.3 g | Sugar: 3.4 g

Easy Cauliflower Rice

Looking for ways to add a little more health (and a few less calories) to each day? You'll love this Easy Cauliflower Rice. Use this dish in place of regular rice in Asian dishes, casseroles, and more!

INGREDIENTS | SERVES 4

1 medium head cauliflower, stem removed, cut into florets
1½ tablespoons nutritional yeast flakes
1 tablespoon rice vinegar

1. Combine all ingredients in a food processor. Pulse in 3-second intervals until mixture is size of rice grains.

2. Place a large skillet over medium heat and spray with vegetable cooking spray. Add cauliflower rice and cook 10 minutes until tender. Let cool 10 minutes.

3. Transfer to a medium lidded container and refrigerate up to 3 days. To serve, heat in microwave at 30-second intervals until heated through.

PER SERVING Calories: 43 | Fat: 0.3 g | Protein: 3.6 g | Sodium: 46 mg | Fiber: 3.2 g | Carbohydrates: 7.8 g | Sugar: 2.8 g

Glazed Carrots

A sweet ginger sauce makes these tender Glazed Carrots shine. It's an easy-to-make side dish that can be prepared ahead of time for family dinners all week.

INGREDIENTS | SERVES 4

1 (1-pound) bag baby carrots
¼ cup no-pulp orange juice
½ cup water
2 teaspoons olive oil
1 teaspoon agave nectar
1 teaspoon ground ginger
⅛ teaspoon salt
⅛ teaspoon ground black pepper

1. Pour all ingredients into a large saucepan over medium heat. Stir to combine. Bring to a boil, then reduce heat to a simmer and cook 30 minutes until a glaze forms.

2. Remove from heat and let cool about 10 minutes. Transfer to a large lidded container (or individual serving containers) and refrigerate up to 5 days. To serve, heat in microwave in 30-second intervals until heated through.

PER SERVING Calories: 73 | Fat: 2.3 g | Protein: 0.9 g | Sodium: 161 mg | Fiber: 3.4 g | Carbohydrates: 12.8 g | Sugar: 7.9 g

Seared Brussels Sprouts

Make these easy Seared Brussels Sprouts in no time with a few simple ingredients. The flavor combination is amazing, and the health benefits are even better!

INGREDIENTS | SERVES 4

1 pound Brussels sprouts, trimmed and halved

1 tablespoon olive oil

2 cloves garlic, peeled and minced

½ teaspoon salt

2 tablespoons chopped almonds

¼ cup dried cranberries

1. Insert a steamer basket in a large saucepan. Fill pan with water until it comes to just below bottom of steamer basket. Bring water to a boil over high heat, then add Brussels sprouts. Place lid on pan and steam until just tender, about 8 minutes. Set aside.

2. Add olive oil to a large skillet over medium heat. Add steamed sprouts, cut-side down. Cook until cut sides of sprouts are caramelized, about 7 minutes. Reduce heat to low and add garlic, salt, almonds, and cranberries. Stir to coat sprouts. Cook 3 minutes until cranberries are tender.

3. Let cool 10 minutes, then store in a large sealed container and refrigerate up to 5 days. To serve, cook in microwave in 30-second intervals until heated through.

PER SERVING Calories: 99 | Fat: 4.9 g | Protein: 4.4 g | Sodium: 317 mg | Fiber: 4.9 g | Carbohydrates: 12.0 g | Sugar: 2.9 g

Roasted Root Vegetables

This elegant and colorful dish is easy to make. There's nothing quite like fresh vegetables cooked slowly in a savory sauce. It will be a favorite go-to side dish.

INGREDIENTS | SERVES 6

1 tablespoon olive oil

3 cloves garlic, peeled and minced

2 teaspoons dried rosemary

1 tablespoon balsamic vinegar

5 medium red potatoes, cut into wedges

1 pound carrots, peeled and cut into 1" pieces

2 large beets, cut into 1" cubes

1 yellow onion, peeled and cut into 1" pieces

1. Preheat oven to 400°F. Line a baking sheet with parchment paper.

2. In a large bowl combine olive oil, garlic, rosemary and balsamic vinegar. Add chopped vegetable pieces and toss to coat.

3. Place coated vegetables on prepared sheet and roast 50 minutes, stirring occasionally.

4. Remove from oven, let cool 10 minutes, then transfer to a large lidded container (or individual serving containers). Refrigerate up to 5 days To serve, heat in microwave in 30-second intervals until heated through.

PER SERVING Calories: 204 | Fat: 2.5 g | Protein: 4.9 g | Sodium: 94 mg | Fiber: 6.1 g | Carbohydrates: 41.2 g | Sugar: 9.1 g

Truck Stop Potatoes

Vegan sour cream and vegan cheese make these Truck Stop Potatoes a creamy and delicious indulgent side dish. It's the perfect comfort food—veganized!

INGREDIENTS | SERVES 6

2 pounds red potatoes, chopped

1 medium yellow onion, peeled and chopped

1 cup vegan sour cream

1 cup vegan Cheddar cheese

½ teaspoon salt

¼ teaspoon cayenne pepper

1 (15-ounce) can diced tomatoes, drained

1. Preheat oven to 350°F. Spray a 9" × 13" pan with vegetable cooking spray.

2. Fill a large pot with water. Bring to a boil over high heat. Add potatoes and onions and cook until tender, about 10 minutes. Once potatoes are done, drain water from pot.

3. In a small bowl combine sour cream, cheese, salt, cayenne pepper, and drained tomatoes. Pour sauce over cooked potatoes. Stir to combine.

4. Pour potato mixture into prepared pan. Cover with aluminum foil and bake 10 minutes until cheese melts. Use tongs to remove foil and bake another 20 minutes until golden brown.

5. Remove from oven and let cool about 15 minutes. Cover and refrigerate up to 5 days. To serve, heat individual servings in microwave in 30-second intervals until heated through.

PER SERVING Calories: 209 | Fat: 11.4 g | Protein: 2.5 g | Sodium: 545 mg | Fiber: 6.2 g | Carbohydrates: 27.5 g | Sugar: 3.6 g

Vegan Scalloped Potatoes

This veganized scalloped potatoes recipe is everything you love in a potato dish: creamy, cheesy, and absolutely delicious. It's a side dish that makes every meal something special.

INGREDIENTS | SERVES 6

3 tablespoons vegan butter

6 tablespoons all-purpose flour

1 teaspoon salt

⅛ teaspoon ground black pepper

2 pounds red potatoes, cut into thin slices

2 cups plain soy milk

½ cup + 2 tablespoons vegan Cheddar shreds, divided

1 medium yellow onion, peeled and thinly sliced

1. Preheat oven to 375°F. Spray a 9" × 9" baking pan with vegetable spray.

2. In a small saucepan over medium heat, add vegan butter. Cook until melted, about 30 seconds. Whisk in flour, salt, and pepper. Still whisking, slowly add milk. Bring to a boil while whisking, until a thick sauce forms.

3. Remove pan from heat. Add ½ cup Cheddar shreds and stir until mostly melted.

4. Place ⅓ potato slices in prepared pan. Cover with ⅓ sliced onions, followed by ⅓ cheese sauce. Repeat until all potatoes, onions, and sauce are used. Top with 2 tablespoons Cheddar shreds.

5. Cover pan with aluminum foil and bake 50 minutes until potatoes are tender. Use tongs to remove foil and bake another 10 minutes to create a golden crust.

6. Remove from oven and let cool about 15 minutes. Cover and refrigerate up to 5 days. To serve, heat individual servings in microwave in 30-second intervals until heated through.

PER SERVING Calories: 240 | Fat: 6.1 g | Protein: 6.6 g | Sodium: 565 mg | Fiber: 3.9 g | Carbohydrates: 39.4 g | Sugar: 3.2 g

Sweet and Savory Baked Beans

Enjoy these Midwest-styled baked beans in a savory sweet sauce, complete with sweet bell peppers, onions, and vegan bacon! It's a must-have recipe for your next backyard barbecue.

INGREDIENTS | SERVES 6

2 teaspoons olive oil

1 large yellow onion, peeled and chopped

½ medium green bell pepper, seeded and chopped

2 tablespoons tamari

2 tablespoons apple cider vinegar

1 tablespoon Dijon mustard

1 teaspoon garlic powder

¼ cup molasses

¼ cup coconut sugar

1 cup barbecue sauce

⅛ teaspoon ground black pepper

4 (15-ounce) cans navy beans, rinsed and drained

4 strips vegan bacon

Add Flavor with Onions!

Cooking with onions is a great way to add flavor to your dishes. Whether simmered, caramelized, or even served raw, onions are the perfect addition for delicious, savory recipes.

1. Preheat oven to 350°F.

2. Add oil to a medium saucepan over medium heat. Add onions and bell peppers and cook until tender, about 7 minutes. Then add tamari, vinegar, mustard, garlic powder, molasses, sugar, barbecue sauce, and black pepper. Stir to combine, then simmer 5 minutes.

3. Pour beans into pot and stir until sauce covers beans. Transfer mixture into an ungreased 9" × 13" baking dish. Top with vegan bacon strips and bake uncovered 40 minutes until bubbly around edges and browned on top.

4. Remove beans from heat and let cool about 15 minutes, then cover and refrigerate up to 7 days. To serve, heat in microwave in 30-second intervals until heated through.

PER SERVING Calories: 552 | Fat: 4.3 g | Protein: 23.4 g | Sodium: 1,780 mg | Fiber: 17.0 g | Carbohydrates: 105.0 g | Sugar: 36.7 g

Steamed Broccoli with Garlic

It's easy to create this steamed dish drizzled with olive oil and minced garlic. Steaming preserves the broccoli's health benefits, making this a go-to healthy side to a variety of main meals and salads.

INGREDIENTS | SERVES 4

3 heads broccoli, trimmed and cut into 2" florets

1 clove garlic, peeled and finely minced

1 tablespoon olive oil

1. Insert a steamer basket in a large saucepan and fill with water until level is just below bottom of steamer basket. Bring water to a boil over high heat, then add broccoli. Place lid on pan and steam until just tender, about 5 minutes.

2. Add garlic and olive oil to a small bowl.

3. Remove steamed broccoli from the steamer basket and while broccoli is still hot, drizzle with garlic mixture. Stir to coat broccoli. Let cool 10 minutes.

4. Transfer broccoli to a large lidded container (or individual serving containers) and refrigerate up to 4 days. To serve, heat broccoli in microwave in 30-second intervals until heated through.

PER SERVING Calories: 65 | Fat: 3.4 g | Protein: 2.9 g | Sodium: 33 mg | Fiber: 2.7 g | Carbohydrates: 7.1 g | Sugar: 1.8 g

Broccoli and Rice Casserole

This vegan Broccoli and Rice Casserole is magical because it's so full of comfort food goodness that it disappears just like that! Ready in less than an hour, this creamy casserole is perfect for potlucks or family dinners.

INGREDIENTS | SERVES 4

1 tablespoon olive oil

1 small yellow onion, peeled and chopped

½ cup diced celery

2 cups sliced white mushrooms

3 cups small broccoli florets

3 tablespoons gluten-free flour

1 cup unsweetened almond milk

1 cup cooked brown rice

⅔ cup vegan sour cream

2 tablespoons Vegan Mayonnaise (see Chapter 7 for recipe)

2 tablespoons nutritional yeast flakes

¼ teaspoon dried thyme

½ cup vegan Cheddar cheese

Is Brown or White Rice Best?

Brown rice is the healthier option, so opt for it in your recipes when possible. Most of the nutrients found in brown rice are also found in white rice, but in lower amounts, since the outer layer is removed. A lot of the plant's nutrients are found in this layer. Brown rice is packed with fiber, which keeps you fuller for longer and can also lower your cholesterol. Brown rice also delivers tons of minerals and nutrients like iron, magnesium, and selenium.

1. Preheat oven to 350°F. Spray a 2-quart casserole dish with vegetable cooking spray.

2. Pour oil, onions, and celery into a large pot. Cook over medium heat until tender, about 7 minutes.

3. Add mushrooms and broccoli to pot. Cook until mushrooms are tender, about 5 minutes.

4. Sprinkle flour over mixture and stir to incorporate. Cook about 2 minutes. Gradually add milk, cooking and stirring another 2 minutes until a sauce forms.

5. Stir in brown rice, vegan sour cream, Vegan Mayonnaise, nutritional yeast, and thyme.

6. Transfer mixture to baking dish and sprinkle with vegan Cheddar cheese. Cover with aluminum foil and bake 15 minutes until cheese melts. Use tongs to remove foil. Bake another 10 minutes until golden brown on top.

7. Remove from oven and let cool about 10 minutes. Cover and refrigerate up to 7 days. To serve, heat in microwave in 30-second increments until warmed through.

PER SERVING Calories: 245 | Fat: 12.4 g | Protein: 6.7 g | Sodium: 185 mg | Fiber: 7.1 g | Carbohydrates: 30.6 g | Sugar: 3.1 g

CHAPTER 9

Burgers, Wraps, and Sandwiches

Sweet Potato Black Bean Burgers

These vegan Sweet Potato Black Bean Burgers will rock your world! The sweet potatoes add colorful flavor and texture to the healthy burgers. The burgers are also gluten-free. Make a double batch and freeze half for a week of meals! Make your burgers pop even more with fresh crunchy lettuce and slices of onion.

INGREDIENTS | SERVES 6

1 medium sweet potato, perforated with a fork

1 cup rolled oats

¼ cup chopped walnuts

1 (15-ounce) can black beans, rinsed and drained

1 tablespoon dehydrated onions

1 teaspoon garlic powder

1 tablespoon taco seasoning

1 tablespoon nutritional yeast flakes

1 tablespoon ground flaxseed

¼ cup frozen corn kernels

6 dairy-free hamburger buns

Sweet Potatoes for Your Health

Sweet potatoes provide many nutrients, including fiber, beta-carotene, and potassium—just to name a few. Many people wrongly assume that they're loaded with calories. However, sweet potatoes are actually a low-calorie food (approximately 103 calories per medium potato) that you can enjoy regularly!

1. Place potato in microwave and cook 2 minutes. Use oven mitts to remove from oven and let cool about 5 minutes. Once cooled, chop into large cubes.

2. Place oats and walnuts in a food processor and pulse until a coarse flour is formed. Add cubed sweet potatoes, black beans, onions, garlic powder, taco seasoning, nutritional yeast flakes, and flaxseed. Pulse 3 seconds and then use a spatula to push ingredients back down sides of bowl. Pulse again 3 seconds.

3. Add frozen corn and use a spatula to stir. Let mixture sit about 5 minutes, then form into 6 patties.

4. Preheat oven to 200°F and spray a large skillet with vegetable cooking spray. Place skillet over medium heat. Place patties in skillet and cook 5 minutes.

5. Flip patties, and cook on other side another 5 minutes until patties have firmed up and are brown on both sides.

6. Place cooked burgers on an ungreased 9" × 13" baking dish and place in heated oven. Cook patties in oven 10 minutes.

7. Let cool 10 minutes, then place cooked patties in a large sealed container and refrigerate up to 7 days, or freeze up to 2 months. To serve, cook in microwave in 30-minute intervals until heated through. Serve on buns.

PER SERVING Calories: 316 | Fat: 6.3 g | Protein: 12.7 g | Sodium: 484 mg | Fiber: 9.2 g | Carbohydrates: 52.0 g | Sugar: 4.8 g

Ultimate Veggie Burgers

Take a bite of one of these Ultimate Veggie Burgers and you'll understand why it's a favorite! Tested with vegans and non-vegans alike, it's been a winner to everyone! This recipe is loaded with vegan cheese, vegan bacon, the best veggie burger ever, and avocados—you'll be surprised it's vegan.

INGREDIENTS | SERVES 6

1 (13-ounce) package Field Roast hand-formed veggie burgers

1 (5.5-ounce) package vegan bacon

2 tablespoons vegan butter

6 dairy-free hamburger buns

1 (7.1-ounce) package vegan Cheddar-style block, sliced

1 medium avocado, peeled, pitted, and sliced

1. In a large skillet over medium heat add veggie burgers, 1–2 at a time. Cook on both sides, about 5 minutes per side. Repeat until all patties are cooked, then set patties aside on a large plate.

2. Place vegan bacon in same skillet and cook 5 minutes per side. Cut cooked bacon strips in half and set aside with patties.

3. Spread vegan butter on cut sides of buns and place butter-side down on skillet to brown, about 5 minutes. Remove from heat.

4. Assemble sandwiches by placing veggie burgers on bottom buns, then topping each with a cheese slice. Place in skillet over medium heat, 1–2 burgers at a time, for 2 minutes to melt cheese.

5. Remove from heat and top each with a few vegan bacon strips, sliced avocado, and top buns.

6. Let cool 10 minutes, then place burgers in a large sealed container and refrigerate up to 7 days, or freeze up to 2 months. To serve, cook in microwave in 30-second intervals until heated through.

PER SERVING Calories: 548 | Fat: 32.6 g | Protein: 24.3 g | Sodium: 1,223 mg | Fiber: 5.1 g | Carbohydrates: 41.7 g | Sugar: 3.0 g

Pesto Veggie Burgers

These flavorful Pesto Veggie Burgers are a great addition (or main dish) in any vegan meal. Serve with Sun-Dried Tomato Aioli (see Chapter 7 for recipe).

INGREDIENTS | SERVES 10

¼ cup pine nuts

¼ cup walnuts

1½ cups rolled oats

½ cup chopped green onion

¾ cup chopped de-stemmed kale

¼ cup nutritional yeast flakes

½ teaspoon salt

½ cup fresh basil, chopped

1 tablespoon ground flaxseed

1 tablespoon cornstarch

1 clove garlic, peeled and chopped

1 (15-ounce) can chickpeas, rinsed and drained

1 (15-ounce) can cannellini beans, rinsed and drained, divided

¼ cup vegan Parmesan

¼ teaspoon ground black pepper

10 dairy-free hamburger buns

1. Add pine nuts, walnuts, and oats to a food processor and pulse about 8 seconds until a coarse flour forms. Add green onions, kale, nutritional yeast flakes, salt, basil, flaxseed, cornstarch, and garlic. Pulse 3 seconds until combined. Add both beans, except ½ cup cannellini beans, in a food processor and pulse 3 seconds until ingredients are well combined.

2. Add reserved cannellini beans and pulse 2 seconds until evenly disbursed throughout mixture.

3. Preheat oven to 250°F. Line a 9" × 13" baking dish with parchment paper.

4. Heat a medium skillet over medium heat and spray with a light coating of vegetable cooking spray.

5. Make patties by measuring out heaping ½-cup measures of mixture and forming into balls. Press each ball to flatten into a patty. Pour vegan Parmesan and pepper in a small plate and dredge each patty through Parmesan mixture on both sides.

6. Place patties 1–2 at a time in heated skillet. Sprinkle with pepper. Cook 5 minutes on each side.

7. Transfer patties to baking dish and cook about 10 minutes in oven.

8. Let cool 10 minutes, then place burgers in a large sealed container and refrigerate up to 7 days, or freeze up to 2 months. To serve, cook patties in microwave in 30-second intervals until heated through and place on buns.

PER SERVING Calories: 267 | Fat: 4.9 g | Protein: 10.3 g | Sodium: 622 mg | Fiber: 3.7 g | Carbohydrates: 43.1 g | Sugar: 4.1 g

Black Bean Pecan Burgers

Busy days mean easy recipes are a must, but there's no need to sacrifice flavor. These Black Bean Pecan Burgers are a filling, satisfying, and delicious meal.

INGREDIENTS | SERVES 8

1½ cups rolled oats

½ cup pecans

2 (15-ounce) cans black beans, rinsed and drained, divided

1 cup cooked brown rice

1 tablespoon ground flaxseed

3 tablespoons nutritional yeast flakes

3 tablespoons dehydrated onions

2 teaspoons garlic powder

½ teaspoon salt

1 tablespoon chili powder

8 dairy-free hamburger buns

Making the Perfect Bean Burgers

Bean burgers are more than a healthy addition to your diet: they also taste great. Using nuts or seeds to your burgers will increase healthy fats and add flavor. In addition, try different herbs and spices for more flavor. Grains like oats and cornmeal also help bind the ingredients together.

1. Preheat oven to 250°F and line a 9" × 13" baking dish with parchment paper.

2. Add oats and pecans in a food processor. Pulse until a coarse flour forms. Add in 1 can black beans, rice, ground flaxseed, nutritional yeast flakes, dehydrated onions, garlic powder, salt, and chili powder. Pulse 3 seconds, then use a spatula to push ingredients down. Pulse again 3 seconds. Add second can black beans and pulse again to combine. Mixture should be a spreadable consistency.

3. Spray a large skillet with vegetable spray and place over medium heat. Form bean mixture into 8 patties and place 3–4 patties in skillet. Cook 6 minutes on each side.

4. Place patties in baking dish and bake 10 minutes. Set cooked patties aside and repeat process with remaining patties. Once done, let patties cool about 5 minutes.

5. Place burgers in a large sealed container and refrigerate up to 7 days, or freeze up to 2 months. To serve, cook patties in microwave in 30-second intervals until heated through. Serve on buns.

PER SERVING Calories: 375 | Fat: 7.9 g | Protein: 15.6 g | Sodium: 625 mg | Fiber: 12.2 g | Carbohydrates: 60.4 g | Sugar: 4.3 g

Lentil Burgers

This recipe lets you enjoy restaurant-quality veggie burgers right at home! Inspire guests with healthy burgers that are high in fiber, folate, and flavor!

INGREDIENTS | SERVES 6

1 cup chopped peeled yellow onion
1 cup dried brown lentils
2½ cups water
1 cup extra-firm tofu, pressed
2 tablespoons ground flaxseed, divided
1¼ cups rolled oats, divided
1 tablespoon cashews
2 teaspoons Better Than Bouillon Seasoned Vegetable Base
1 tablespoon nutritional yeast flakes
1 teaspoon rubbed sage
¼ teaspoon ground turmeric
1 teaspoon paprika
1 teaspoon ground black pepper
6 dairy-free hamburger buns

1. Add onions and lentils to a medium saucepan. Add water. Bring to a boil over high heat, then reduce heat to low, cover, and cook 25 minutes.

2. In a food processor add tofu, 1 tablespoon flaxseed, ½ cup rolled oats, cashews, Better Than Bouillon, nutritional yeast, sage, turmeric, and paprika. Pulse until combined.

3. When lentils are done, drain any excess liquid in a strainer. Add 2 cups lentil mixture to tofu mixture and pulse to combine.

4. Add remaining lentil mixture into food processing bowl and use a spatula to stir. Add remaining flaxseed and oats and stir to combine. Set aside 5 minutes to allow mixture to thicken.

5. Preheat oven to 375°F. Line two baking sheets with parchment paper.

6. Measure ½ cup dollops of lentil mixture on baking sheets (six total dollops). Use back of cup to press into patties. Sprinkle tops of each with pepper.

7. Bake patties 25 minutes, flipping burgers once halfway through baking.

8. Let cool 10 minutes, then place burgers in a large sealed container and refrigerate up to 7 days, or freeze up to 2 months. To serve, cook in microwave in 30-second intervals until heated through. Serve on buns.

PER SERVING Calories: 410 | Fat: 8.6 g | Protein: 23.1 g | Sodium: 454 mg | Fiber: 9.0 g | Carbohydrates: 61.2 g | Sugar: 4.4 g

Sweet Potato Quinoa Burgers

There's a lot to love with these Sweet Potato Quinoa Burgers, but let's start with the quinoa. It's one of the few grains that is a complete protein, so eat up and feel the benefits!

INGREDIENTS | SERVES 6

1 medium sweet potato, perforated with a fork

1 cup rolled oats

¼ cup pecans

1 (15-ounce) can chickpeas, rinsed and drained

2 tablespoons sliced green onion

1 teaspoon garlic powder

½ teaspoon salt

¼ cup nutritional yeast flakes

½ cup cooked quinoa, drained and pressed

1 tablespoon ground flaxseed

1 tablespoon cornstarch

½ cup chopped baby kale

⅛ teaspoon ground black pepper

6 dairy-free hamburger buns

What Is Quinoa?

Quinoa is a gluten-free grain that's easy to cook and adds a nutty flavor to dishes. It's high in protein and also offers fiber, magnesium, iron, potassium, and more. Quinoa takes only around 30 minutes to cook, making it an easy addition to many recipes. You can find quinoa near the beans and grains section in most grocery stores.

1. Place sweet potato in microwave and cook 2 minutes. Remove with oven mitts and let cool about 5 minutes. Once cooled, chop into large cubes.

2. Place oats and pecans in a food processor and pulse until a coarse flour is formed. Add sweet potatoes, chickpeas, green onions, garlic powder, salt, nutritional yeast flakes, quinoa, ground flaxseed, and cornstarch. Pulse 2 seconds and then use a spatula to push ingredients back down. Pulse again 3 seconds. Let mixture sit about 5 minutes, then stir in chopped kale.

3. Preheat oven to 350°F and use vegetable cooking spray to grease a large skillet over medium-high heat.

4. Form mixture into 6 patties, then place 3–4 patties in skillet and cook about 5 minutes on one side. Flip patties, sprinkle with pepper, and cook another 5 minutes.

5. Place cooked burgers on an ungreased baking sheet, place in oven. Repeat cooking remaining patties, then add to sheet in oven and let sit 10 minutes.

6. Let cool 10 minutes, then place burgers in a large sealed container and refrigerate up to 7 days, or freeze up to 2 months. To serve, cook in microwave in 30-second intervals until heated through. Serve on buns.

PER SERVING Calories: 330 | Fat: 7.0 g | Protein: 12.7 g | Sodium: 564 mg | Fiber: 7.8 g | Carbohydrates: 53.1 g | Sugar: 6.1 g

Crispy Black Bean Burritos

This easy Crispy Black Bean Burritos recipe is made with brown rice, potatoes, corn, and black beans. It's a delicious, fun-to-eat food that you'll want to serve on repeat!

INGREDIENTS | SERVES 10

2 tablespoons vegetable oil

1 small yellow onion, peeled and diced

2 cups frozen hash brown potatoes

2 (15-ounce) cans black beans, rinsed and drained

1 (15-ounce) can pinto beans, rinsed and drained

1 (15-ounce) can corn kernels, drained

1 cup cooked brown rice

1 tablespoon chili powder

1 teaspoon ground black pepper

2 teaspoons garlic powder

1 teaspoon cumin

1 teaspoon paprika

10 (12") flour tortillas

Cooking Brown Rice

You can buy precooked brown rice in most grocery stores for convenience, but you can also make your own in just a few easy steps. Add 1 cup rice to 2 cups water in a large pot. Bring to a boil over high heat, then reduce heat to medium-low and simmer 45 minutes. Turn off heat and let rice sit 10 minutes. Transfer to a large sealable container and refrigerate up to 7 days, or freeze up to 2 months.

1. Add vegetable oil to a large skillet over medium heat. Add onions and potatoes and sauté about 7 minutes until tender.

2. Add beans, corn, rice, and spices to skillet with potato mixture. Stir to combine, reduce heat to low, and simmer 15 minutes.

3. Let cool 10 minutes, then store in a large sealed container in refrigerator up to 7 days or freezer up to 2 months.

4. To serve, place one tortilla on a large plate and warm in microwave 20 seconds. Cook black bean mixture in microwave in 30-second intervals until heated through. Add mixture to tortilla. Roll up tortilla to form a burrito.

5. Place a large skillet over medium-high heat. Place burrito in skillet and cook 5 minutes, until tortilla is crispy.

PER SERVING Calories: 565 | Fat: 10.1 g | Protein: 19.0 g | Sodium: 1,119 mg | Fiber: 10.8 g | Carbohydrates: 98.6 g | Sugar: 6.1 g

Vegan Chick'n Taquitos

A crispy shell on the outside is combined with creamy ingredients on the inside and an avocado dipping sauce to finish it off. Vegan Chick'n Taquitos are super easy to make and will have your family begging for more!

INGREDIENTS | SERVES 10

½ cup dairy-free cream cheese

3 tablespoons chopped peeled white onion

⅓ cup mild green salsa

3 tablespoons chopped fresh cilantro

2 tablespoons lime juice

2 teaspoons taco seasoning

1 (10-ounce) package Beyond Meat Beyond Chicken Strips (Grilled), thawed and thinly sliced

1 cup vegan Mexican blend shredded cheese

10 (8") flour tortillas

1 medium avocado, peeled, pitted, and cubed

1. Preheat oven to 400°F. Line a baking sheet with aluminum foil.

2. In a medium bowl add vegan cream cheese. Place in microwave and heat 20 seconds to soften. Add onion, salsa, cilantro, lime juice, and taco seasoning. Stir to combine. Reserve two tablespoons of this mixture in a separate small bowl.

3. Add vegan chicken strips and Mexican cheese to cream cheese mixture. Stir to combine.

4. Place tortillas in microwave and warm 15 seconds.

5. Add ⅒ filling mixture to one tortilla. Spread mixture in a line across tortilla and then roll up tortilla tightly. Place it seam-side down on prepared baking sheet. Repeat until all vegan chicken mixture is used up and 10 taquitos are made.

6. Place taquitos in oven and bake 20 minutes until tortillas are crisp and browned on edges.

7. Make avocado dipping sauce by adding cubed avocado to small bowl with reserved cilantro filling. Stir together to combine. Cover and refrigerate up to 5 days.

8. When taquitos are done, remove from oven and let cool, about 5 minutes.

9. Individually wrap taquitos in foil, then place in a large sealed container and refrigerate up to 7 days, or freeze up to 2 months.

10. To serve, unwrap from foil and cook in microwave in 30-second intervals until heated through. Serve with avocado dipping sauce.

PER SERVING Calories: 349 | Fat: 12.9 g | Protein: 12.5 g | Sodium: 912 mg | Fiber: 4.3 g | Carbohydrates: 45.6 g | Sugar: 3.2 g

Vegetable Lettuce Wraps

You're going to love these delicious Vegetable Lettuce Wraps made with blackberry hoisin sauce. This 30-minute dish is full of healthy and flavorful ingredients. Enjoy!

INGREDIENTS | SERVES 10

For Wraps

1 tablespoon sesame oil

1 (15-ounce) package extra-firm tofu, pressed and broken into chunks

2 cloves garlic, peeled and minced

1 medium yellow onion, peeled and diced

¼ cup hoisin sauce

2 tablespoons tamari

1 tablespoon rice wine vinegar

1 (8-ounce) can whole water chestnuts, drained and chopped

¼ cup chopped seeded red bell pepper

1 green onion, chopped

10 leaves butter lettuce

For Sauce

2 tablespoons blackberry jam

1 tablespoon tamari

1 teaspoon garlic powder

1 teaspoon powdered ginger

1 teaspoon rice vinegar

1. **To make Wraps:** heat sesame oil in a small saucepan over medium-high heat 30 seconds. Add tofu. Use a spatula to continue breaking tofu down into a crumbly mixture as it cooks (about 10 minutes).

2. Reduce heat to medium and stir in garlic, onion, hoisin sauce, tamari, and rice wine vinegar. Cook until onions are tender, about 5 minutes. Stir in water chestnuts, bell peppers, and green onions. Cook 3 more minutes, until peppers begin to become tender.

3. Let cool 10 minutes, then transfer mixture to a large lidded container and store in refrigerator up to 7 days.

4. **To make Sauce:** combine ingredients in a small sealable container. Refrigerate up to 7 days.

5. Store lettuce leaves in a small sealable container in refrigerator up to 5 days.

6. To serve, scoop a spoonful of vegan tofu mixture into center of each butter lettuce leaf. Serve topped with blackberry sauce.

PER SERVING Calories: 96 | Fat: 3.9 g | Protein: 5.6 g | Sodium: 412 mg | Fiber: 1.3 g | Carbohydrates: 10.7 g | Sugar: 5.2 g

Ground or Fresh Ginger?

Oftentimes you're encouraged to use fresh ingredients. However, there are times when fresh isn't best. For example, if you're not used to working with fresh ginger, the strong flavor can take a few rounds of trial and error to master. Ground ginger has a more mellow flavor and the packaging makes it easy to add to your dishes.

Vegan Egg Salad Sandwiches

Now you can simulate the color, flavor, and even feel of egg salad with this Vegan Egg Salad recipe. Use it to make sandwiches, top leafy salads, and more! Think you never could like tofu? Think again, because this recipe transforms tofu into a dish you won't believe is vegan. Add fresh lettuce to each sandwich for a bit more crunch.

INGREDIENTS | SERVES 10

1 (15-ounce) package extra-firm tofu, pressed and crumbled

½ cup Vegan Mayonnaise (see Chapter 7 for recipe)

1 teaspoon dried parsley

2 tablespoons chopped green onion

1 teaspoon garlic powder

¾ teaspoon salt

¼ teaspoon ground turmeric

½ teaspoon paprika

½ teaspoon dried thyme

1½ tablespoons yellow mustard

10 whole-wheat hamburger buns

1. Add tofu to a medium lidded bowl. Push tofu to one side and stir in remaining ingredients. Then combine with tofu.

2. Place lid on bowl and refrigerate up to 7 days. To serve, spread on whole-wheat buns.

PER SERVING Calories: 63 | Fat: 4.0 g | Protein: 5.4 g | Sodium: 315 mg | Fiber: 0.6 g | Carbohydrates: 2.0 g | Sugar: 0.6 g

Vegan Tuna Salad Sandwiches

These Vegan Tuna Salad Sandwiches are a vegan twist on a popular recipe. The chickpeas are full of healthy ingredients, including fiber, so you'll be satisfied and energized!

INGREDIENTS | SERVES 10

1 (15-ounce) can chickpeas, rinsed and drained

1 tablespoon yellow mustard

2 tablespoons sweet mild miso paste

½ cup Vegan Mayonnaise (see Chapter 7 for recipe)

¼ cup finely chopped green onion

½ cup finely chopped seeded red bell pepper

1 clove garlic, peeled and minced

½ cup finely chopped sweet pickle relish

1 teaspoon celery seeds

1 teaspoon salt

20 slices whole-wheat bread

1. In a medium sealable bowl mash chickpeas with a fork. Set aside.

2. In a small bowl combine mustard, miso paste, and Vegan Mayonnaise. Add remaining ingredients (except bread) and stir well.

3. Stir mayonnaise mixture into mashed chickpeas. Cover and refrigerate up to 7 days. To serve, sandwich portioned spread between slices whole-wheat bread.

PER SERVING Calories: 246 | Fat: 4.3 g | Protein: 11.4 g | Sodium: 949 mg | Fiber: 6.3 g | Carbohydrates: 39.9 g | Sugar: 8.5 g

Barbecue Lentil Meatball Sandwiches

You'll love these Barbecue Lentil Meatball Sandwiches, featuring a simple, smoky tomato sauce over savory, garlicky lentil meatballs. The sauce is smothered with sweet cabbage coleslaw and served on soft rolls. You can also toast the buns for crispier goodness.

INGREDIENTS | SERVES 10

1 cup ketchup

¼ cup packed light brown sugar

1 tablespoon molasses

4 tablespoons apple cider vinegar, divided

2 teaspoons dry mustard

1 teaspoon nutmeg

2 teaspoons liquid smoke

1 batch Cocktail Lentil Meatballs (see Chapter 14 for recipe)

½ cup Vegan Mayonnaise (see Chapter 7 for recipe)

2 tablespoons mild miso paste

2 tablespoons agave nectar

⅛ teaspoon celery seeds

⅓ teaspoon ground turmeric

½ teaspoon salt

2 tablespoons chia seeds

3 cups coleslaw mix

10 dairy-free hamburger buns

1. Combine ketchup, brown sugar, molasses, vinegar, dry mustard, nutmeg, and liquid smoke in a small bowl. Pour over meatballs in a large sealed container and refrigerate up to 7 days.

2. To make coleslaw stir together mayonnaise, vinegar, miso paste, agave nectar, celery seeds, turmeric, salt, and chia seeds in a medium lidded bowl. Add coleslaw mix and stir until coated. Cover and refrigerate up to 7 days.

3. To serve, heat meatballs in microwave in 30-second intervals until heated through. Place 3 meatballs on each bun and top with creamy coleslaw.

PER SERVING Calories: 810 | Fat: 18.4 g | Protein: 44.4 g | Sodium: 1,290 mg | Fiber: 18.6 g | Carbohydrates: 120.8 g | Sugar: 21.6 g

Vegan French Dip Sandwiches

Enjoy these savory Vegan French Dip Sandwiches, made in 30 minutes with minimal ingredients and ready to tempt your taste buds! Include this recipe in your easy vegan recipes repertoire, and garnish with fresh parsley for an extra eye-catching presentation.

INGREDIENTS | SERVES 6

2 tablespoons olive oil, divided

2 (10-ounce) packages Gardein Beefless Tips, thawed

1 tablespoon soy sauce

2 cups water

1 tablespoon all-purpose flour

¼ cup dry minced onions

1 tablespoon Better Than Bouillon No Beef Base

¼ teaspoon dried thyme

2 bay leaves

6 dairy-free French rolls

12 slices vegan provolone cheese

Where Do I Find Vegan Beefless Tips?

Vegan faux meats have come a long way over the years, both in flavor and accessibility. You don't have to travel for miles to remote health food stores to find products like these Gardein Beefless Tips: you can find these tasty and texture-friendly tips in many popular store chains and the health food sections of most grocery stores.

1. Heat 1 tablespoon olive oil in a large skillet over medium-high heat. Place beefless tips in skillet and brown on all sides (about 3 minutes per side).

2. In a medium bowl combine 1 tablespoon olive oil, soy sauce, water, flour, onions, Better Than Bouillon, and dried thyme. Pour mixture over beefless tips. Top with bay leaves.

3. Place lid on skillet, turn heat down to low, and simmer about 15 minutes. Use a spatula to divide beefless tips into smaller pieces.

4. Preheat oven to 350°F and line a 9" × 13" baking pan with parchment paper.

5. Split rolls and place bottoms on prepared pan. Top each bottom with vegan beef followed by 2 slices vegan cheese. Bake 10 minutes until cheese is melted.

6. Place top side of bun on each sandwich. Allow sandwiches to cool about 3 minutes. Place in a large sealed container and refrigerate up to 7 days. Place pan sauce in a small sealable container and refrigerate up to 5 days. To serve, preheat oven to 300°F, top sandwiches with pan sauce, and cook 10 minutes.

PER SERVING Calories: 448 | Fat: 17.6 g | Protein: 24.6 g | Sodium: 1,225 mg | Fiber: 4.4 g | Carbohydrates: 49.0 g | Sugar: 4.5 g

Vegan Chicken Avocado Sandwiches

Take a bite out of one of these Vegan Chicken Avocado Sandwiches with vegan bacon strips. It's an easy vegan recipe that will have you coming back for more!

INGREDIENTS | SERVES 4

1 tablespoon olive oil

4 vegan chicken patties, thawed

1 tablespoon McCormick Brown Sugar Bourbon Seasoning

4 slices vegan bacon

4 slices vegan Cheddar cheese

4 dairy-free hamburger buns

1 medium avocado, peeled and pitted

1 tablespoon lime juice

1 cup shredded field greens

Speak Up!

Are you discouraged at the lack of vegan products at your local grocery store? Speak up! Many stores have customer request forms where you can request specific products by name. The more people who speak up, the more these stores will start stocking more vegan products!

1. Pour olive oil into a large skillet over medium-high heat. Place vegan chicken patties in skillet. Sprinkle ½ bourbon seasoning among tops of patties. Cook about 5 minutes, then flip and coat top with remaining seasoning. Add vegan bacon to pan and cook an additional 5 minutes.

2. Top each vegan chicken patty with 1 slice vegan cheese and allow cheese to melt before removing from skillet (about 1 minute). Set patties and vegan bacon aside.

3. Add buns to skillet, cut sides down and toast about 5 minutes, until golden brown. Add chicken patties on top of bottom buns, followed by vegan bacon slices and top buns. Let cool about 3 minutes.

4. In a small bowl, mash avocado with lime juice.

5. Place sandwiches in a large sealed container and refrigerate up to 7 days. Separately seal and refrigerate mashed avocado in a small lidded container (up to 3 days).

6. To serve, preheat oven to 300°F and cook sandwiches 10 minutes. Top with mashed avocado and field greens.

PER SERVING Calories: 411 | Fat: 18.4 g | Protein: 15.3 g | Sodium: 1,497 mg | Fiber: 5.9 g | Carbohydrates: 47.0 g | Sugar: 4.4 g

Vegan Philly Cheesesteak Sandwiches

These Vegan Philly Cheesesteak Sandwiches are made with marinated and braised tofu, caramelized onions, and dairy-free cheese. They're so good that you'll want to make the recipe every week!

INGREDIENTS | SERVES 4

2 medium green onions, roughly chopped

1 teaspoon garlic powder

⅓ cup soy sauce

3 tablespoons olive oil, divided

4 tablespoons agave nectar

4 tablespoons rice vinegar

1 (15-ounce) block extra-firm tofu, pressed and thinly sliced

1 cup sliced seeded red bell pepper

1 cup peeled, sliced, yellow onions

1 cup white mushrooms

1 medium avocado, peeled and pitted

1 teaspoon minced garlic

1 cup dairy-free mozzarella cheese

4 dairy-free hoagie buns

1. Preheat oven to 200°F.

2. Add green onion, garlic powder, soy sauce, 1 tablespoon olive oil, agave nectar, and vinegar to a food processor. Pulse 3 seconds until ingredients are combined. Pour ½ mixture into bottom of a 9" × 9" ungreased baking dish.

3. Place tofu strips in marinade. Cover with a bit more marinade and add another layer of tofu strips until all tofu and mixture is in dish. Tilt dish slowly from side to side to allow marinade to saturate all tofu.

4. Bake 1½ hours.

5. Place 1 tablespoon olive oil in a medium skillet over medium-high heat. Add bell peppers, onions, and mushrooms. Cook until tender and caramelized along edges, about 7 minutes. Remove from skillet, let cool 10 minutes, then transfer to a small sealable container and refrigerate up to 7 days.

6. Pour 1 tablespoon olive oil in same skillet over medium-high heat. Add several slices baked tofu at a time and cook until browned on both sides—about 5 minutes. Pour any remaining marinade mixture from baking dish over top of tofu as it's cooking. Repeat this step until all tofu has been browned. Remove from skillet, transfer to a large sealable container, let cool 10 minutes, then refrigerate up to 7 days.

7. Mash avocado in a small sealable bowl with minced garlic. Refrigerate up to 7 days.

8. To serve, preheat oven to 250°F and tear off four slices of aluminum foil large enough to wrap individual sandwiches.

9. Place one bun on each strip of aluminum foil. Spread both sides of each bun with avocado mixture. Add several tofu strips, followed by sautéed vegetables and ¼ cup cheese.

10. Place top bun on each serving, wrap sandwiches in foil, and bake 10 minutes until cheese melts. Remove from oven and let cool about 5 minutes. Place sandwiches in a large sealed container and refrigerate up to 7 days. To serve, preheat oven to 250°F and cook sandwiches 10 minutes.

PER SERVING Calories: 417 | Fat: 26.4 g | Protein: 15.3 g | Sodium: 1,463 mg | Fiber: 5.4 g | Carbohydrates: 29.7 g | Sugar: 12.9 g

Vegan Chicken Salad Sandwich

This Vegan Chicken Salad Sandwich is easy to make and reminiscent of the recipe you've enjoyed for years—except this one is made without meat or dairy! But don't worry: there's lots of flavor, protein, and creaminess to keep you coming back for more!

INGREDIENTS | SERVES 4

1 (8-ounce) package tempeh, cut into ½" cubes

½ medium Granny Smith apple, diced

1 large carrot, peeled and diced

1 stalk celery, finely chopped

¼ cup diced green onion

2 tablespoons dried cranberries

¼ cup walnuts, chopped

⅓ cup Vegan Mayonnaise (see Chapter 7 for recipe)

1 tablespoon white vinegar

2 tablespoons strawberry preserves

⅛ teaspoon salt

⅛ teaspoon ground black pepper

8 slices whole-wheat bread

What Is Tempeh?

Tempeh is a soy-based product that uses fermentation to bind soybeans together in a loaf. Tempeh has a nutty flavor and is high in protein and other nutrients. It's recommended to steam the tempeh first to help bind it together more and prevent crumbling.

1. Place a steamer basket in a small pot and add water to just below bottom of basket. Steam tempeh in covered pot over medium heat about 20 minutes until tender.

2. In a medium bowl add apples, carrots, celery, green onions, dried cranberries, and walnuts and mix well.

3. Once tempeh is done steaming, carefully remove steamer basket from pan, drain any excess liquid, and pour hot tempeh cubes into bowl with apple mixture. Set aside.

4. In a small bowl combine mayonnaise, vinegar, and preserves. Add mayonnaise mixture to cooled tempeh and season with salt and pepper.

5. Place mixture in a large sealed container and refrigerate up to 7 days. To serve, sandwich portions between slices of whole-wheat bread.

PER SERVING Calories: 407 | Fat: 14.3 g | Protein: 21.8 g | Sodium: 578 mg | Fiber: 6.4 g | Carbohydrates: 47.5 g | Sugar: 11.6 g

Vegan "Big Macs"

You don't have to abandon all your favorite foods in order to become vegan—just veganize them. Case in point: these Vegan "Big Mac" sandwiches are made with all of your favorite burger trimmings!

INGREDIENTS | SERVES 4

1 (15-ounce) can pinto beans, rinsed and drained

1 tablespoon ground flaxseed

1 tablespoon cornstarch

1 tablespoon dried minced onion

1 tablespoon garlic powder

½ teaspoon celery seeds

1 teaspoon paprika

3 tablespoons cornmeal

1 tablespoon nutritional yeast flakes

1 tablespoon soy sauce

1 cup cooked red quinoa

2 tablespoons water

4 dairy-free hamburger buns

1 batch Vegan Special Sauce (see Chapter 7 for recipe)

8 large leaves leaf lettuce

4 slices vegan Cheddar

4 dairy-free thin sandwich rounds

12 hamburger dill pickle chips

½ yellow onion, peeled and sliced into 4 slices

1. Add pinto beans, flaxseed, cornstarch, dried onions, garlic powder, celery seeds, paprika, cornmeal, nutritional yeast flakes, and soy sauce to a food processor. Pulse 3 seconds, then use a spatula to push ingredients down from side of bowl. Pulse again 3 seconds. Repeat this process until ingredients are well combined.

2. Add cooked red quinoa to processor and pulse again 3 seconds. Add water and stir, then form mixture into 8 patties and set aside.

3. Place a large skillet over medium heat and spray with vegetable cooking spray. Add patties 1–2 at a time to skillet and cook until browned, about 5 minutes per side.

4. Let cool about 5 minutes then transfer to a large lidded container. Refrigerate up to 7 days or freeze up to 2 months.

5. To serve, remove patties from refrigerator and cook in microwave in 30-second intervals until heated through. Place bottom half of each bun on a plate. Place divided amounts of the following on each bottom bun in this order: Vegan Special Sauce, lettuce, 1 slice vegan Cheddar cheese, 1 patty, 1 side of thin sandwich bun, lettuce, Vegan Special Sauce, pickles, 1 slice onion, 1 patty, top side of bun.

PER SERVING Calories: 570 | Fat: 14.8 g | Protein: 26.9 g | Sodium: 1,521 mg | Fiber: 11.8 g | Carbohydrates: 109.9 g | Sugar: 11.2 g

Carrot "Dogs"

You will be amazed at how good carrots can taste with these vegan Carrot "Dogs." You'll forget all about processed meats when you've got these flavorful delights ready to go! Serve with your favorite toppings.

INGREDIENTS | SERVES 8

1 tablespoon olive oil
2 tablespoons agave nectar
2 tablespoons tamari
1 teaspoon yellow miso paste
½ cup hot water
⅛ teaspoon ground black pepper
½ teaspoon garlic powder
½ teaspoon smoked paprika
1 teaspoon liquid smoke
8 medium carrots, peeled and ends trimmed
8 dairy-free hot dog buns

Swapping Non-Vegan Classics for Vegan Ingredients

It's hard to believe you can make so many tasty vegan versions of classic dishes from whole plants like carrots. Plant-based versions offer all the nutritional benefits of plants without the cholesterol and saturated fats from animal products! You can use jackfruit to create a texture similar to pulled pork or cauliflower to create delicious fried rice.

1. In a small bowl combine olive oil, agave nectar, tamari, miso paste, water, pepper, garlic powder, paprika, and liquid smoke. Pour into a 9" × 9" baking pan.

2. Add carrots to pan and use tongs to coat in mixture. Cover with aluminum foil and set aside to marinate 30 minutes.

3. Preheat oven to 400°F. Place covered dish in oven as it heats. Once temperature is reached, roast carrots 30 minutes.

4. Use tongs to remove foil. Cook another 20 minutes uncovered. Carrots should be slightly tender when pierced with a fork.

5. Remove from oven and let cool 10 minutes. Place in a medium sealed container in refrigerator up to 5 days. To serve, heat carrot dogs in microwave in 30-second intervals until heated through. Place carrots in hot dog buns.

PER SERVING Calories: 176 | Fat: 3.2 g | Protein: 5.4 g | Sodium: 540 mg | Fiber: 3.0 g | Carbohydrates: 31.3 g | Sugar: 8.6 g

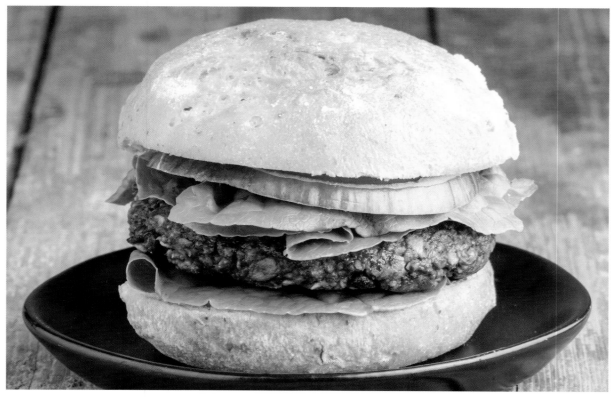

Sweet Potato Black Bean Burgers (Chapter 9)

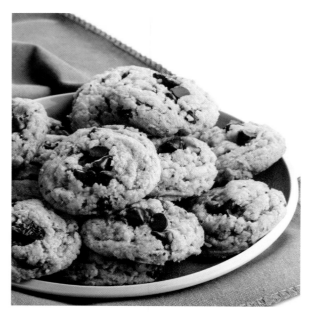

Chocolate Chip Cookies (Chapter 15)

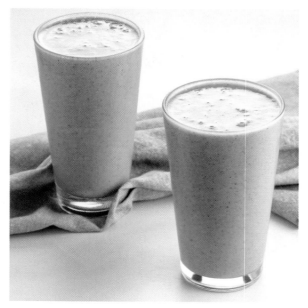

Green Tea Banana Smoothies (Chapter 5)

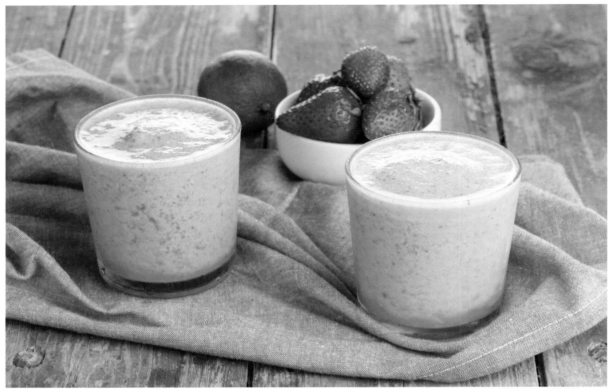

Vanilla Strawberry Lime Smoothies (Chapter 5)

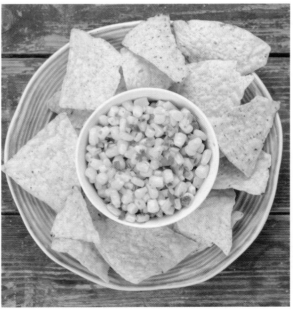

Fresh Corn Salsa (Chapter 8)

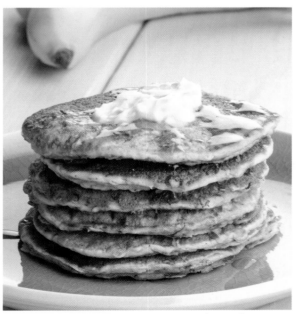

Banana Pancakes (Chapter 3)

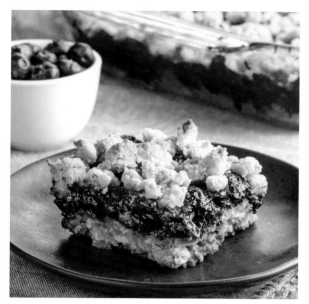

Healthy Blueberry Crumble Bars (Chapter 15)

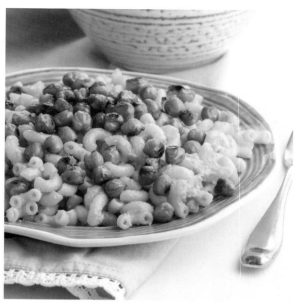

Vegan Mac and Cheese with Smoky Chickpeas (Chapter 17)

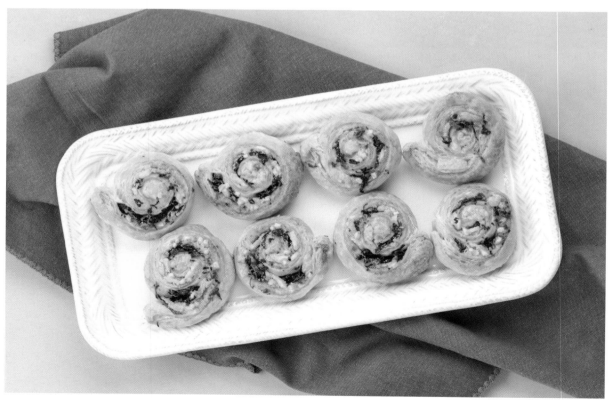

Vegan Spinach Cheese Pinwheels (Chapter 14)

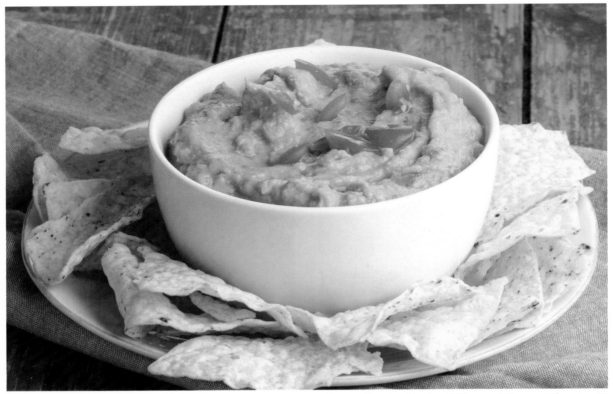
Sweet Potato Nacho "Cheese" Sauce (Chapter 7)

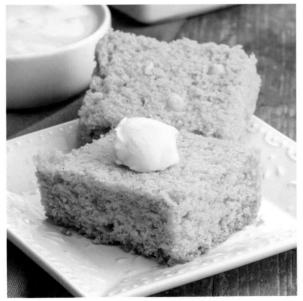
Easy Corn Bread (Chapter 4)

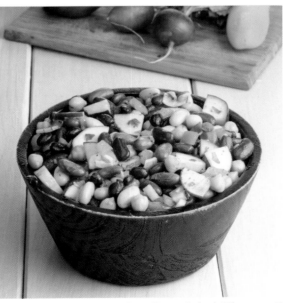
Five-Bean Salad (Chapter 6)

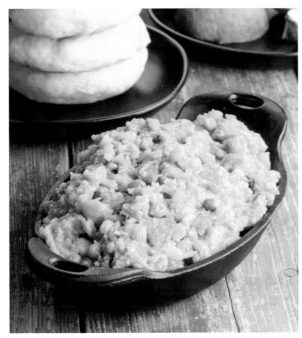

One-Pot Chickpea Coconut Curry (Chapter 12)

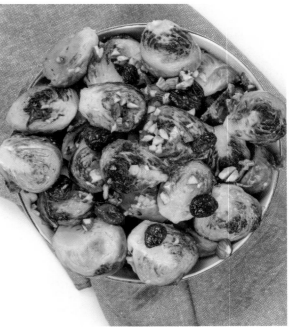

Seared Brussels Sprouts (Chapter 8)

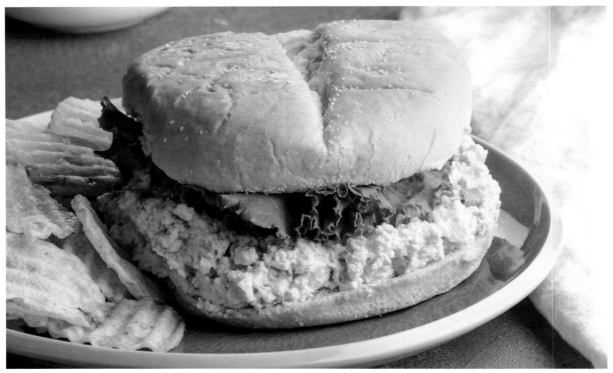

Vegan Egg Salad Sandwiches (Chapter 9)

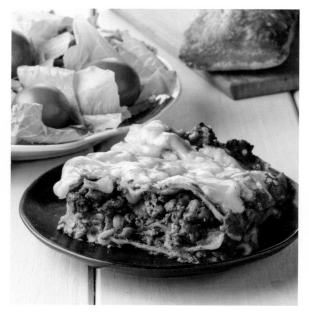

Easy Vegan Lasagna (Chapter 13)

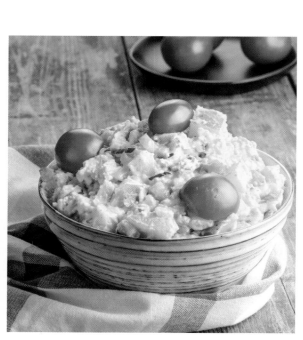

Vegan Potato Salad (Chapter 6)

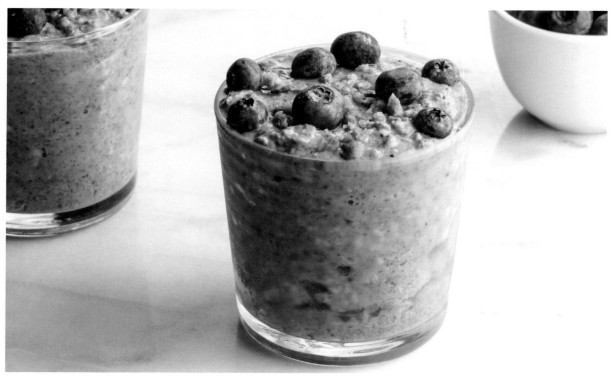

Blueberry Overnight Oats (Chapter 3)

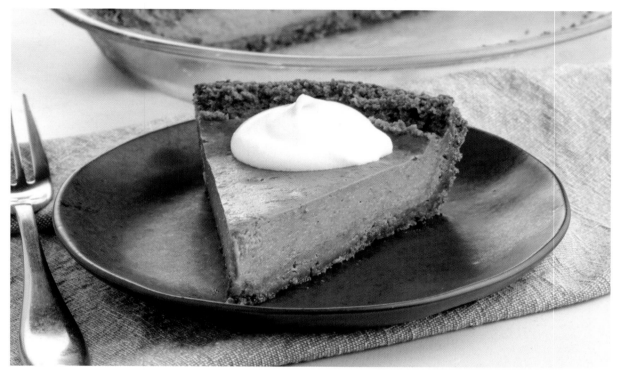

Pumpkin Pie (Chapter 16)

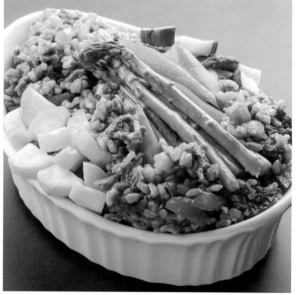

Vegan Jambalaya (Chapter 12)

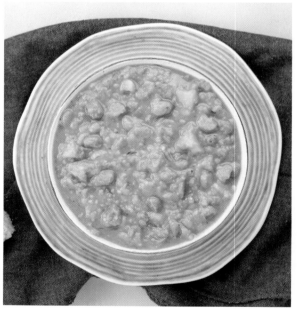

Pinto Bean Soup (Chapter 10)

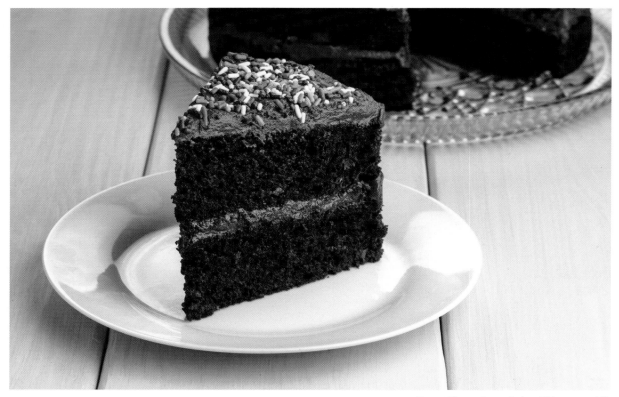

Easy Chocolate Cake (Chapter 16)

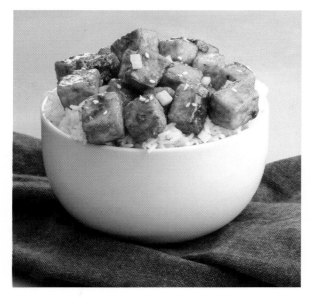

Sticky Sweet Tofu and Rice (Chapter 11)

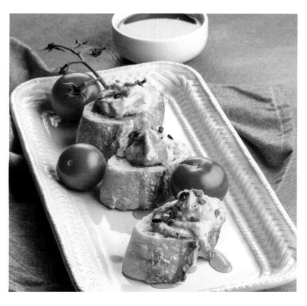

Vegan Bacon Ricotta Crostini (Chapter 14)

Lentil Sloppy Joes

Try these delicious Lentil Sloppy Joes on the next Meatless Monday—or any day of the week—for a satisfying, healthy meal. Place on hamburger buns and serve with your favorite sides.

INGREDIENTS | SERVES 12

½ cup chopped peeled carrots

1 tablespoon olive oil

1 medium yellow onion, peeled and chopped

½ cup chopped seeded yellow bell pepper

2 cloves garlic, peeled and minced

3 cups cooked brown lentils, divided

1 (15-ounce) can diced tomatoes

½ cup tomato paste

2 tablespoons chili powder

1 teaspoon dried oregano

1 teaspoon dried basil

1 tablespoon liquid smoke

1 tablespoon paprika

½ cup cornmeal

1 cup cooked brown rice

12 dairy-free hamburger buns

Cooking Lentils

Lentils are relatively easy to cook from scratch because they don't require soaking. Cook one part lentils with two parts water and do not salt the water. One cup of dried lentils will yield 2½ cups cooked lentils.

1. Place carrots in a small microwave-safe container with enough water to cover and cook 2 minutes. Let sit about 5 minutes until carrots become tender.

2. Add oil to a medium skillet over medium heat. Add onions, cooked carrots, bell peppers, and garlic. Sauté until vegetables are tender and onions are translucent, about 5 minutes.

3. Add cooked lentils (reserving 1 cup), diced tomatoes, tomato paste, spices, and cornmeal. Stir and cook another 10 minutes.

4. Add reserved cup lentil mixture and brown rice to a food processor. Pulse until mixture is consistency of paste. Stir paste into lentil mixture. Remove from heat and let cool about 10 minutes.

5. Place in a medium sealed container in refrigerator up to 7 days, or freeze up to 2 months. To serve, heat in microwave in 30-second intervals until heated through and place on buns.

PER SERVING Calories: 258 | Fat: 3.2 g | Protein: 10.8 g | Sodium: 324 mg | Fiber: 7.5 g | Carbohydrates: 47.0 g | Sugar: 6.7 g

Vegan Baked Hot Dogs

Enjoy these comfort-food Vegan Baked Hot Dogs made with vegetarian chili, onions, and vegan cheese on top.

INGREDIENTS | SERVES 8

½ cup Vegan Mayonnaise (see Chapter 7 for recipe)

8 dairy-free hot dog buns

8 vegan hot dogs

2 cups Easy Vegan Chili (see Chapter 10 for recipe)

1 cup vegan Cheddar shreds

4 green onions, chopped

1. Preheat oven to 350°F.

2. Spread Vegan Mayonnaise across insides of each hot dog bun. Place 1 vegan hot dog in each prepared bun and place hot dogs in a 2-quart oblong baking pan. Spoon chili mixture on top of each hot dog, followed by shredded vegan cheese and chopped onions.

3. Cover pan with aluminum foil and bake 30 minutes. Remove from oven. Let cool about 10 minutes before covering and refrigerating up to 5 days.

4. To serve, heat individual portions in microwave in 30-second intervals until cooked through.

PER SERVING Calories: 276 | Fat: 7.6 g | Protein: 14.9 g | Sodium: 1,083 mg | Fiber: 4.9 g | Carbohydrates: 37.3 g | Sugar: 6.3 g

Vegan Deviled Ham Sandwich Spread

Did you grow up eating Deviled Ham? The stuff in the little cans? If you thought your devilish deviled ham days were over because of your vegan diet, you're in for a surprise. This Vegan Deviled Ham Sandwich Spread is even better (and cheaper) than the kind you used to buy in those cans!

INGREDIENTS | SERVES 4

1 cup Spicy Roasted Chickpeas (see Chapter 14 for recipe)

¼ cup sun-dried tomatoes

6 tablespoons Vegan Mayonnaise (see Chapter 7 for recipe)

1 green onion, finely chopped

1 teaspoon yellow mustard

¼ teaspoon garlic powder

1 teaspoon liquid smoke

1. Add chickpeas and sun-dried tomatoes to a food processor. Pulse until mixture is broken down into small bits. Add Vegan Mayonnaise, green onions, mustard, garlic powder, and liquid smoke. Pulse until combined.

2. Place in a small sealed container and refrigerate up to 7 days or freeze up to 2 months.

PER SERVING Calories: 103 | Fat: 4.5 g | Protein: 4.9 g | Sodium: 506 mg | Fiber: 3.0 g | Carbohydrates: 11.1 g | Sugar: 3.3 g

Vegan Chopped Cheese Sandwiches

These easy, cheesy vegan sandwiches, are a meat- and dairy-free version of the famous NYC sandwich! They are also ready in just 10 minutes.

INGREDIENTS | SERVES 4

1 (13.7-ounce) package vegan crumbles

1 green onion, chopped

4 dairy-free hoagie buns

8 slices vegan Cheddar

¼ cup Vegan Mayonnaise (see Chapter 7 for recipe)

¼ cup ketchup

1. Place vegan crumbles in a medium skillet over medium heat. Add green onions. Stir and cook about 5 minutes.

2. Place hoagie buns in a toaster oven and toast about 3 minutes.

3. Use a spatula to mold vegan crumbles into 4 rows about the size of hoagie buns. Place 2 cheese slices over each row and cook covered 5 minutes until cheese starts to melt.

4. Add vegan mayonnaise and ketchup to top and bottom of each bun. Then use spatula to place one row vegan meat and cheese mixture on each bun.

5. Allow sandwiches to cool about 5 minutes before placing in a large sealed container and refrigerating up to 5 days. To serve, bake individual sandwiches 10 minutes in toaster oven set to 200°F.

PER SERVING Calories: 541 | Fat: 18.6 g | Protein: 29.7 g | Sodium: 1,400 mg | Fiber: 8.1 g | Carbohydrates: 64.7 g | Sugar: 9.6 g

Vegan Spring Rolls

Eat your greens, your reds, your yellows, and more with these easy and tasty Vegan Spring Rolls.

INGREDIENTS | SERVES 4

¼ cup all-natural peanut butter

1 tablespoon sesame oil

1 teaspoon tamari

1 tablespoon hoisin sauce

1 tablespoon sriracha

½ teaspoon garlic powder

½ teaspoon ground ginger

½ cup water

1 medium zucchini, peeled and julienned

1 medium red bell pepper, seeded and julienned

1 medium yellow bell pepper, seeded and julienned

2 leaves purple cabbage, chopped

1 bunch watercress, chopped (approximately 4 ounces)

½ medium avocado, peeled, pitted, and thinly sliced

1 cup warm water

10 spring roll rice wraps

1 cup cooked rice noodles

1 (8-ounce) package Nasoya Sesame Ginger TofuBaked (organic), sliced

2 tablespoons chopped peanuts

Meal Prepping Hacks

When it comes to meal prepping, having the right equipment matters. For example, a food processor will make homemade sauces a breeze. Also invest in a knife sharpener so you can keep your knives sharp for slicing and dicing ingredients.

1. To make peanut dipping sauce, combine peanut butter, sesame oil, tamari, hoisin sauce, sriracha, garlic powder, and ginger in a medium bowl. Stir well. Add water and stir to combine. Place mixture in a medium sealed container and refrigerate up to 5 days.

2. Lay out chopped and sliced vegetables in assembly-line order. Place a cutting board in center of cooking station.

3. Pour warm water into a 9" round cake pan. Place one spring roll rice wrap in water, making sure entire wrap gets wet. When you remove it from water it should collapse in the middle just a little.

4. Place wet wrap on cutting board. Place a few pieces of each vegetable and rice noodles in center of rice wrap. Finish it with TofuBaked slices. Drizzle with peanut sauce and chopped peanuts.

5. Turn bottom and top edges of rice wrap up over vegetables. Beginning on left side, turn wrap very tightly and roll it (very similar to a burrito). Place finished vegetable roll in a large sealable container and repeat with remaining wraps and ingredients.

6. Refrigerate container up to 5 days. For serving, slice each vegetable roll in half for dipping in peanut sauce.

PER SERVING Calories: 600 | Fat: 21.6 g | Protein: 24.2 g | Sodium: 861 mg | Fiber: 7.3 g | Carbohydrates: 74.9 g | Sugar: 7.3 g

Freezer-Ready Vegan Club Sandwiches

Enjoy these all-American layered sandwiches, made vegan and with all the trimmings—including vegan bacon! Meal prepping takes a delicious turn with this freezer-ready recipe!

INGREDIENTS | SERVES 8

1 tablespoon olive oil

12 slices vegan bacon

4 tablespoons vegan butter, softened

8 dairy-free whole-wheat buns

16 slices vegan deli slices

½ cup Vegan Mayonnaise (see Chapter 7 for recipe)

¼ cup Dijon mustard

1 medium avocado, peeled, pitted, and sliced

8 slices vegan Cheddar cheese

1 (8-ounce) package Tofurky Slow Roasted Chick'n

Freeze or Refrigerate?

If you think you'll be eating the food right away, storing meals or individual servings in the refrigerator is a great idea. However, if you may not get through the dish in less than a week, freezing might be a better option. Not every recipe is freezer-friendly, so be sure to check recipe instructions to ensure it can be frozen!

1. Pour olive oil in a medium skillet over medium heat. Cook vegan bacon according to package directions. Set aside on a piece of paper towel to cool 5 minutes, then slice each strip in half.

2. Spread softened butter across top and bottom slice of each bun. Place 2 vegan deli slices on bottom half of each bun. Top with a slathering of Vegan Mayonnaise, followed by divided amounts of Dijon mustard and avocado slices, 1 slice Cheddar, 3 bacon halves, and a portion Slow Roasted Chick'n. Finish with top bun, buttered side down.

3. Place two long toothpicks down center of each sandwich. Wrap each sandwich in plastic wrap, place in a large freezer bag and freeze up to 2 months.

4. To serve, remove wrapping and place sandwiches on an ungreased baking sheet. Place pan in a cold oven and preheat to 350°F. Once oven is heated, cook 20 minutes until sandwiches are heated through and tops of buns are toasted.

PER SERVING Calories: 44 | Fat: 23.0 g | Protein: 26.5 g | Sodium: 1,276 mg | Fiber: 5.7 g | Carbohydrates: 35.2 g | Sugar: 4.6 g

CHAPTER 10

Soups, Stews, and Chilis

Vegan Cheeseburger Soup

Sit yourself down to a bowl of this creamy, cheesy, savory Vegan Cheeseburger Soup. This flavorful dish is an American classic veganized and transformed into a soup perfect for adding a little warmth to a cold week ahead.

INGREDIENTS | SERVES 4

2 teaspoons olive oil

1 small yellow onion, peeled and chopped

1 cup chopped peeled carrots

4 cups unpeeled chopped red potatoes

3 cups vegetable broth

1 bay leaf

1 cup cashews

1 cup water

½ cup unsweetened almond milk

½ cup nutritional yeast flakes

1 teaspoon garlic powder

2 cups vegan crumbles, thawed

1 cup vegan Cheddar cheese

Meal Prepping Tip

On meal prepping day, fill a sink or a large bowl with hot, sudsy water. Then drop used utensils, measuring cups, and dishes in the hot water as you cook. This will make clean-up even easier, as the used items will be soaking, rather than creating a mess on your kitchen surfaces.

1. Heat olive oil 30 seconds in a large pot over medium heat, then add onions and cook 5 minutes until tender. Add carrots and potatoes. Stir to coat, then simmer about 10 minutes.

2. Add vegetable broth and bay leaf and bring back to a simmer about 10 minutes.

3. Place cashews in a small saucepan and add water. Simmer over medium heat 5 minutes until cashews are tender and most of water is gone. Remove from heat.

4. Pour cashews and remaining liquid into a food processor along with almond milk, nutritional yeast flakes, and garlic powder. Pulse until completely smooth. Push down contents from sides and pulse again until smooth.

5. Use a fork to test tenderness of potatoes and carrots. Once tender, remove bay leaf and stir in cashew cream. Then stir in vegan crumbles and vegan Cheddar shreds. Remove from heat and let cool about 10 minutes.

6. Transfer to a large lidded container (or individual serving containers), and refrigerate up to 7 days. To serve, cook in microwave in 30-second intervals until heated through.

PER SERVING Calories: 557 | Fat: 27.5 g | Protein: 22.8 g | Sodium: 981 mg | Fiber: 11.6 g | Carbohydrates: 58.2 g | Sugar: 6.6 g

Vegan Broccoli Cheese Soup

This extra creamy Vegan Broccoli Cheese Soup is the perfect comfort food any day of the year! Serve it as a side dish or as a main course with a salad on the side.

INGREDIENTS | SERVES 4

6 tablespoons vegan butter

1 cup finely chopped peeled yellow onion

1 clove garlic, peeled and finely minced

¼ cup all-purpose flour

3 cups plain soy milk

2 cups vegetable broth

¼ cup nutritional yeast flakes

½ cup vegan sour cream

3 cups broccoli florets

2 cups vegan Cheddar shreds

½ teaspoon salt

½ teaspoon ground black pepper

1. Place a medium saucepan over medium heat. Add vegan butter, using a spatula to break into pieces. Add onions and cook 5 minutes until tender. Add garlic and cook another 1 minute, stirring occasionally. Sprinkle in flour, stirring constantly. Cook another 1 minute until mixture thickens.

2. Gradually add milk while stirring. Add vegetable broth, nutritional yeast flakes, and vegan sour cream. Stir to combine. Stir in broccoli and cook 10 minutes until broccoli is tender, stirring throughout.

3. Add vegan Cheddar shreds. Stir another 2 minutes until cheese melts. Remove from heat. Season with salt and pepper.

4. Let cool about 10 minutes before transferring to a large sealable container. Refrigerate up to 7 days. To serve, pour into individual bowls and cook in microwave in 30-second intervals until heated through.

PER SERVING Calories: 458 | Fat: 29.5 g | Protein: 11.5 g | Sodium: 1,350 mg | Fiber: 9.2 g | Carbohydrates: 40.7 g | Sugar: 4.2 g

Easy Vegan Chicken Noodle Soup

This simply delicious Easy Vegan Chicken Noodle Soup is made with minimal ingredients and lots of flavor!

INGREDIENTS | SERVES 6

1 cup sliced peeled carrot

2 tablespoons water

1 tablespoon olive oil

½ cup chopped peeled yellow onion

½ cup chopped celery

5 cups vegetable broth

1 (10-ounce) package Gardein Chick'n Strips, thawed and chopped

1½ cups egg-free wide noodles

½ teaspoon dried Italian seasoning

1 bay leaf

Egg-Free Noodles

Some store brands offer wide noodles that are egg-free. Double-check ingredients before purchase. If you need egg-free noodles and can't find them, break egg-free lasagna noodles into pieces.

1. In a small microwave-safe bowl add carrots with 2 tablespoons water, stirring to coat carrots. Cover and cook in microwave 3 minutes until tender. Let cool about 5 minutes during next step.

2. In a large pot over medium heat add olive oil, onion, and celery. Cook until just tender, about 5 minutes.

3. Add vegetable broth, vegan chicken pieces, and noodles. Add cooked carrots (including liquid). Sprinkle top with Italian seasoning and add bay leaf.

4. Bring to a boil over high heat, then reduce heat to medium-low and simmer about 15 minutes.

5. Remove from heat and allow soup to cool about 10 minutes. Remove bay leaf and transfer soup to a large sealed container. Refrigerate up to 7 days.

PER SERVING Calories: 156 | Fat: 5.9 g | Protein: 9.3 g | Sodium: 615 mg | Fiber: 2.2 g | Carbohydrates: 16.5 g | Sugar: 3.1 g

Pinto Bean Soup

Hearty, nourishing and easy to make, this vegan Pinto Bean Soup boasts rich flavors and vibrant colors. You'll love that you can prepare this satisfying comfort food with simple ingredients. Serve with Easy Corn Bread (see Chapter 4 for recipe)!

INGREDIENTS | SERVES 8

1 teaspoon olive oil

½ cup chopped peeled yellow onion

½ cup chopped celery

2 large carrots, peeled and chopped

2 medium red potatoes, chopped

3 (15-ounce) cans pinto beans, including liquid

1 teaspoon garlic powder

1 teaspoon marjoram

1 teaspoon dried thyme

1 tablespoon liquid smoke

1 tablespoon Better Than Bouillon Seasoned Vegetable Base

4 cups water

1 bay leaf

½ teaspoon salt

½ teaspoon ground black pepper

1. Place a large pot over medium heat. Add olive oil, then add onions, celery, carrots, and potatoes. Cook until vegetables are tender, about 10 minutes.

2. Add beans, spices, and liquid smoke. Stir to combine. Add Better Than Bouillon and water. Stir to combine. Place bay leaf on top of broth and then cover and cook 40 minutes.

3. Remove bay leaf. Use a potato masher to mash some beans to create a thicker sauce. Stir in salt and pepper. Remove from heat and let cool about 10 minutes.

4. Transfer soup to a large lidded container (or individual serving containers), cover, and refrigerate up to 10 days or freeze up to 3 months.

5. To serve, cook in microwave in 30-second intervals until heated through.

PER SERVING Calories: 194 | Fat: 1.3 g | Protein: 9.2 g | Sodium: 856 mg | Fiber: 9.4 g | Carbohydrates: 37.2 g | Sugar: 3.4 g

Curried Lentil Soup

This Curried Lentil Soup is hearty and full of spices, but it won't make your mouth feel on fire, although you can certainly add more heat if that's your thing. This soup takes only 10 minutes of prep work and a little simmering to make.

INGREDIENTS | SERVES 6

1 teaspoon olive oil

1 cup chopped peeled yellow onion

2 cups chopped peeled carrots

2 medium red potatoes, chopped into ½" cubes

1 clove garlic, peeled and minced

2 teaspoons curry powder

2 tablespoons soy sauce

½ teaspoon ground turmeric

⅛ teaspoon crushed red pepper flakes

4 cups low-sodium vegetable stock

4 cups water

1 (14.5-ounce) can stewed tomatoes

2 cups dried brown lentils

1 cup cooked brown rice

⅛ teaspoon ground black pepper

1. Combine olive oil and onion in a large pot over medium heat. Sauté onion until tender, about 3 minutes. Add carrots and potatoes and cook until vegetables begin to become tender, about 7 minutes.

2. Add remaining ingredients and turn up heat to high until soup comes to a boil. Reduce heat to low, cover, and simmer until lentils are tender, about 40 minutes.

3. Remove from heat and let cool for about 10 minutes. Transfer to a large lidded container (or individual serving containers) and refrigerate up to 10 days. To serve, cook in microwave in 30-second intervals until heated through.

PER SERVING Calories: 386 | Fat: 1.8 g | Protein: 20.5 g | Sodium: 564 mg | Fiber: 12.9 g | Carbohydrates: 74.7 g | Sugar: 9.8 g

What Is Curry?

Curry is sold as a single ingredient, but it's actually made up of several different spices. Traditional curry is made from turmeric, cumin, coriander, chili peppers, and often ground ginger. Curry can be added to a variety of dishes, like soups, rice dishes, vegetables, and more.

Beefless Stew

You'll love this savory, easy-to-prepare Beefless Stew for chilly nights. Enjoy leftovers throughout the week!

INGREDIENTS | SERVES 10

2 tablespoons olive oil, divided

1 medium yellow onion, peeled and chopped

2 cups chopped baby carrots

4 medium red potatoes, chopped into ½" cubes

1 (32-ounce) container vegetable broth

1 (15-ounce) can corn kernels, drained

1 (15-ounce) can stewed tomatoes, juice included

1 bay leaf

1 (10-ounce) package Gardein Beefless Tips

1. Pour 1 tablespoon olive oil in a Dutch oven and heat over medium heat and add onions, carrots, and potatoes. Cook about 10 minutes, until vegetables are just starting to become tender.

2. Add vegetable broth, corn, stewed tomatoes, and bay leaf. Bring to a boil over high heat, then reduce to a simmer over medium heat and cook 10 minutes.

3. Add remaining tablespoon oil to a medium skillet over medium heat. Add Gardein Beefless Tips and stir until each piece is coated with oil. Cook until each side is browned, about 5 minutes per side.

4. Add browned beefless tips to Dutch oven and continue simmering another 10 minutes to allow flavors to combine.

5. Remove bay leaf, let cool 10 minutes, then transfer stew to a large lidded container (or individual serving containers), and refrigerate up to 7 days. To serve, cook in microwave in 30-second intervals until heated through.

PER SERVING Calories: 185 | Fat: 4.7 g | Protein: 8.0 g | Sodium: 523 mg | Fiber: 4.9 g | Carbohydrates: 30.0 g | Sugar: 6.4 g

Red Beans and Rice

Red Beans and Rice is a traditional New Orleans dish full of flavor. This vegan version is healthy and filling. Be sure to serve it with corn bread and hot sauce!

INGREDIENTS | SERVES 8

1 tablespoon olive oil

1 medium yellow onion, peeled and chopped

2 cups chopped peeled carrots

3 cloves garlic, peeled and chopped

1 cup vegetable broth

2 cups TVP (textured vegetable protein)

3 (15-ounce) cans red beans, including juice

2 tablespoons chili powder

1 tablespoon ground cumin

1 teaspoon ground turmeric

1 (15-ounce) can stewed tomatoes

½ teaspoon salt

¼ teaspoon ground black pepper

2 cups cooked brown rice

1. Place olive oil in a large pot over medium-high heat. Add onions and carrots and cook 5 minutes until vegetables are just tender.

2. Reduce heat to medium and add remaining ingredients. Stir to combine, then bring to a boil. Reduce heat to a simmer and cook 40 minutes. Set aside to cool about 15 minutes.

3. Transfer to a large lidded container (or individual serving containers) and refrigerate up to 7 days or freeze up to 3 months. To serve, cook in microwave in 30-second intervals until heated through.

PER SERVING Calories: 323 | Fat: 3.2 g | Protein: 22.9 g | Sodium: 812 mg | Fiber: 14.8 g | Carbohydrates: 51.9 g | Sugar: 10.5 g

What Is TVP?

TVP stands for Textured Vegetable Protein. The process involves removing the oil from soybeans. What remains is dried and processed. TVP is oftentimes used in place of meat in recipes. It's high in protein, cooks quickly, and has a texture similar to ground beef. You can find TVP in the health food section of most grocery stores and in health food stores.

Easy Vegan Chili

Nothing showcases just how easy vegan cooking can be like this Easy Vegan Chili recipe. It's made with minimal ingredients and is ready in less than 30 minutes. Store it in the refrigerator or freezer to serve throughout the week!

INGREDIENTS | SERVES 6

1 tablespoon olive oil

1 cup chopped peeled yellow onion

2 cups vegan crumbles

1 clove garlic, peeled and minced

1 (15-ounce) can black beans, drained and rinsed

1 (15-ounce) can kidney beans, drained and rinsed

2 (15-ounce) cans diced tomatoes with green chilies

2 tablespoons chili powder

1. Add olive oil and onion to a large pot over medium-high heat. Cook 5 minutes until onions are tender. Add vegan crumbles and cook another 5 minutes until crumbles are browned.

2. Add garlic, beans, tomatoes with chilies, and chili powder. Bring to a boil over high heat, then then reduce heat to medium-low and cook 15 minutes. Remove from heat and let cool about 15 minutes.

3. Transfer to a large lidded container (or individual serving containers) and refrigerate up to 10 days or freeze up to 3 months. To serve, cook in microwave in 30-second intervals until heated through.

PER SERVING Calories: 245 | Fat: 4.9 g | Protein: 15.8 g | Sodium: 954 mg | Fiber: 12.3 g | Carbohydrates: 35.1 g | Sugar: 6.7 g

Vegan Beer Cheese Soup

This easy Vegan Beer Cheese Soup recipe is rich and creamy and made with only a few ingredients. Enjoy it topped with sourdough bread croutons and fresh chives.

INGREDIENTS | SERVES 6

2 cups dairy-free sourdough bread, cut into 1" cubes
2 tablespoons olive oil, divided
1 teaspoon salt, divided
1 cup chopped peeled yellow onion
1 cup chopped peeled carrots
2 cloves garlic, peeled and chopped
¼ cup all-purpose flour
2 cups plain soy milk
2 cups vegetable broth
1 (12-ounce) bottle pale lager beer
1 tablespoon Dijon mustard
1½ cups vegan Cheddar shreds
⅛ teaspoon ground black pepper
2 teaspoons fresh chopped chives

Soup As a Condiment

Finding ways to be versatile with your recipes will add diversity to you meal prepping. For example, a creamy soup can be served as it was intended in bowls, but it can also be drizzled over baked potatoes or steamed vegetables.

1. Preheat oven to 300°F.

2. Add sourdough cubes, 1 tablespoon olive oil, and ½ teaspoon salt to a large bowl. Toss to coat.

3. Place coated bread cubes on an ungreased baking pan and bake 20 minutes until toasted. Let cool 10 minutes, then transfer to a medium sealed container and refrigerate up to 7 days.

4. Add remaining olive oil in a medium pot over medium heat. Add onions and carrots and cook until vegetables are tender, about 7 minutes. Add garlic and cook another 1 minute.

5. Add flour and stir to combine. Continue cooking over medium heat until flour begins to turn a golden brown, about 5 minutes.

6. Pour milk, mixture from pot, broth, beer, mustard, and vegan Cheddar shreds into a blender. Don't fill blender more than halfway full, and remove lid insert to allow heat to escape. Place a kitchen towel over top and blend at low speed in short bursts until mixture is smooth.

7. Transfer mixture back to pot. Cook and stir over medium heat until cheese is melted, about 10 minutes. Remove from heat and stir in remaining ½ teaspoon of salt and pepper.

8. Let cool 10 minutes, then transfer to a large sealed container and refrigerate up to 7 days. To serve, cook in microwave in 30-second intervals until heated through. Top with sourdough bread croutons and chives.

PER SERVING Calories: 244 | Fat: 13.4 g | Protein: 5.0 g | Sodium: 777 mg | Fiber: 3.4 g | Carbohydrates: 25.6 g | Sugar: 3.7 g

Simple Vegan Minestrone

This Simple Vegan Minestrone is made with carrots, potatoes, beans, and quinoa. It's a great go-to for meal prepping because it's easy to make on the weekend and yields a lot of leftovers for the coming week.

INGREDIENTS | SERVES 10

1 tablespoon olive oil

1 medium yellow onion, peeled and chopped

4 cloves garlic, peeled and chopped

6 cups vegetable broth

2 cups + 4 tablespoons water, divided

3 cups chopped peeled carrots

5 medium russet potatoes, chopped into ½" cubes

1 (28-ounce) can diced tomatoes

1 cup uncooked quinoa, rinsed

2 bay leaves

1 (15-ounce) can corn kernels, including liquid

2 (15-ounce) cans light red kidney beans, rinsed and drained

1 tablespoon dried basil

2 teaspoons dried oregano

½ teaspoon salt

1 teaspoon ground black pepper

1 tablespoon cornstarch

4 tablespoons water

1. Heat olive oil in a Dutch oven over medium heat, about 30 seconds. Add onions and cook until translucent, about 5 minutes. Add garlic and cook another 1 minute. Stir in vegetable broth, 2 cups water, carrots, potatoes, tomatoes, and quinoa. Add bay leaves.

2. Bring pot to a boil, then reduce heat to low and cook about 20 minutes until carrots are tender. Add corn, kidney beans, basil, oregano, salt, and pepper.

3. Combine cornstarch and remaining water in a small bowl. Add to soup. Turn heat to medium-high and bring soup back to a simmer 2 minutes.

4. Discard bay leaf. Remove from heat and let cool about 15 minutes before transferring to a large lidded container (or individual serving containers). Refrigerate up to 7 days or freeze up to 3 months.

5. To serve, place individual servings in bowls. Cook in microwave in 30-second intervals until heated through.

PER SERVING Calories: 321 | Fat: 3.3 g | Protein: 11.6 g | Sodium: 882 mg | Fiber: 10.6 g | Carbohydrates: 63.3 g | Sugar: 8.7 g

Vegan Tomato Bisque

This thick, creamy Vegan Tomato Bisque recipe is seasoned with a hint of basil and made hearty with chickpeas. Serve with croutons for added flavor and texture.

INGREDIENTS | SERVES 10

2 tablespoons olive oil

2 cups chopped peeled yellow onion

4 cups chopped peeled carrots

2 cloves garlic, peeled and minced

1 tablespoon dried basil

3 (28-ounce) cans whole tomatoes, including liquid

3 cups vegetable broth

1 (15-ounce) can chickpeas, rinsed and drained

1 cup Ripple Original Plant-Based Half & Half

1 cup croutons

1. In a large pot, heat olive oil 30 seconds over medium heat. Stir in onions and carrots and cook 10 minutes until slightly tender. Add garlic and cook another 3 minutes.

2. Stir in basil, tomatoes, broth, and chickpeas. Bring to a boil over high heat, then reduce heat to a simmer on medium-low, stirring occasionally, 20 minutes. Remove from heat and let cool 3 minutes.

3. Transfer soup along with half-and-half into a blender. Never fill blender more than halfway full. Remove lid insert to allow heat to escape. Place a kitchen towel over top and blend at low speed until mixture is smooth.

4. Transfer to a large sealable container (or individual serving containers) and refrigerate up to 5 days. To serve, pour soup into bowls and cook in microwave in 30-second intervals until heated through. Top with croutons.

PER SERVING Calories: 199 | Fat: 6.2 g | Protein: 4.1 g | Sodium: 917 mg | Fiber: 6.2 g | Carbohydrates: 31.2 g | Sugar: 17.0 g

Simple Potato Soup

This simple recipe features hearty potatoes as the star ingredient. It's a creamy soup, made with minimal ingredients and lots of flavor.

INGREDIENTS | SERVES 4

2 tablespoons vegan butter

¾ cup finely chopped peeled yellow onion

1 clove garlic, peeled and minced

2 cups ½"-cubed red potatoes

1½ cups vegetable broth

1 bay leaf

½ teaspoon salt

¼ teaspoon ground black pepper

1¾ cups plain soy milk

3 tablespoons McCormick Bac'n Pieces Bacon Flavored Bits

3 tablespoons chopped green onion

1. Place a large saucepan over medium heat. Add vegan butter and onion. Cook 5 minutes until onions are tender. Add garlic and cook another 1 minute. Add potatoes and cook another 3 minutes.

2. Add vegetable broth, bay leaf, salt, and pepper. Bring to a boil over high heat, then reduce to a simmer over medium-low heat. Cover and cook 20 minutes, stirring occasionally, until potatoes are fork tender.

3. Remove bay leaf. Stir in soy milk and use a potato masher to mash some potatoes. Remove from heat.

4. Let soup cool about 10 minutes before transferring to a large sealed container (or individual serving containers). Store in refrigerator up to 5 days.

5. To serve, pour into individual bowls and cook in microwave in 30-second intervals until heated through. Top with vegan bacon bits and chopped green onions.

PER SERVING Calories: 158 | Fat: 4.9 g | Protein: 7.3 g | Sodium: 713 mg | Fiber: 3.2 g | Carbohydrates: 21.2 g | Sugar: 2.8 g

Moroccan Chickpea Turmeric Stew

This is a hearty stew, featuring chickpeas and mouthwatering flavors.
Serve with warm bread to heat up a cold evening.

INGREDIENTS | SERVES 6

1 tablespoon olive oil

½ cup chopped peeled red onion

2 cloves garlic, peeled and minced

2 medium sweet potatoes, cut into 1" cubes

1 (15-ounce) can chickpeas, rinsed and drained

1 (15-ounce) can diced tomatoes, including liquid

1 teaspoon ground ginger

1 teaspoon ground turmeric

½ teaspoon ground cumin

3 cups vegetable broth

3 cups Easy Cauliflower Rice (see Chapter 8 for recipe)

1 tablespoon chopped fresh parsley

1. In a large saucepan over medium-high heat add olive oil and onions. Cook 5 minutes until onions are tender. Reduce heat to medium and add garlic. Cook 1 minute. Add sweet potatoes and stir until coated. Cook 3 minutes.

2. Add chickpeas, tomatoes, ginger, turmeric, cumin, and vegetable broth. Simmer until sweet potatoes are tender, about 20 minutes.

3. Remove from heat and use a potato masher to mash some potatoes and chickpeas to create a thick sauce. Let cool about 10 minutes, then transfer to a large sealed container (or individual serving containers) and refrigerate up to 7 days.

4. To serve, pour cauliflower rice in serving bowls. Spoon scoops of stew over top of each bowl. Cook in microwave in 30-second intervals until heated through. Garnish with fresh parsley.

PER SERVING Calories: 174 | Fat: 3.2 g | Protein: 6.5 g | Sodium: 540 mg | Fiber: 7.8 g | Carbohydrates: 30.0 g | Sugar: 7.9 g

Creamy Pumpkin Soup

A delicious way to get that immunity-boosting beta-carotene in your diet. This Creamy Pumpkin Soup is a supereasy, savory soup perfect for chilly nights!

INGREDIENTS | SERVES 6

1 teaspoon olive oil

½ cup chopped peeled yellow onion

2 cups pumpkin purée

1 (15-ounce) can chickpeas, rinsed and drained

4 cups vegetable broth

2 teaspoons Better Than Bouillon Seasoned Vegetable Base

1 clove garlic, peeled and minced

2 medium unpeeled red potatoes, diced

1 cup Ripple Original Plant-Based Half & Half

1 cup croutons

2 tablespoons chopped green onion

1. Combine olive oil and onion in a large saucepan over medium-high heat. Cook 5 minutes until onions are tender. Stir in pumpkin, chickpeas, vegetable broth, bouillon, garlic, and potatoes and bring to a boil over high heat. Reduce to a simmer over medium-low heat and cook 20 minutes until potatoes are tender. Remove from heat.

2. Transfer soup to a blender along with half-and-half. Never fill blender more than halfway. Remove lid insert to allow heat to escape. Place a kitchen towel over top and blend at low speed until mixture is smooth.

3. Transfer soup to a large sealable container (or individual serving containers) and refrigerate up to 5 days. To serve, pour soup into bowls and cook in microwave in 30-second intervals until heated through. Top with croutons and green onions.

PER SERVING Calories: 220 | Fat: 4.5 g | Protein: 6.4 g | Sodium: 417 mg | Fiber: 7.7 g | Carbohydrates: 37.7 g | Sugar: 7.6 g

Green Goddess Soup

This Green Goddess Soup is wellness in a bowl. Full of wholesome, healthy herbs and plant-based ingredients, this refreshing recipe is perfect for a quick, energizing lunch or dinner during the week.

INGREDIENTS | SERVES 6

1 tablespoon olive oil

2 cups chopped peeled yellow onion

3 cloves garlic, peeled and minced

3 cups broccoli florets

3 cups chopped fresh kale

5 cups vegetable broth

⅔ cup green lentils, rinsed and drained

1 (15-ounce) can chickpeas, rinsed and drained

1 bay leaf

1 teaspoon dried tarragon

1 tablespoon dried chives

1 tablespoon dried parsley

1 (10-ounce) container frozen chopped spinach, thawed

1 cup plain soy milk

1 cup croutons

2 tablespoons chopped green onion

Recycling Aluminum Cans

When you use a recipe that calls for canned goods, recycling those cans can result in energy savings, helping to reduce your carbon footprint. Many cities offer curbside pickup or recycling drop-off points. Recycle those cans!

1. Add olive oil and onion to a large pot over medium-high heat. Cook onions 5 minutes until tender. Reduce heat to medium and add garlic. Cook 1 minute.

2. Add broccoli florets and kale and stir to coat in oil. Add broth, lentils, chickpeas, bay leaf, tarragon, chives, and parsley. Bring to a boil over high heat.

3. Reduce to a simmer over medium-low heat and cook covered 30 minutes until lentils are tender. Remove from heat. Discard bay leaf and stir in spinach and soy milk.

4. Transfer soup to a blender. Never fill blender more than halfway full. Remove lid insert to allow heat to escape. Place a kitchen towel over top and blend at low speed until mixture is smooth.

5. Transfer soup to a large sealable container (or individual serving containers) and refrigerate up to 5 days or freeze up to 3 months. To serve, pour soup into bowls and cook in microwave in 30-second intervals until heated through. Top with croutons and chopped green onions.

PER SERVING Calories: 259 | Fat: 4.2 g | Protein: 14.3 g | Sodium: 651 mg | Fiber: 10.3 g | Carbohydrates: 42.1 g | Sugar: 6.8 g

Mexican "Meatballs" and Black Bean Soup

This is a savory soup made with black beans, vegan meatballs, and the perfect Mexican spices. You'll want to double and freeze this recipe to always have on hand. Serve with brown rice and corn bread for extra goodness.

INGREDIENTS | SERVES 6

2 teaspoons olive oil

1 medium yellow onion, peeled and finely chopped

2 cloves garlic, peeled and minced

1 (12-ounce) package Gardein Meatless Meatballs

2 tablespoons tomato paste

1 tablespoon smoked paprika

2 cups vegetable broth

2 (14.5-ounce) cans diced tomatoes, including liquid

1 (15-ounce) can black beans, rinsed and drained

1 (10-ounce) package frozen corn kernels

½ cup vegan sour cream

2 tablespoons chopped green onion

1. Add olive oil and onion to a large pot over medium-high heat. Cook 5 minutes until onions are tender. Reduce heat to medium and add garlic. Cook 1 minute. Add vegan meatballs and cook 7 minutes, turning frequently, until browned. Transfer meatballs to a medium plate.

2. Add tomato paste, paprika, and vegetable broth to pot with remaining onions and garlic. Stir and cook 1 minute. Add tomatoes, black beans, and corn.

3. Bring to a boil over high heat, then reduce heat to a simmer on medium-low and cook 15 minutes until sauce thickens. Return meatballs to pot and gently stir to coat.

4. Let cool 10 minutes, then transfer soup to a large sealable container (or individual serving containers) and refrigerate up to 5 days or freeze up to 3 months.

5. To serve, pour soup into bowls and cook in microwave in 30-second intervals until heated through. Top with sour cream and green onions.

PER SERVING Calories: 301 | Fat: 9.8 g | Protein: 16.9 g | Sodium: 824 mg | Fiber: 13.3 g | Carbohydrates: 40.6 g | Sugar: 7.3 g

Vegan White Chili

For a fun twist on a classic, try this creamy Vegan White Chili, made with all the spices you'd expect from a delicious traditional chili.

INGREDIENTS | SERVES 6

1 tablespoon olive oil

1 cup chopped peeled yellow onion

1 clove garlic, peeled and minced

1 jalapeño, seeded and minced

1 (10-ounce) package vegan chicken strips, thawed

1 teaspoon chili powder

2 teaspoons ground cumin

2 (4-ounce) cans green chilies

1 cup frozen corn kernels, thawed

2 cups vegetable broth

2 (15-ounce) cans cannellini beans, rinsed and drained

½ cup vegan sour cream

3 tablespoons chopped green onions

1. In a large pot over medium-high heat, add olive oil, onions, garlic, and jalapeños. Stir to coat vegetables, then cook 5 minutes until vegetables are just tender.

2. Add vegan chicken strips, using a spatula to break into smaller, bite-sized pieces. Cook until heated through, about 5 minutes.

3. Stir in chili powder, cumin, green chilies, corn, vegetable broth, and beans. Bring to a boil over high heat, then reduce heat to medium-low and simmer 20 minutes.

4. Use a potato masher to mash some beans to create a thicker chili sauce, then remove pot from heat and let cool about 10 minutes.

5. Transfer to a large lidded container (or individual serving containers) and refrigerate up to 7 days or freeze up to 3 months.

6. To serve, pour into individual bowls and cook in microwave in 30-second intervals until heated through. Top with sour cream and green onions.

PER SERVING Calories: 266 | Fat: 9.4 g | Protein: 16.1 g | Sodium: 921 mg | Fiber: 11.9 g | Carbohydrates: 36.6 g | Sugar: 2.9 g

Vegan Lasagna Soup

This Vegan Lasagna Soup is everything you love about lasagna—veganized and served in a bowl! It's an easy recipe that you can refrigerate or freeze and simply heat up for a quick meal.

INGREDIENTS | SERVES 6

2 teaspoons olive oil

1 cup chopped peeled yellow onion

3 cloves garlic, peeled and minced

1 (24-ounce) jar dairy-free marinara sauce

5 cups vegetable broth

1 (14.5-ounce) can crushed tomatoes, including liquid

2 tablespoons tomato paste

1 teaspoon dried basil

1 teaspoon dried oregano

2 cups vegan crumbles

1 bay leaf

10 uncooked lasagna noodles, broken into 2" pieces

½ cup Ripple Original Plant-Based Half & Half

Vegan Cream

You can find vegan cream in a variety of sources. For example, canned coconut milk adds perfect creaminess to most recipes, as well as a distinct flavor. Most grocery stores also carry nondairy creamers that are intended for coffee, but they can be used in vegan cooking as well. In addition, certain brands create vegan creams for cooking.

1. Place a large pot over medium-high heat. Add olive oil and onion and cook 5 minutes, stirring occasionally, until onions are tender. Reduce heat to medium and add garlic. Stir and cook 1 minute.

2. Add sauce, broth, crushed tomatoes, tomato paste, spices, vegan crumbles, bay leaf, and lasagna noodle pieces. Stir and bring to a boil over high heat, then reduce to medium-low and simmer about 20 minutes, stirring occasionally, until lasagna noodles are tender.

3. Discard bay leaf and stir in half-and-half. Remove from heat and let cool about 10 minutes.

4. Transfer to a large lidded container (or individual serving containers) and refrigerate up to 7 days or freeze up to 3 months. To serve, pour into bowls and cook in microwave in 30-second intervals until heated through.

PER SERVING Calories: 286 | Fat: 6.7 g | Protein: 14.4 g | Sodium: 1,171 mg | Fiber: 8.2 g | Carbohydrates: 44.2 g | Sugar: 11.4 g

One Pot Vegan Beef and Beer Chili

This hearty One Pot Vegan Beef and Beer Chili is made with beans. Rich in chili flavors, this recipe is easy to make and then reheat on cold nights.

INGREDIENTS | SERVES 12

1 tablespoon olive oil

2 cups chopped peeled yellow onion

1 cup chopped seeded red bell pepper

½ cup chopped seeded yellow bell pepper

7 tablespoons chili powder

1 teaspoon ground cumin

1 teaspoon dried oregano

1 teaspoon ground coriander

¼ teaspoon ground black pepper

1 (28-ounce) can crushed tomatoes, including liquid

1 (28-ounce) can petite diced tomatoes, including liquid

2 (15-ounce) cans dark red kidney beans, rinsed and drained

1 (12-ounce) bottle dark ale

2 cups vegan crumbles

1 cup vegan sour cream

½ cup pickled jalapeño peppers

1. In a large pot on medium-high heat, cook olive oil, onions, and bell peppers, stirring occasionally, about 5 minutes until vegetables are tender. Stir in chili powder, cumin, oregano, coriander, black pepper, tomatoes, beans, ale, and vegan crumbles.

2. Bring to a boil over high heat. Reduce heat to medium-low and simmer 15 minutes, stirring occasionally.

3. Remove from heat and let cool about 15 minutes. Transfer to a large sealable container (or individual serving containers) and refrigerate up to 7 days or freeze up to 2 months.

4. To serve, pour into bowls and cook in microwave in 30-second intervals until heated through. Top with sour cream and pickled jalapeño peppers.

PER SERVING Calories: 208 | Fat: 6.8 g | Protein: 10.5 g | Sodium: 711 mg | Fiber: 10.5 g | Carbohydrates: 30.3 g | Sugar: 9.4 g

CHAPTER 11

Grilled and Stir-Fried

Grilled Reuben "Brats" with Special Sauce

Warm-weather grilling meets cool-weather favorites with these vegan Grilled Reuben "Brats" with Special Sauce. Made in less than 30 minutes, this dish will be ready for you to enjoy in no time!

INGREDIENTS | SERVES 4

1 (12-ounce) bottle pale lager beer

4 vegan sausages

4 dairy-free hot dog buns

¼ cup peeled thin-sliced red onion

½ cup sauerkraut, drained

½ cup shredded vegan mozzarella

1 batch Vegan Special Sauce (see Chapter 7 for recipe)

1. Bring beer to a boil in a large saucepan over high heat. Add vegan sausages and reduce heat to medium-low. Simmer 15 minutes.

2. Heat gas or charcoal grill. When sausages are ready, place on heated grill and cook 10 minutes, turning to brown all sides.

3. When sausages are browned, place one sausage in each bun. Top with onion slices, sauerkraut and vegan cheese. Place on grill 3 minutes until cheese begins to melt. Remove from heat and allow to cool 5 minutes before transferring to a large sealed container. Refrigerate up to 5 days.

4. To serve, place in a toaster oven set to 350F and cook until heated through, about 5 minutes. Drizzle with Vegan Special Sauce.

PER SERVING Calories: 429 | Fat: 19.0 g | Protein: 19.1 g | Sodium: 1,288 mg | Fiber: 4.2 g | Carbohydrates: 37.0 g | Sugar: 9.1 g

Grilled Lemon Cauliflower Steaks

These Grilled Lemon Cauliflower Steaks transform the common cauliflower into a "meaty," caramelized meal. The herbed lemon dressing adds flavor and zest to this delicious recipe that's perfect for summer (but can be served all year long).

INGREDIENTS | SERVES 2

3 tablespoons olive oil, divided

Zest and juice from 1 large lemon

¼ cup chopped green onion

1 teaspoon salt

⅛ teaspoon ground black pepper

1 clove garlic, peeled and minced

1 large head cauliflower, trimmed and cut into 2½"-thick "steaks"

1. Combine 1 tablespoon olive oil, lemon zest, lemon juice, green onions, salt, pepper, and garlic in a small bowl.

2. Lay cauliflower steaks in a large, ungreased pan and drizzle with 1 tablespoon olive oil. Use a brush to coat steaks on both sides.

3. Heat grill to medium-high. Use remaining olive oil to oil grill grates. Place cauliflower steaks on grill. Cook until tender and grill lines form, about 10 minutes. Flip and repeat cooking on other side.

4. Drizzle lemon mixture over cauliflower steaks. Let cool 10 minutes, then store in a large sealed container in refrigerator up to 5 days. To serve, cook steaks in microwave in 30-second intervals until heated through.

PER SERVING Calories: 229 | Fat: 14.0 g | Protein: 8.3 g | Sodium: 125 mg | Fiber: 8.8 g | Carbohydrates: 23.0 g | Sugar: 8.6 g

Kung Pao Cauliflower

This stir-fried cauliflower recipe is seasoned with a sweet and spicy kung pao sauce. It is a classic Chinese take-out dish, transformed into healthier (yet still delicious) fare thanks to the cauliflower.

INGREDIENTS | SERVES 4

½ cup all-purpose flour
1 teaspoon baking soda
¾ cup unsweetened almond milk
1 head cauliflower, cut into florets
½ cup crumbled Kellogg's Corn Flakes
3 tablespoons tamari
3 tablespoons agave nectar
1 tablespoon sesame oil
1 teaspoon rice vinegar
1 teaspoon garlic powder
1 teaspoon ground ginger
1 tablespoon cornstarch
4 cups cooked brown rice
1 tablespoon finely chopped fresh cilantro
2 tablespoons sesame seeds

1. Preheat oven to 400°F. Line a baking sheet with parchment paper.

2. Combine flour, baking soda, and almond milk in a large bowl. Add cauliflower florets. Stir until florets are coated. Sprinkle with Corn Flakes crumbs. Place coated cauliflower florets on prepared baking sheet, allowing space between each piece.

3. Place in oven and bake 15 minutes. Remove from oven and transfer to a large bowl. Set aside.

4. In a small microwave-safe bowl combine tamari, agave nectar, sesame oil, rice vinegar, garlic powder, ginger, and cornstarch. Heat in microwave 30 seconds. Remove and stir. Repeat until sauce begins to bubble.

5. Pour sauce over cauliflower. Stir gently to coat cauliflower. Pour cauliflower back onto baking sheet and bake 15 minutes.

6. Remove from oven and set aside to cool 10 minutes. Store covered in refrigerator up to 5 days.

7. To serve, heat in microwave in 30-second intervals until heated through. Next heat rice in 30-second intervals until heated through. Serve cauliflower over rice and topped with cilantro and sesame seeds.

PER SERVING Calories: 404 | Fat: 7.5 g | Protein: 10.7 g | Sodium: 1,132 mg | Fiber: 7.6 g | Carbohydrates: 74.3 g | Sugar: 12.5 g

Vegan Sausage and Red Bell Pepper Skewers

It's time to get out of the kitchen and enjoy the great outdoors! You'll love the perfect vegan recipe for warm-weather grilling: "sausage" and pepper skewers!

INGREDIENTS | SERVES 10

1 (14-ounce) package vegan Italian sausages, cut into 1" pieces

1 medium red bell pepper, seeded and cut into 1" pieces

1 medium yellow bell pepper, seeded and cut into 1" pieces

1 medium orange bell pepper, seeded and cut into 1" pieces

1 medium red onion, peeled and cut into 1" pieces

20 cherry tomatoes

10 small white mushrooms

2 tablespoons olive oil

1 teaspoon soy sauce

1 teaspoon liquid smoke

Tricks for Vegan Grilling

Most vegan dishes that you'll be grilling don't require high temperatures: you're basically cooking them on the grill to get that smoky flavor and a few grill marks. You can use foil, or spray the grill with vegetable spray before placing food directly on top. In addition, consider purchasing a grill basket for vegetables.

1. Soak ten wooden skewers in water 20 minutes.

2. Thread vegan sausage slices and assorted vegetables onto prepared wooden skewers, alternating between sausage and different vegetables.

3. In a small bowl stir together olive oil, soy sauce, and liquid smoke. Brush each prepared skewer with oil mixture.

4. Heat your grill to medium heat.

5. Place skewers on heated grill. Cook until vegetables are tender, about 10 minutes, turning occasionally throughout cook time.

6. Transfer skewers to a serving platter. Brush with leftover olive oil mixture. Transfer to a large sealed container and refrigerate up to 5 days. To serve, heat skewers in microwave in 30-second intervals until heated through.

PER SERVING Calories: 160 | Fat: 8.3 g | Protein: 13.2 g | Sodium: 280 mg | Fiber: 1.8 g | Carbohydrates: 8.5 g | Sugar: 3.8 g

Tofu Kebabs

Imagine your favorite vegetables, like bell peppers, onions, and mushrooms, skewered and cooked on the grill and marinated with Italian dressing. Build your own delicious vegan kebabs!

INGREDIENTS | SERVES 12

1 cup Italian dressing

1 (15-ounce) package extra-firm tofu, pressed and cut into 1" cubes

1 medium red bell pepper, seeded and cut into 1" pieces

1 medium yellow bell pepper, seeded and cut into 1" pieces

1 medium orange bell pepper, seeded and cut into 1" pieces

1 medium red onion, peeled and cut into 1" pieces

12 cherry tomatoes

12 small white mushrooms

1. Soak twelve wooden skewers in water 20 minutes. Pour Italian dressing into a 9" × 9" baking dish.

2. Place tofu in dish with Italian dressing and allow to marinate 30 minutes.

3. Heat your grill to medium heat.

4. Thread cubed tofu and assorted vegetables onto prepared skewers. Alternate tofu with vegetables as you thread.

5. Place skewers on heated grill. Cook, turning occasionally, until vegetables are tender, about 10 minutes.

6. Let cool 10 minutes, then transfer skewers to a large sealed container and refrigerate up to 5 days. To serve, heat skewers in microwave in 30-second intervals until heated through.

PER SERVING Calories: 76 | Fat: 3.3 g | Protein: 6.8 g | Sodium: 27 mg | Fiber: 1.9 g | Carbohydrates: 6.0 g | Sugar: 2.2 g

Pineapple Fried Rice

This veganized fried rice favorite uses diced pineapple to add a hint of sweetness and tropical flavor to every bite. It also includes tofu for added protein. Fried rice is a perfect go-to meal when you're in a hurry but still want to tickle your taste buds with an ultra-tasty, satisfying meal.

INGREDIENTS | SERVES 8

1 tablespoon olive oil

1 cup chopped peeled white onion

1 cup extra-firm tofu

2 packets Tasty Bite Garlic Brown Rice

2 cups diced fresh pineapple

3 tablespoons soy sauce

½ teaspoon ground ginger

2 tablespoons sesame oil

1 cup frozen peas and carrots mixture, thawed

1. Place a large skillet over medium heat. Pour in olive oil, then add onions and cook until tender, about 5 minutes.

2. Add tofu to skillet and use a spatula to mash tofu, stirring to coat with oil. Cook until tofu begins to brown, about 4 minutes.

3. Add rice and pineapple. Stir to combine.

4. In a small bowl combine soy sauce, ginger, and sesame oil. Pour over rice mixture and stir to incorporate.

5. Add frozen peas and carrots, stir, and cook another 1 minute until vegetables have heated through.

6. Remove from heat and let cool about 10 minutes, then transfer to a large sealed container (or individual serving containers) and refrigerate up to 5 days.

7. To serve, cook in microwave in 30-second intervals until heated through.

PER SERVING Calories: 218 | Fat: 8.7 g | Protein: 6.6 g | Sodium: 563 mg | Fiber: 2.9 g | Carbohydrates: 29.1 g | Sugar: 5.6 g

Vegan Tex-Mex Hot Dogs

*Simple, delicious vegan hot dogs are grilled and prepared with five different toppings.
Create your own vegan hot dog bar—this is vegan comfort food at its finest!*

INGREDIENTS | SERVES 8

1 package vegan hot dogs
(approximately 8)

1 package dairy-free hot dog buns
(approximately 8)

3 green onions, chopped

1 (15-ounce) can seasoned black beans,
drained

1 cup chopped cherry tomatoes

1 cup Fresh Corn Salsa (see Chapter 8
for recipe)

2 cups vegan Cheddar cheese shreds

1. Turn gas or charcoal grill on medium heat. Spray grill with vegetable cooking spray.

2. Use a fork or tongs to place vegan hot dogs and buns on heated grill and cook 10 minutes, turning hot dogs to brown all sides. Let cool 10 minutes.

3. Refrigerate hot dogs, buns, green onions, black beans, tomatoes, salsa, and cheese in separate containers up to 5 days.

4. To serve, place hot dog in bun and top with cheese. Heat in microwave about 30 seconds until cheese begins to melt. Top with green onions, black beans, tomatoes, and salsa.

PER SERVING Calories: 344 | Fat: 9.0 g | Protein: 15.5 g | Sodium: 1,131 mg | Fiber: 7.8 g | Carbohydrates: 51.4 g | Sugar: 11.2 g

Easy Garlic Noodles

*This is an easy Chinese noodle dish, made with garlic and other great
flavors, as well as savory tofu. It's a perfect meal.*

INGREDIENTS | SERVES 6

2 tablespoons sesame oil

6 cloves garlic, peeled and minced

3 tablespoons low-sodium soy sauce

2 tablespoons agave nectar

¼ teaspoon dried basil

½ teaspoon ground ginger

1 batch Air-Fried Tofu (see Chapter 14
for recipe)

1 (12-ounce) package soba noodles,
cooked according to package
instructions

1. In a large skillet over medium heat add oil and minced garlic. Cook 2 minutes until garlic is tender. Add soy sauce, agave nectar, basil, and ginger. Stir in tofu until coated. Add noodles and stir to coat.

2. Let cool 10 minutes, then transfer to a large sealed container (or individual serving containers) and refrigerate up to 5 days. To serve, heat in a microwave in 30-second intervals until heated through.

PER SERVING Calories: 359 | Fat: 10.0 g | Protein: 16.2 g | Sodium: 825 mg | Fiber: 0.5 g | Carbohydrates: 55.6 g | Sugar: 4.8 g

Vegan Grilled Chorizo Burgers

If you're looking for a grill-worthy homemade veggie burger, look no further than these Vegan Grilled Chorizo Burgers.

INGREDIENTS | SERVES 8

10 ounces vegan chorizo

1 (14-ounce) package vegan sausage

1 teaspoon liquid smoke

½ cup bread crumbs

3 tablespoons dried minced onion

1 tablespoon dried parsley

3 cloves garlic, peeled and roughly minced

½ teaspoon ground cumin

½ teaspoon paprika

½ teaspoon dried thyme

½ teaspoon salt

8 dairy-free hamburger buns

What Is Chorizo?

Traditional chorizo is a spicy concoction made from pork. Vegan versions are now widely available and are usually made from soy or other plant-based ingredients. Look in your health food store or in the health food section of your grocery store for this flavorful addition to your recipes!

1. Add all ingredients except buns to a large bowl and combine. Use a spatula to break larger pieces down.

2. Make mixture into 8 patties and place them on a large plate or in a large lidded container. Cover and refrigerate until ready to grill.

3. Heat grill to medium heat. Spray with vegetable cooking spray.

4. Cook burgers about 5 minutes and then flip and repeat cooking on other side. Set aside to cool about 5 minutes.

5. Transfer burgers to a large lidded container and refrigerate up to 7 days or freeze up to 2 months. To serve, cook in microwave in 30-second intervals until heated through. Serve on buns.

PER SERVING Calories: 343 | Fat: 11.1 g | Protein: 21.1 g | Sodium: 1,111 mg | Fiber: 4.8 g | Carbohydrates: 36.5 g | Sugar: 5.5 g

Zesty Sesame Zoodles

These Zesty Sesame Zoodles are drizzled in a creamy sesame sauce. Forget calorie-loaded flour noodles and opt for these zucchini zoodles instead!

INGREDIENTS | SERVES 2

2 medium zucchini, ends removed and spiralized (about 3 cups zoodles)

1 tablespoon sesame oil

3 tablespoons gluten-free tamari

2 tablespoons rice vinegar

2 tablespoons tahini

1 tablespoon agave nectar

1 tablespoon finely grated fresh ginger

1 teaspoon dried minced garlic

1 teaspoon sriracha

1 green onion, thinly sliced

1 tablespoon sesame seeds

What Exactly Are Zoodles?

Zoodles are zucchini noodles that are made using a spiralizer. You can use a spiralizer to make noodles out of many different vegetables, including carrots and sweet potatoes. You can eat vegetable noodles raw, but cooking them for even a few minutes results in a flavor and texture more consistent with flour noodles. Vegetable noodles are a low-calorie, gluten-free addition to your everyday meals.

1. Bring a large pot filled halfway with water to boil over high heat. Add zucchini noodles and cook until barely tender, about 5 minutes. Drain and rinse with cold water. Set aside.

2. In a medium bowl combine sesame oil, tamari, rice vinegar, tahini, agave nectar, ginger, garlic, and sriracha. Pour over cooked zoodles and toss.

3. Place zoodles in a large lidded container (or individual serving containers) and refrigerate up to 3 days. To serve, cook in microwave in 30-second intervals until heated through, or serve cold, topped with green onions and sesame seeds.

PER SERVING Calories: 225 | Fat: 13.8 g | Protein: 8.0 g | Sodium: 1,585 mg | Fiber: 3.8 g | Carbohydrates: 18.7 g | Sugar: 10.8 g

10-Minute Pad Thai Zoodles

These delicious vegan 10-Minute Pad Thai Zoodles are a healthy, low-calorie, and fast meal. And they are incredibly tasty!

INGREDIENTS | SERVES 2

¼ cup water

1 tablespoon almond butter

1 tablespoon tamari

1 teaspoon mild yellow miso paste

1 teaspoon agave nectar

1 teaspoon lime juice

1 teaspoon sriracha

1 medium green onion, chopped

1 clove garlic, peeled and minced

¼ medium red bell pepper, seeded and cut into slivers

1 medium zucchini, ends removed and spiralized

1 medium carrot, spiralized

1 tablespoon chopped peanuts

1. Combine water, almond butter, tamari, miso paste, agave nectar, lime juice, and sriracha in a medium bowl.

2. Place a large skillet over medium heat. Add onions, garlic, and bell pepper slices, and cook about 30 seconds. Add sauce mixture and continue cooking about 5 minutes, until peppers are tender.

3. Add zucchini and carrot noodles to pan and cook until noodles are tender, about 5 minutes.

4. Let cool 10 minutes, then place in a large lidded container (or individual serving containers) and refrigerate up to 3 days. To serve, drain excess water from container and cook in microwave in 30-second intervals until heated through, or serve cold. Top with peanuts.

PER SERVING Calories: 148 | Fat: 6.6 g | Protein: 5.8 g | Sodium: 724 mg | Fiber: 4.7 g | Carbohydrates: 18.2 g | Sugar: 10.1 g

Vegan Grilled Corn on the Cob with Herbed Mayonnaise

Corn on the cob has never tasted better than when it's grilled over an open flame. This recipe makes it easy to make your own delicious corn on the cob slathered in savory herbed mayonnaise sauce!

INGREDIENTS | SERVES 4

4 cups cold water

4 ears corn, in husk

½ cup Vegan Mayonnaise (see Chapter 7 for recipe)

½ teaspoon salt

½ teaspoon paprika

½ teaspoon dried thyme

½ teaspoon dried rosemary

1 teaspoon dried basil

1. Pour water into a large bowl. Add corn and cover with a second bowl to keep corn underwater. Allow to sit in water 25 minutes.

2. Heat your grill to medium heat.

3. Place unpeeled corn on grill and cook 20 minutes, using tongs to turn occasionally. Remove grilled corn from heat.

4. Let cool 3 minutes until cool enough to handle, then peel husks and remove silks. Cut corncobs in half.

5. In a small bowl combine Vegan Mayonnaise with salt and herbs. Brush mayonnaise sauce over corn, reserving some for serving.

6. Place corn in a large sealed container and refrigerate up to 3 days. Cover leftover mayonnaise sauce and refrigerate up to 5 days. To serve, heat corn in microwave in 30-second intervals until heated through. Serve with leftover mayonnaise sauce.

PER SERVING Calories: 142 | Fat: 5.4 g | Protein: 5.9 g | Sodium: 583 mg | Fiber: 2.7 g | Carbohydrates: 20.9 g | Sugar: 7.1 g

Cauliflower Fried Rice

If you love fried rice, but not the calories, this cauliflower fried rice will be your new go-to. It's infused with flavorful sesame oil and tossed with the best vegetables.

INGREDIENTS | SERVES 6

2 tablespoons sesame oil

1 small yellow onion, peeled and finely chopped

1 (12-ounce) package firm tofu, pressed

1 batch Easy Cauliflower Rice (see Chapter 8 for recipe)

3 cups frozen stir-fry vegetables, thawed

1 cup frozen peas

3 tablespoons soy sauce

1 tablespoon agave nectar

1 teaspoon ground ginger

1 teaspoon garlic powder

2 tablespoons chopped green onion

2 tablespoons sesame seeds

Cauliflower for Your Health

Cauliflower is another vegetable in the very important cruciferous family. This means it is packed with healthy nutrients, including vitamin C, fiber, omega-3s, and folate. You can use cauliflower rice in place of regular rice in most recipes!

1. Heat sesame oil 30 seconds in a large skillet over medium heat. Add onions and cook until onions are tender, about 5 minutes.

2. Add tofu to skillet with cooked onions. Use a spatula to break tofu into bite-sized pieces. Stir to coat tofu in oil and cook about 5 minutes. Add cauliflower rice, stir-fry vegetables, and peas. Stir and cook until vegetables are heated through, about 5 minutes.

3. In a small bowl combine soy sauce, agave nectar, ginger, and garlic powder. Pour over tofu mixture. Stir to coat vegetables and tofu.

4. Let cool 10 minutes, then transfer mixture to a large sealed container (or individual serving containers) and refrigerate up to 4 days. To serve, heat rice in microwave in 30-second intervals until heated through. Top with green onions and sesame seeds.

PER SERVING Calories: 174 | Fat: 8.3 g | Protein: 10.4 g | Sodium: 508 mg | Fiber: 5.3 g | Carbohydrates: 16.6 g | Sugar: 5.7 g

Sticky Sweet Tofu and Rice

This tofu is served over rice and tastes better than takeout! Make this dish on the weekends and serve throughout the week along with some steamed broccoli! For the finishing touch, sprinkle each serving with chopped green onion.

INGREDIENTS | SERVES 4

1 (15-ounce) package extra-firm tofu, pressed and cut into ½" cubes

2 tablespoons cornstarch

¼ cup agave nectar

¼ cup soy sauce

1 teaspoon ground ginger

1 teaspoon garlic powder

1 tablespoon lime juice

1 tablespoon olive oil

4 cups cooked brown rice

1 tablespoon sesame seeds

1. Place tofu in a large bowl. Toss with cornstarch until coated.

2. In a small bowl add agave nectar, soy sauce, ginger, garlic powder, and lime juice. Stir to combine.

3. Pour olive oil in a large skillet over medium-high heat. Add coated tofu cubes. Cook 5 minutes on each side.

4. Reduce heat to medium and pour in soy sauce mixture, making sure each piece is coated. Cook until sauce thickens, about 3 minutes.

5. Place tofu in a large sealed container with any extra sauce and refrigerate up to 5 days. To serve, heat tofu and brown rice together in microwave in 30-second intervals until heated through. Top with sesame seeds.

PER SERVING Calories: 427 | Fat: 11.7 g | Protein: 16.9 g | Sodium: 886 mg | Fiber: 4.5 g | Carbohydrates: 64.6 g | Sugar: 10.1 g

Vegan Chimichurri Steak Skewers

Grilled vegan steak skewers are basted with a chimichurri sauce and threaded with bell peppers, red onions, cherry tomatoes, and mushrooms in this mouthwatering recipe.

INGREDIENTS | SERVES 10

¼ cup finely chopped fresh cilantro leaves

½ cup finely chopped fresh flat-leaf parsley leaves

½ teaspoon garlic powder

1 teaspoon dried oregano

1 tablespoon white wine vinegar

1 tablespoon lime juice

⅓ cup + 2 tablespoons olive oil, divided

2 (10-ounce) packages Gardein Beefless Tips

3 medium red bell peppers, seeded and cut into 1½" pieces

1 medium red onion, peeled and cut into 10 wedges

20 cherry tomatoes

20 small white mushrooms

What Is Chimichurri?

Chimichurri is a South American sauce. It's typically made with parsley, oregano, and garlic. You can freeze chimichurri sauce up to 1 month to savor the bright flavors in different dishes.

1. Soak ten wooden skewers in water 20 minutes.

2. Place cilantro and parsley in a small lidded bowl. Add garlic powder, oregano, vinegar, lime juice, and ⅓ cup olive oil. Stir to combine. Set aside.

3. Add beefless tips, peppers, onions, tomatoes, and mushrooms to a separate medium bowl. Drizzle with 2 tablespoons chimichurri sauce and 1 tablespoon olive oil. Toss to coat.

4. Heat your grill to medium-high. Brush grates with remaining oil.

5. Thread soaked skewers evenly with vegan beef pieces and vegetables. Brush a little chimichurri sauce over each skewer.

6. Place skewers on grill. Cook 10 minutes, turning occasionally, until vegetables are tender and grill marks appear.

7. Let cool 10 minutes, then transfer skewers and chimichurri sauce to separate sealed containers. Refrigerate skewers up to 5 days and sauce up to 3 days. To serve, heat skewers in microwave in 30-second intervals until heated through. Drizzle with chimichurri sauce.

PER SERVING Calories: 188 | Fat: 12.0 g | Protein: 11.0 g | Sodium: 322 mg | Fiber: 3.2 g | Carbohydrates: 10.2 g | Sugar: 3.8 g

Vegan Fried Rice

This vegan twist on fried rice is served with lots of vegetables and uses tofu instead of eggs.

INGREDIENTS | SERVES 8

1 tablespoon olive oil
1 cup chopped peeled white onion
1 cup firm tofu
3 cups cooked brown rice
3 tablespoons soy sauce
½ teaspoon ground ginger
1 tablespoon sesame oil
2 cups frozen Asian vegetables, thawed
1 cup frozen peas, thawed
2 tablespoons chopped green onion
2 tablespoons sesame seeds

Sesame Seeds for Your Health

Compared to chia and flaxseed, sesame seeds have taken a back seat over the years. However, that doesn't mean they should be ignored! They are a powerful source of important nutrients like protein, iron, and fiber—just to name a few. Sprinkle sesame seeds over fried rice, salads, or stir it into sauces and dressings. You can also find it in a paste form.

1. Preheat a large skillet over medium heat. Pour olive oil in skillet. Add onions and cook until tender, about 5 minutes.

2. Add tofu to skillet and use a spatula to mash tofu, stirring to coat with oil. Cook until tofu begins to brown, about 4 minutes. Add rice and stir to combine.

3. In a small bowl combine soy sauce, ginger, and sesame oil. Pour over rice mixture and stir to incorporate.

4. Add frozen vegetables and cook until vegetables are heated through, about 5 minutes.

5. Let cool 10 minutes, then store rice in a large sealed container (or individual serving containers) in refrigerator up to 7 days. To serve, heat servings in microwave in 30-second intervals until heated through. Top with green onions and sesame seeds.

PER SERVING Calories: 175 | Fat: 6.2 g | Protein: 6.5 g | Sodium: 354 mg | Fiber: 3.4 g | Carbohydrates: 23.8 g | Sugar: 1.6 g

CHAPTER 12

One Pot and Slow Cooker Meals

One Pot Vegan Mac and Cheese

The ultimate comfort food meets convenience in this One Pot Vegan Mac and Cheese recipe. This delicious and creamy mac and cheese is made with just a handful of ingredients.

INGREDIENTS | SERVES 4

1 (12-ounce) box elbow pasta

1¼ cups water

2 cups plain cashew milk

1 tablespoon vegan butter

1 teaspoon garlic powder

2 cups vegan shredded Cheddar cheese, divided

½ teaspoon salt

¼ teaspoon ground black pepper

1. Place macaroni, water, and cashew milk in a medium saucepan over medium heat. Bring to a boil, stirring frequently to keep pasta from clumping. Reduce to a simmer over medium-low heat and cook 10 minutes until noodles are tender and a thick consistency is achieved. Add vegan butter and garlic powder and stir.

2. Add ½ vegan cheese and stir until melted. Add remaining cheese, stirring until melted. Season with salt and pepper.

3. Let cool 10 minutes, then transfer to a large sealable container (or individual serving containers) and refrigerate up to 7 days. To serve, cook in microwave in 30-second intervals until heated through.

PER SERVING Calories: 502 | Fat: 17.0 g | Protein: 11.4 g | Sodium: 936 mg | Fiber: 4.8 g | Carbohydrates: 76.7 g | Sugar: 2.3 g

Slow Cooker Vegan Bulgogi Jackfruit

Bulgogi jackfruit is a delicious vegan alternative to pulled pork. The sweet and spicy bulgogi sauce is made with pears, ginger, and spices.

INGREDIENTS | SERVES 12

2 (20-ounce) cans young green jackfruit in brine, rinsed and drained

½ cup tamari

¼ cup soy sauce

½ cup agave nectar

1 cup white wine

2 tablespoons peeled minced fresh ginger

8 cloves garlic, peeled and chopped

1 medium yellow onion, peeled and sliced

1 medium green pear, cored and chopped

4 tablespoons sesame oil

½ cup water

1. Place jackfruit in a slow cooker. Add remaining ingredients and stir to combine. Cover and cook on low 6 hours.

2. Remove cover, turn heat to high, and cook another 1 hour to help absorb any remaining liquid.

3. Use a firm spatula to break apart jackfruit into pieces. Let cool 10 minutes, then transfer to a large sealable container (or individual serving containers) and refrigerate up to 7 days or freeze up to 2 months.

4. To serve, cook in microwave in 30-second intervals until heated through.

PER SERVING Calories: 119 | Fat: 4.4 g | Protein: 2.7 g | Sodium: 1,135 mg | Fiber: 2.8 g | Carbohydrates: 16.6 g | Sugar: 8.4 g

One Pot Chickpea Coconut Curry

This delicious One Pot Chickpea Coconut Curry is made with basmati rice and a splash of lime. It's so easy—and so delicious! Serve with steamed broccoli and baked naan bread.

INGREDIENTS | SERVES 6

1 (15-ounce) can unsweetened coconut milk

Water to fill coconut milk can 3 times

2 cups uncooked basmati rice

4 cloves garlic, peeled and minced

1 cup finely chopped peeled carrots

1 medium red potato, chopped into small cubes

1 (15-ounce) can chickpeas, drained and rinsed

3 tablespoons curry seasoning

1 tablespoon soy sauce

Juice of 1 lime

2 tablespoons finely chopped fresh cilantro

1 cup frozen corn kernels

1 cup frozen peas

1. Combine coconut milk, water, rice, garlic, carrots, potatoes, and chickpeas in a large pot over medium-high heat. Bring pot to a boil, then reduce heat to medium and add curry and soy sauce. Cook about 20 minutes. Basmati rice should be tender and sauce should be very thick.

2. Add lime juice, cilantro, corn, and peas and stir until combined.

3. Let cool 10 minutes, then transfer to a large sealable container (or individual serving containers) and refrigerate up to 7 days or freeze up to 2 months.

4. To serve, dish out into small bowls and cook in microwave in 30-second intervals until heated through.

PER SERVING Calories: 508 | Fat: 16.0 g | Protein: 12.2 g | Sodium: 289 mg | Fiber: 8.0 g | Carbohydrates: 79.8 g | Sugar: 3.9 g

What Is One Pot Cooking?

Anytime you can minimize ingredients or instruments used in the kitchen, you'll make meal prepping more achievable. One pot meals simplify the steps involved in making a dish, including the cleanup. Most one pot recipes have been calibrated to combine starches, proteins, and vegetables together.

One Pot Vegan Chili Mac and Cheese

This One Pot Vegan Chili Mac and Cheese combines two favorite comfort foods in a delicious, easy meal that everyone will love!

INGREDIENTS | SERVES 6

1 tablespoon olive oil

1 medium yellow onion, peeled and diced

2 cloves garlic, peeled and minced

1 (13.7-ounce) package vegan crumbles

4 cups vegetable broth

1 (14.5-ounce) can diced tomatoes, including liquid

2 (15-ounce) cans dark red kidney beans, rinsed and drained

1 tablespoon chili powder

1 teaspoon ground cumin

1 teaspoon paprika

1¾ cups elbow pasta

2 tablespoons nutritional yeast flakes

1 cup vegan Cheddar shreds

½ teaspoon salt

¼ teaspoon ground black pepper

1. In a large pot, add olive oil and onions over medium-high heat. Cook 5 minutes until onions are tender. Add remaining ingredients, stirring to combine. Bring to a boil, then reduce heat to medium-low and simmer, covered, 15 minutes until pasta is tender. Remove from heat and let cool about 10 minutes.

2. Transfer to a large sealable container (or individual serving containers) and refrigerate up to 7 days or freeze up to 2 months. To serve, pour into bowls and cook in microwave in 30-second intervals until heated through.

PER SERVING Calories: 446 | Fat: 10.2 g | Protein: 26.9 g | Sodium: 1,422 mg | Fiber: 14.1 g | Carbohydrates: 63.1 g | Sugar: 8.4 g

One Pot Taco Quinoa Soup

This taco quinoa soup is so hearty and flavorful and made with favorite taco seasonings. Throw everything together in one pot to make cleanup a breeze.

INGREDIENTS | SERVES 10

1 medium yellow onion, peeled and chopped

1 tablespoon olive oil

2 cloves garlic, peeled and minced

2 (15-ounce) cans pinto beans, rinsed and drained

2 (15-ounce) cans light red kidney beans, rinsed and drained

2 (15-ounce) cans stewed tomatoes, including liquid

1 (15-ounce) can corn kernels, drained

2 cups vegetable broth

1 (10-ounce) can green chili enchilada sauce

1 (4.5-ounce) can green chilies, chopped

1 cup uncooked red quinoa

1 cup Gardein Beefless Ground

2 tablespoons taco seasoning

3 tablespoons nutritional yeast flakes

1 cup vegan sour cream

2 tablespoons chopped fresh cilantro

1. Place onions and olive oil in a large pot. Stir to combine. Cook 5 minutes over medium heat until onions are tender. Add garlic, beans, tomatoes, corn, vegetable broth, enchilada sauce, green chilies, and red quinoa. Bring pot to a simmer and cook about 20 minutes until quinoa is tender.

2. Add vegan crumbles, taco seasoning, and nutritional yeast flakes and stir to combine. Remove from heat to cool about 10 minutes.

3. Transfer to a large lidded container (or individual serving containers) and refrigerate up to 7 days or freeze up to 2 months.

4. Combine vegan sour cream with cilantro in a small lidded bowl. Cover and refrigerate up to 5 days.

5. To serve, pour into bowls and cook in microwave in 30-second intervals until heated through. Top with cilantro mixture.

PER SERVING Calories: 385 | Fat: 9.3 g | Protein: 16.5 g | Sodium: 1,053 mg | Fiber: 10.6 g | Carbohydrates: 61.1 g | Sugar: 8.1 g

Slow Cooker Sweet Potato Chili

This vegan slow cooker chili is also gluten-free. You'll love the extra nutrition provided from the sweet potatoes and black beans.

INGREDIENTS | SERVES 10

1 medium yellow onion, peeled and chopped

2 cloves garlic, peeled and minced

1 tablespoon olive oil

2 medium sweet potatoes, chopped

2 (15-ounce) cans black beans, rinsed and drained

2 (15-ounce) cans diced tomatoes, including liquid

1 (8-ounce) can tomato sauce

1 cup vegetable broth

3 tablespoons chili seasoning

1 cup vegan crumbles

2 tablespoons nutritional yeast flakes

1. Place onions and minced garlic in a slow cooker and drizzle with olive oil. Stir to combine. Set temperature to high and cook about 10 minutes.

2. Turn heat to low and add sweet potatoes, beans, tomatoes, tomato sauce, vegetable broth, and chili seasoning. Cook 8 hours.

3. About 30 minutes before serving, add vegan crumbles and nutritional yeast flakes. Stir to combine. Turn heat off and let cool about 10 minutes.

4. Transfer to a large sealable container (or individual serving containers) and refrigerate up to 7 days or freeze up to 2 months.

5. To serve pour into bowls and cook in microwave in 30-second intervals until heated through.

PER SERVING Calories: 163 | Fat: 2.0 g | Protein: 9.0 g | Sodium: 624 mg | Fiber: 9.4 g | Carbohydrates: 27.7 g | Sugar: 5.0 g

Vegan Two Bean Enchilada Casserole

This Vegan Two Bean Enchilada Casserole is an inexpensive and easy recipe for meal prepping. Simply make it on the weekend and reheat for a quick meal throughout the week. Be sure to serve with your favorite tortilla chips and salsa!

INGREDIENTS | SERVES 6

1 tablespoon olive oil

1 tablespoon all-purpose flour

1 (8-ounce) can tomato sauce

1 cup vegetable broth

1 tablespoon taco seasoning

1 (15-ounce) can black beans, drained

1 (15-ounce) can pinto beans, drained

½ cup chopped seeded red bell pepper

½ cup frozen corn kernels

1 (4-ounce) can green chilies

1 small yellow onion, peeled and chopped

5 (6") soft corn tortillas, quartered

2 cups vegan Cheddar shreds

1. Preheat oven to 375°F. Coat a 9" × 9" square baking dish with vegetable cooking spray.

2. Place a medium saucepan over medium heat and add olive oil and flour, stirring and cooking about 1 minute. Add tomato sauce, vegetable broth, and taco seasoning and continue stirring and cooking 3 minutes until thickened.

3. In a medium bowl stir together black beans, pinto beans, bell peppers, corn, green chilies, and onions. Set aside.

4. Spread 2 tablespoons red sauce in prepared baking dish. Top with tortilla pieces, followed by 1½ cups bean mixture. Drizzle ½ remaining sauce over top. Sprinkle with ½ Cheddar shreds. Repeat layers until all ingredients are used, ending with remaining cheese on top.

5. Bake 15 minutes until cheese is melted.

6. Let cool 10 minutes, then transfer to a large sealable container (or individual serving containers) and refrigerate up to 7 days or freeze up to 2 months. To serve, cook in microwave in 30-second intervals until heated through.

PER SERVING Calories: 336 | Fat: 12.4 g | Protein: 10.3 g | Sodium: 1,079 mg | Fiber: 9.5 g | Carbohydrates: 48.8 g | Sugar: 3.6 g

Wild Rice and Sweet Potato Skillet Dinner

This Wild Rice and Sweet Potato Skillet Dinner is easy, affordable, and delicious. It will be a go-to meal prep favorite!

INGREDIENTS | SERVES 6

1 (6.2-ounce) box fast cook long grain & wild rice

1½ cups water

1 tablespoon olive oil

1 medium sweet potato, cut into ½" cubes

1 (15-ounce) can northern beans, rinsed and drained

1 cup vegan mozzarella shreds

Wild Rice

When compared to both white and brown rice, wild rice has fewer calories and more protein than both white and brown rice, and a similar amount of fiber as brown rice. It is naturally gluten-free as well!

1. Combine rice, water, and olive oil in a large skillet. Bring to a boil over high heat, then reduce to simmer over medium-low heat about 10 minutes.

2. Place sweet potatoes in a medium microwave-safe bowl. Cook in microwave 4 minutes until tender.

3. Add potatoes to simmering rice, along with beans. Sprinkle top with vegan mozzarella shreds. Cover and simmer another 7 minutes, then remove from heat and allow to sit covered about 1 minute until cheese melts.

4. Let cool 10 minutes, then transfer mixture to a large sealable container (or individual serving containers) and refrigerate up to 7 days. To serve, cook in microwave in 30-second intervals until heated through.

PER SERVING Calories: 289 | Fat: 6.7 g | Protein: 11.0 g | Sodium: 367 mg | Fiber: 6.9 g | Carbohydrates: 47.0 g | Sugar: 2.7 g

Vegan Chorizo with Lentils and Brown Rice

In this one pot Vegan Chorizo with Lentils and Brown Rice, the vegan chorizo adds a smoky flavor. Reheat the leftovers of this hearty, healthy dinner all week.

INGREDIENTS | SERVES 6

2 tablespoons olive oil

1 (14-ounce) package tempeh, chopped into ½" cubes

1 medium white onion, peeled and chopped

5 cloves garlic, peeled and minced

¼ cup sun-dried tomatoes, chopped

3 cups vegetable broth

1 cup dried brown lentils

2 bay leaves

3 tablespoons tomato paste

3 tablespoons soy sauce

2 tablespoons chipotle seasoning

1 cup cooked brown rice

½ medium green bell pepper, seeded and roughly chopped

½ medium red bell pepper, seeded and roughly chopped

1 (15-ounce) can stewed tomatoes, including liquid

2 teaspoons liquid smoke

1. In a large saucepan add olive oil, tempeh, and onions. Cook over medium heat until onions are tender, about 5 minutes. Add garlic and sun-dried tomatoes. Cook another 1 minute.

2. Add vegetable broth, lentils, and bay leaves. Lower heat to medium-low and simmer 25 minutes until lentils are tender. Use a spatula to break up tempeh into smaller pieces while cooking.

3. Remove bay leaves and add tomato paste, soy sauce, chipotle seasoning, brown rice, bell peppers, stewed tomatoes, and liquid smoke to pan. Cook another 10 minutes until peppers are tender.

4. Let cool 10 minutes, then transfer to a large lidded container (or individual serving containers) and refrigerate up to 7 days or freeze up to 2 months.

5. To serve, spoon into bowls and cook in microwave in 30-second intervals until heated through.

PER SERVING Calories: 372 | Fat: 11.0 g | Protein: 23.3 g | Sodium: 1,032 mg | Fiber: 7.1 g | Carbohydrates: 46.4 g | Sugar: 7.3 g

Vegan Jambalaya

Bring the flavors of New Orleans home with this Vegan Jambalaya! It is bursting with brown rice, Creole-inspired seasonings, vegan chorizo, and steamed vegetables.

INGREDIENTS | SERVES 4

1 tablespoon olive oil

1 medium yellow onion, peeled and chopped

1 teaspoon agave nectar

1 (12-ounce) package Tofurky Chorizo Plant-Based Crumbles

3 cloves garlic, peeled and minced

¼ cup chopped seeded red bell pepper

¼ cup chopped celery

2 cups cooked brown rice

1 tablespoon paprika

½ teaspoon cayenne pepper

1 teaspoon dried oregano

1 teaspoon dried thyme

½ cup chopped Roma tomatoes

1 tablespoon tamari

1 cup vegetable broth

10 asparagus spears, ends removed

1 medium yellow summer squash, ends removed, sliced

1 medium zucchini, ends removed, sliced

1. Pour oil in a large pot over medium-high heat. Add onion and cook until translucent, about 7 minutes. Stir in agave nectar and cook until onions are caramelized, about 5 minutes.

2. Stir chorizo crumbles into onions and cook 5 minutes until chorizo has browned. Reduce heat to medium and add garlic, peppers, and celery and cook and stir another 3 minutes until vegetables are slightly tender.

3. Stir in cooked rice, seasonings, tomatoes, tamari, and vegetable broth. Bring mixture back to a simmer then reduce heat to low and cook another 10 minutes.

4. Remove pot from heat and let cool about 10 minutes before transferring to a large lidded container (or individual serving containers).

5. Place a steamer basket in a medium saucepan and fill with water up to just below bottom of basket. Place asparagus, squash, and zucchini in basket, cover, and steam 5 minutes, leaving some crispiness to vegetables.

6. Add steamed vegetables to jambalaya and refrigerate up to 7 days. To serve, cook in microwave in 30-second intervals until heated through.

PER SERVING Calories: 465 | Fat: 16.9 g | Protein: 30.6 g | Sodium: 818 mg | Fiber: 12.0 g | Carbohydrates: 45.6 g | Sugar: 8.6 g

Slow Cooker Smoky Black Bean Soup

Packed with fiber, protein, and a smoky, savory sauce, this Slow Cooker Smoky Black Bean Soup is sure to win a spot in your weekly dinner rotation.

INGREDIENTS | SERVES 6

1 cup chopped peeled yellow onion

1 tablespoon olive oil

1 medium red bell pepper, seeded and chopped

2 cups chopped peeled carrots

2 cups chopped red potatoes

3 cloves garlic, peeled and minced

1 jalapeño, seeded and diced

4 cups vegetable broth

4 (15-ounce) cans black beans, rinsed and drained

2 bay leaves

1 teaspoon cumin powder

1 tablespoon chili powder

1 tablespoon liquid smoke

1 medium avocado, peeled and sliced

Does the Bay Leaf Really Do Anything?

A lot of soups and stews call for a bay leaf, but why? Although the bay leaf won't be the star flavor of your soup or stew, it does add just enough subtle herbal flavor to make a difference. You can buy fresh or dried bay leaves in most grocery stores.

1. Combine onions and olive oil in a slow cooker on high heat. Cook 10 minutes.

2. Reduce heat to low and add remaining ingredients except avocado. Cook 7 hours until potatoes and carrots are tender. When done, turn heat off and remove bay leaf.

3. Transfer soup to a blender. Never fill blender more than halfway full. Remove lid insert to allow heat to escape. Place a kitchen towel over top and blend at low speed until mixture is smooth.

4. Transfer soup to a large sealable container (or individual serving containers) and refrigerate up to 10 days or freeze up to 2 months. Refrigerate avocado in a separate sealable container up to 4 days.

5. To serve, pour soup into bowls and cook in microwave in 30-second intervals until heated through. Serve each bowl with avocado slices.

PER SERVING Calories: 399 | Fat: 6.3 g | Protein: 19.5 g | Sodium: 1,075 mg | Fiber: 25.0 g | Carbohydrates: 67.5 g | Sugar: 6.2 g

Vegan Barbecue Pulled Pork

Enjoy this easy-to-make Kansas City–style slow cooker "pork" (a.k.a. jackfruit) any time of the week. Serve on a bun with coleslaw, or on soft tacos.

INGREDIENTS | SERVES 8

2 (20-ounce) cans young green jackfruit in brine, drained

1 cup fresh cranberries

1 medium green pear, cored and chopped

½ cup ketchup

½ cup packed light brown sugar

1 tablespoon apple cider vinegar

1 tablespoon liquid smoke

½ teaspoon ground nutmeg

1 cup water

1. Place drained jackfruit in a slow cooker and turn heat to high. Add fresh cranberries and chopped pear.

2. In a small bowl combine ketchup, brown sugar, vinegar, liquid smoke, nutmeg, and water. Pour over jackfruit mixture and stir to distribute evenly.

3. Place lid on slow cooker and cook about 15 minutes until simmering. Once simmering, turn heat to low and cook 5 hours. Use a spatula to break jackfruit into pieces.

4. Let cool 10 minutes, then transfer "pork" to a sealable container (or individual serving containers) and refrigerate up to 7 days or freeze up to 2 months. To serve, cook in microwave in 30-second intervals until heated through.

PER SERVING Calories: 101 | Fat: 0.1 g | Protein: 0.8 g | Sodium: 255 mg | Fiber: 2.7 g | Carbohydrates: 25.7 g | Sugar: 19.2 g

Vegan Cheeseburger Zucchini Boats

These Vegan Cheeseburger Zucchini Boats are filled with vegan crumbles and drizzled with a special sauce. This recipe is a healthy go-to perfect for meal prepping.

INGREDIENTS | SERVES 4

2 medium zucchini, ends removed and sliced lengthwise

1 teaspoon olive oil

½ cup chopped peeled red onion

½ teaspoon garlic powder

1 cup vegan crumbles

½ cup chopped white mushrooms

2 tablespoons ketchup

1 cup vegan Cheddar shreds, divided

½ teaspoon salt

⅛ teaspoon ground black pepper

½ cup chopped field greens

½ cup chopped cherry tomatoes

½ cup Vegan Special Sauce (see Chapter 7 for recipe)

1. Preheat oven to 350°F. Line a baking sheet with parchment paper.

2. Use a teaspoon to scoop out zucchini pulp, leaving approximately ½" pulp in zucchini. Chop scooped-out pulp and set aside.

3. Place zucchini boats on a large microwave-safe plate and microwave 3 minutes. Set aside.

4. In a large skillet over medium-high heat, add olive oil and onion. Cook 5 minutes until onion is tender.

5. Reduce heat to medium and add garlic powder, vegan crumbles, mushrooms, and zucchini pulp. Cook another 5 minutes until mushrooms are tender. Stir in ketchup, ½ vegan Cheddar shreds, salt, and pepper. Remove from heat.

6. Spoon filling equally into each zucchini boat. Top with remaining cheese and bake 20 minutes on prepared pan until cheese is melted and zucchini is tender.

7. Let cool about 10 minutes, then transfer to a sealed container and refrigerate up to 4 days.

8. To serve, place zucchini boats on a large plate and cook in microwave in 30-second intervals until heated through. Top with field greens and cherry tomatoes, and drizzle with Vegan Special Sauce.

PER SERVING Calories: 162 | Fat: 12.9 g | Protein: 7.8 g | Sodium: 951 mg | Fiber: 4.0 g | Carbohydrates: 18.6 g | Sugar: 7.3 g

Vegan Skillet Enchiladas

These easy one-pan enchiladas are veganized and ready to eat in 15 minutes! Imagine the flavors of enchiladas coming together with tortillas and a zesty tomato sauce.

INGREDIENTS | SERVES 6

1 teaspoon olive oil

1 (10-ounce) package Gardein Chick'n Strips

1 teaspoon taco seasoning

½ teaspoon dried cumin

½ teaspoon dried oregano

1 (16-ounce) jar mild chunky salsa

1 (15-ounce) can black beans, rinsed and drained

1 cup vegan sour cream, divided

4 (6") corn tortillas, cut into 1" strips

1 cup vegan Cheddar shreds, divided

2 tablespoons sliced green onion

½ cup guacamole

1. Place a large skillet over medium heat. Add olive oil and vegan chicken. Cook 5 minutes. As it cooks, use a spatula to break pieces down into bite-sized bits. Sprinkle with taco seasoning, cumin, and oregano and stir to coat. Stir in salsa, black beans, and ½ sour cream. Continue cooking 5 minutes.

2. Add tortilla strips and ½ Cheddar shreds. Stir to combine. Top with remaining Cheddar shreds, cover, and remove from heat. Set aside 10 minutes to let cheese melt.

3. Let cool 10 minutes, then transfer to a large sealable container (or individual serving containers) and refrigerate up to 7 days.

4. To serve, transfer to plates and cook in microwave in 30-second intervals until heated through. Top with remaining sour cream, green onions, and guacamole.

PER SERVING Calories: 358 | Fat: 20.2 g | Protein: 14.6 g | Sodium: 1,304 mg | Fiber: 11.4 g | Carbohydrates: 36.0 g | Sugar: 4.0 g

Mexican Rice Skillet

This Mexican Rice Skillet can be either a side dish or a full meal. Cooked in one pan, it makes for easy cleanup and features favorite Mexican flavors.

INGREDIENTS | SERVES 6

2 teaspoons olive oil

1 cup chopped peeled red onion

1 cup chopped seeded red bell pepper

2 teaspoons taco seasoning

1 teaspoon smoked paprika

1 teaspoon dried oregano

1 (10-ounce) can diced tomatoes, including liquid

1 cup frozen corn kernels, thawed

1 (15-ounce) can black beans, rinsed and drained

1 (10-ounce) can mild enchilada sauce

1½ cups cooked brown rice

¼ cup nutritional yeast flakes

2 tablespoons chopped green onion

1. Place a large skillet over medium heat. Add oil, onions, and bell peppers. Stir to coat vegetables with oil. Cook 5 minutes until onions are tender. Stir in taco seasoning, paprika, and oregano and cook another 3 minutes.

2. Stir in tomatoes, corn, black beans, enchilada sauce, rice, and yeast flakes. Cook another 3 minutes until heated through. Remove from heat and let cool 10 minutes.

3. Once cooled, transfer to a large sealed container (or individual serving containers) and refrigerate up to 7 days or freeze up to 2 months.

4. To serve, cook in microwave in 30-second intervals until heated through. Top with green onions.

PER SERVING Calories: 179 | Fat: 2.2 g | Protein: 8.6 g | Sodium: 732 mg | Fiber: 9.1 g | Carbohydrates: 32.0 g | Sugar: 8.4 g

Slow Cooker Caribbean Black Bean Soup

This spicy Slow Cooker Caribbean Black Bean Soup is made in a slow cooker, so the flavors simmer together for hours.

INGREDIENTS | SERVES 8

1 tablespoon olive oil

1 cup chopped peeled yellow onion

½ cup chopped seeded red bell pepper

2 cups chopped peeled carrots

5 cloves garlic, peeled and minced

1 jalapeño, seeded and diced

5 cups vegetable broth

1 (15-ounce) can diced tomatoes, including liquid

4 (15-ounce) cans black beans, rinsed and drained

1 bay leaf

1 teaspoon dried thyme

2 tablespoons chili powder

½ teaspoon salt

½ teaspoon ground ginger

½ teaspoon ground allspice

1 cup vegan sour cream

½ cup fresh cilantro, chopped

1 lime, wedged

1. Stir together all ingredients except vegan sour cream, cilantro, and lime in a slow cooker. Cook on high 4 hours, or on low 8 hours.

2. Remove bay leaf and use a potato masher to mash some beans to create a thick base.

3. Let cool 10 minutes, then transfer to a large sealed container (or individual serving containers) and refrigerate up to 5 days or freeze up to 2 months. To serve, cook individual servings in a microwave in 30-second intervals until heated through. Top with sour cream, cilantro, and lime wedges.

PER SERVING Calories: 312 | Fat: 7.5 g | Protein: 14.2 g | Sodium: 1,160 mg | Fiber: 20.3 g | Carbohydrates: 49.8 g | Sugar: 5.4 g

CHAPTER 13

Pizzas and Pastas

Go-To Pizza Crust

This easy pizza crust recipe tastes just as good as pizza crusts made in your favorite restaurants. Make a full batch and freeze one of the dough balls to make a second pizza later.

INGREDIENTS | MAKES 2 CRUSTS

1½ cups water

4 teaspoons fast-acting yeast

2 tablespoons agave nectar

3 cups + ¼ cup all-purpose flour, divided

1 cup whole-wheat pastry flour

1 tablespoon cornstarch

2 teaspoons salt

2 tablespoons olive oil

Double It!

If you've found a favorite meal for meal prepping, go ahead and double the recipe. If you can cook something once that lasts twice as long, you've saved yourself a lot of time. It's also a bonus if the dish is freezer-friendly, as the recipe will last even longer.

1. Pour water in a medium microwave-safe bowl and microwave 11 seconds. Stir in yeast and agave nectar and set aside 10 minutes to become frothy.

2. In a large bowl whisk together flours (except ¼ cup all-purpose flour), cornstarch, and salt. Set aside.

3. Pour olive oil into yeast mixture, then pour yeast mixture into flour mixture and stir to combine. This will result in a sticky dough.

4. Next, sprinkle top of dough with a little remaining all-purpose flour and grab far edge of dough. Turn half of dough back toward you, like you're folding a towel. Sprinkle in a little bit more flour and continue, pressing down on dough ball between each turn, about 5 minutes until dough is no longer sticky.

5. Remove dough from bowl and spray ball with vegetable cooking spray. Place back in bowl and cover with a kitchen towel. Place bowl in a slightly warm place and let rise 1 hour until doubled in size.

6. When dough is ready, punch it down in bowl, then cut in half. Roll each half into a ball. Cover each in plastic wrap and refrigerate up to 5 days, or freeze up to 1 month.

7. When ready to use, roll dough ball into desired size and place on ungreased pizza pan. Pre-baking crust 7 minutes at 400°F will create a crispier crust.

PER SERVING (1 crust) Calories: 1,161 | Fat: 14.9 g | Protein: 30.2 g | Sodium: 2,333 mg | Fiber: 15.7 g | Carbohydrates: 218.5 g | Sugar: 9.9 g

Gluten-Free Vegan Pizza with Herbed Quinoa

Make this delicious and easy gluten-free pizza crust topped with pizza sauce, vegan cheese, and a savory herbed quinoa.

INGREDIENTS | MAKES 1 PIZZA

¾ cup warm water
1 teaspoon granulated sugar
2 teaspoons fast-acting yeast
2 tablespoons olive oil, divided

1 tablespoon ground flaxseed
2 cups gluten-free baking flour
1 teaspoon salt, divided
1 teaspoon dried basil
1 cup cooked quinoa

½ teaspoon dried sage
1 teaspoon dried thyme
½ teaspoon dried fennel seeds
1½ cups dairy-free pizza sauce
1½ cups vegan mozzarella shreds

1. Combine water, sugar, and yeast in a small bowl and let stand 3 minutes to allow yeast to proof. Add 1 tablespoon olive oil and flaxseed to mixture and stir.

2. In a medium bowl add flour, ¾ teaspoon salt, and basil. Stir to combine. Pour yeast mixture into flour mixture and stir until well combined.

3. Mold dough into a ball and spray with light coating vegetable cooking spray. Return to medium bowl, cover dough with a kitchen towel, set in a warm place, and let rise 20 minutes.

4. In a large skillet over medium heat, combine remaining olive oil, quinoa, sage, thyme, fennel seeds, and remaining salt. Cook 5 minutes. Remove from heat and set aside.

5. Preheat oven to 400°F. Spray a pizza pan with a light coat of vegetable cooking spray.

6. Tear off a piece of plastic wrap and place dough ball on top. Tear off another piece of plastic wrap and place on top of dough. Use a rolling pin to roll dough out.

7. Place dough on pizza pan and bake 10 minutes. Remove from oven and set aside.

8. Top pizza crust with pizza sauce. Sprinkle cooked quinoa over top of sauce, distributing evenly across pizza. Top with mozzarella. Place pizza in oven and bake until pizza crust is cooked and cheese has melted, about 20 minutes. Remove from oven and cool about 15 minutes.

9. Slice pizza and transfer slices to a large lidded container. Refrigerate up to 7 days or freeze up to 1 month.

10. To serve, cook slices in a toaster oven 5 minutes until heated through.

PER SERVING (⅛ pizza) Calories: 236 | Fat: 9.8 g | Protein: 5.6 g | Sodium: 667 mg | Fiber: 5.2 g | Carbohydrates: 32.2 g | Sugar: 3.3 g

Deep Dish Vegan Pepperoni Pizza

Even if you traveled to Chicago, you may be hard-pressed to find a vegan deep dish pepperoni pizza. Thanks to this recipe, you can make it right at home!

INGREDIENTS | MAKES 1 PIZZA

1 cup warm water

2 teaspoons fast-acting yeast

1 teaspoon granulated sugar

2 cups all-purpose flour

½ cup whole-wheat pastry flour

1½ teaspoons salt

1 tablespoon ground flaxseed

2 tablespoons olive oil

1 (7.8-ounce) container vegan provolone slices

3 cups vegan mozzarella shreds

2 cups dairy-free pizza sauce

24 slices Vegan Pepperoni (see this chapter for recipe)

2 tablespoons vegan Parmesan

1. Spray bottom and sides of a 12" deep dish pizza pan with vegetable cooking spray.

2. In a large bowl combine yeast, sugar, flours, salt, and flaxseed. Create a well in middle of flour. Pour water and olive oil into well then stir together, slowly incorporating flour. Knead dough in bowl 3 minutes. Cover with a damp kitchen towel and set aside to rise one hour.

3. Once dough is ready, turn out onto a floured surface and use a rolling pin to roll to size of pizza pan, then fit in pan.

4. Preheat oven to 450°F.

5. Place vegan provolone slices across dough. Cover with mozzarella, distributing evenly across dough. Spread pizza sauce over cheese. Distribute vegan pepperoni slices evenly over sauce. Sprinkle with Parmesan.

6. Bake 25 minutes until crust is golden. Remove from oven and let cool about 20 minutes.

7. Slice cooled pizza and transfer slices to a large lidded container. Refrigerate up to 7 days or freeze up to 1 month.

8. To serve, cook slices in a toaster oven 5 minutes until heated through.

PER SERVING (⅛ pizza) Calories: 444 | Fat: 20.3 g | Protein: 9.3 g | Sodium: 1,395 mg | Fiber: 5.3 g | Carbohydrates: 53.2 g | Sugar: 3.1 g

Basic Vegan Pepperoni Pizza

Forget all of the oil and indigestion of traditional pepperoni pizza. This vegan pepperoni pizza is easy on the stomach and absolutely delicious, topped with vegan crumbles and vegan pepperoni. Have another slice!

INGREDIENTS | MAKES 2 PIZZAS

1 batch Go-To Pizza Crust (see this chapter for recipe)

2 cups dairy-free pizza sauce

2 cups Gardein Beefless Ground

2 cups Vegan Pepperoni, divided

½ cup chopped red peeled onion

2 cups vegan mozzarella cheese shreds

10 fresh basil leaves, chopped

1. Preheat oven to 400°F. Grease 2 pizza pans with vegetable cooking spray.

2. Use a rolling pin to roll prepared dough balls into size required for pans. Place on prepared pans and bake 10 minutes. Remove from oven.

3. Top crusts with equal amounts pizza sauce, followed by equal amounts beefless grounds, ½ pepperoni slices, onions, and mozzarella.

4. Place pizzas back in oven and bake 20 minutes until cheese has melted. Remove from oven.

5. Top pizzas immediately with remaining pepperoni slices and basil. Let cool 15 minutes.

6. Slice cooled pizzas and transfer to a large lidded container. Refrigerate up to 7 days or freeze up to 1 month.

7. To serve, cook slices in a toaster oven 5 minutes until pizza is heated through.

PER SERVING (1 pizza) Calories: 1,253 | Fat: 42.3 g | Protein: 60.5 g | Sodium: 3,631 mg | Fiber: 29.7 g | Carbohydrates: 197.3 g | Sugar: 26.5 g

Vegan Pizza Pot Pie

This Vegan Pizza Pot Pie is easy to make and works great for a meal prepping schedule. Make it on the weekend and reheat for a crispy, savory dish throughout the week.

INGREDIENTS | SERVES 12

1 (24-ounce) jar dairy-free pizza sauce

2 cups vegan crumbles

2 cups broccoli florets

1 cup frozen corn kernels

1 (4-ounce) package vegan pepperoni, divided

1 teaspoon fast-acting yeast

1 teaspoon packed light brown sugar

2 cups all-purpose flour

1½ teaspoons baking powder

½ teaspoon baking soda

1 tablespoon ground flaxseed

1 tablespoon cornstarch

1½ teaspoons salt

3 tablespoons vegan margarine, sliced and softened

⅔ cup warm water

2 cups vegan mozzarella shreds

3 tablespoons vegan Parmesan

1 cup sliced Roma tomatoes

6 fresh basil leaves, chopped

Is Cornstarch Bad for You?

Cornstarch is a highly processed food but will not impact your health if consumed in minimal amounts. Some people opt for less processed alternatives like potato starch, tapioca starch, or arrowroot powder. You can also use ground chia seeds as a natural thickener.

1. Preheat oven to 350°F. Spray a 9" × 13" baking pan with a light coating of vegetable cooking spray.

2. Pour pizza sauce across bottom of prepared baking dish. Top with vegan crumbles, broccoli florets, frozen corn, and ½ vegan pepperoni.

3. In a large bowl stir together yeast, brown sugar, flour, baking powder, baking soda, flaxseed, cornstarch, and salt. Add sliced margarine and stir. Add water and stir again to create a sticky dough.

4. Drop dough by spoonfuls across baking pan. Sprinkle top of dough with vegan mozzarella cheese and top with vegan Parmesan. Add sliced tomatoes and remaining vegan pepperoni.

5. Bake 30 minutes until crust is golden brown around edges. Remove from oven and top with basil leaves.

6. Let cool 15 minutes, then cover and refrigerate up to 10 days. To serve, cook slices in a toaster oven 5 minutes until heated through.

PER SERVING Calories: 253 | Fat: 7.6 g | Protein: 11.0 g | Sodium: 1,007 mg | Fiber: 4.6 g | Carbohydrates: 34.2 g | Sugar: 3.8 g

Easy Vegan Pizzas

Hungry? Make yourself two Easy Vegan Pizzas! This is a cheap, easy, and yummy recipe to satisfy your desire for pizza!

INGREDIENTS | SERVES 16

2 store-bought dairy-free pizza crusts
1 (24-ounce) jar dairy-free pizza sauce
1 cup vegan crumbles
½ cup chopped red peeled onions
½ cup chopped black olives
1 (8-ounce) package vegan mozzarella shreds

1. Preheat oven to 450°F.

2. Place pizza crusts on large ungreased pizza pans and bake 5 minutes to create a crispy crust.

3. Remove crusts from oven and spread equal amounts pizza sauce over each crust. Evenly distribute vegan crumbles, onions, black olives, and mozzarella across crusts.

4. Bake pizzas 20 minutes until crust is golden on edges and cheese has melted. Remove pizzas from oven and set aside to cool about 15 minutes.

5. Slice cooled pizzas and transfer to a large lidded container. Refrigerate up to 7 days or freeze up to 1 month.

6. To serve, cook slices in a toaster oven 5 minutes until heated through.

PER SERVING Calories: 160 | Fat: 5.5 g | Protein: 4.6 g | Sodium: 508 mg | Fiber: 2.8 g | Carbohydrates: 22.3 g | Sugar: 2.5 g

Vegan Pepperoni

Top your pizzas, Italian dishes, sandwiches, and even salads with this delicious, gluten-free, and slightly spicy Vegan Pepperoni.

INGREDIENTS | MAKES 5 CUPS PEPPERONI

¾ cup water

½ cup sun-dried tomatoes (not packed in oil)

1 (10-ounce) package extra-firm tofu, pressed and cut into 1" cubes

1 (15-ounce) can chickpeas, including liquid

1½ teaspoons salt

1½ teaspoons ground black pepper

1 teaspoon dry mustard powder

1 teaspoon fennel seeds

1 tablespoon smoked paprika

2 tablespoons paprika

2 teaspoons garlic powder

1 teaspoon onion powder

1 teaspoon olive oil

2 teaspoons coconut sugar

½ teaspoon crushed red pepper flakes

½ cup beet purée

2 tablespoons liquid smoke

1. Preheat oven to 400°F. Line two baking sheets with parchment paper.

2. Add water to a small microwave-safe bowl. Heat 2 minutes. Add sun-dried tomatoes to bowl and set aside.

3. Place tofu and chickpeas in a food processor. Pulse until mostly smooth. Add remaining ingredients except tomatoes. Pulse until combined. Add tomatoes and pulse again, leaving bits of tomato throughout batter.

4. Pour batter onto prepared baking sheets and use a spatula to press out to about 1¼" thickness. Spray top with a light coating of vegetable cooking spray.

5. Bake 30 minutes. Remove from oven and cool about 10 minutes.

6. Use a small round cookie cutter to cut into pepperoni, then transfer to a large lidded container. Refrigerate up to 5 days or freeze up to 3 months.

PER SERVING Calories: 90 | Fat: 2.8 g | Protein: 5.7 g | Sodium: 422 mg | Fiber: 3.4 g | Carbohydrates: 11.9 g | Sugar: 3.8 g

Easy Penne Pasta with Red Peppers

Serve this Easy Penne Pasta with Red Peppers along with "Cheesy" Pull-Apart Bread (see Chapter 4 for recipe) for a memorable dinner.

INGREDIENTS | SERVES 6

1 teaspoon olive oil

1 large yellow onion, peeled and chopped

1 medium red bell pepper, seeded and chopped

1 (14-ounce) package vegan Italian sausage, cut into 1" pieces

1 (14-ounce) can stewed tomatoes, including liquid

1 (8-ounce) can tomato sauce

1 teaspoon garlic powder

1 teaspoon dried basil

1 teaspoon dried oregano

1 (16-ounce) box penne pasta, cooked according to package directions

1 cup vegan mozzarella shreds

1. In a large skillet over medium heat add olive oil, onions, and bell peppers. Cook 5 minutes until onions and peppers are tender. Add vegan sausage, followed by tomatoes, tomato sauce, and seasonings. Stir to combine and cook about 10 minutes until heated through.

2. Add pasta to skillet, stirring until pasta is coated. Sprinkle top with vegan cheese shreds. Remove from heat.

3. Let cool 10 minutes, then transfer to a large lidded container (or individual serving containers) and refrigerate up to 7 days or freeze up to 1 month.

4. To serve, cook in microwave in 30-second intervals until heated through.

PER SERVING Calories: 348 | Fat: 9.6 g | Protein: 17.9 g | Sodium: 732 mg | Fiber: 4.7 g | Carbohydrates: 41.7 g | Sugar: 4.9 g

Walnut Basil Pesto

This Walnut Basil Pesto can be served many ways, including over pasta and spread on toasted Italian bread. You can also freeze the recipe and enjoy it for even longer.

INGREDIENTS | SERVES 6

3 cloves garlic, peeled and roughly chopped

½ cup olive oil, divided

¼ cup walnuts

1 cup fresh basil leaves

3 tablespoons nutritional yeast flakes

1 tablespoon vegan Parmesan

½ teaspoon salt

1. Place chopped garlic in a medium skillet with 1 tablespoon olive oil. Cook over medium-low heat until garlic is slightly tender, about 2 minutes.

2. Place garlic and remaining ingredients in a food processor and pulse until ingredients are combined to preferred texture.

3. Transfer pesto to a small lidded container and refrigerate up to 10 days or freeze up to 2 months. To serve, allow to warm to room temperature.

PER SERVING Calories: 207 | Fat: 21.0 g | Protein: 2.0 g | Sodium: 220 mg | Fiber: 0.8 g | Carbohydrates: 2.4 g | Sugar: 0.2 g

Spaghetti Pie

A simple recipe with tantalizing flavors is the secret to this crowd-pleasing Spaghetti Pie. Ready in 30 minutes, it's great for meal prepping.

INGREDIENTS | SERVES 8

1 (15-ounce) package firm silken tofu

1 tablespoon olive oil

2 tablespoons nutritional yeast flakes

1 teaspoon dried ground basil

1 teaspoon garlic powder

1½ tablespoons mild yellow miso paste

2 cups vegan mozzarella cheese shreds, divided

6 ounces spaghetti noodles, cooked according to package directions

1 (10-ounce) package frozen spinach, thawed and squeezed dry

1 (12-ounce) package vegan crumbles

1½ cups dairy-free marinara sauce

Spinach for Your Health

A system developed by Dr. Joel Fuhrman measures foods based on their micronutrients; it lists spinach to be one of the top ten nutrient-dense foods, along with kale and Swiss chard. It has high levels of fiber, potassium, iron, calcium, and protein!

1. Preheat oven to 375°F. Spray a 9" pie dish with vegetable cooking spray.

2. Place tofu, olive oil, nutritional yeast, basil, garlic powder, and miso paste in a food processor. Pulse until smooth. Stir in 1 cup vegan mozzarella.

3. Add ½ tofu mixture to cooked pasta in a large bowl. Stir until all pasta is coated. Press mixture into prepared pie dish.

4. Add spinach to remaining tofu mixture in processor. Pulse 3 times until combined, leaving a marbled look. Spoon spinach mixture over pasta in pie dish.

5. In a medium bowl stir together vegan crumbles and marinara sauce. Pour over spinach. Top with remaining mozzarella.

6. Bake 20 minutes until cheese is melted. Remove from oven and let cool about 15 minutes.

7. Cut into slices and transfer to a large lidded container (or individual serving containers) and refrigerate up to 7 days. To serve, cook in microwave in 30-second intervals until heated through.

PER SERVING Calories: 322 | Fat: 11.7 g | Protein: 17.9 g | Sodium: 849 mg | Fiber: 6.1 g | Carbohydrates: 34.2 g | Sugar: 5.1 g

Garlic Pasta Casserole

This easy Garlic Pasta Casserole is a creamy delight covered in red sauce and dripping with melted vegan cheese. It's easy to make and healthy too!

INGREDIENTS | SERVES 12

1 (16-ounce) box penne pasta, cooked according to package directions

1 small sweet potato, perforated with a fork

4 cloves garlic, peeled and chopped

2 tablespoons olive oil

½ cup vegetable broth

2 cups dairy-free marinara sauce

1 cup vegan crumbles

1 cup vegan mozzarella shreds

1. Preheat oven to 375°F.

2. Spread cooked pasta across bottom of an ungreased 9" × 13" baking dish.

3. Microwave potato 3 minutes until slightly tender. Chop into chunks (including peel).

4. Add potato chunks, garlic, and olive oil to a food processor. Pulse until smooth. Add vegetable broth and pulse until combined.

5. Pour sweet potato mixture over pasta and stir to distribute throughout pasta. Pour marinara sauce evenly over top. Spread vegan crumbles over sauce, then sprinkle with vegan mozzarella.

6. Bake 20 minutes until cheese is melted. Once pasta is done, remove from oven and set aside to cool about 15 minutes.

7. Once cool, cover, and refrigerate up to 7 days or freeze up to 1 month. To serve, cook in microwave in 30-second intervals until heated through.

PER SERVING Calories: 235 | Fat: 5.4 g | Protein: 7.8 g | Sodium: 347 mg | Fiber: 3.2 g | Carbohydrates: 37.3 g | Sugar: 4.0 g

Pasta with Roasted Beet Hummus

This light and colorful Pasta with Roasted Beet Hummus is made with simple, accessible ingredients.

INGREDIENTS | SERVES 8

2 tablespoons olive oil, divided
1 medium beet, peeled and chopped
½ cup chopped yellow peeled onion
2 cloves garlic, peeled and chopped
¼ cup red wine
¼ cup almonds
1 (15-ounce) can chickpeas, rinsed and drained
¼ cup fresh basil leaves
½ teaspoon salt
4 tablespoons water
1 (13.25-ounce) box penne pasta, cooked according to package directions
3 tablespoons vegan Parmesan

Cooking and Coloring with Beets

Beets can add a lot of color to your recipes. However, that color can also stain things like countertops, containers, and your hands. Be sure to slice beets on surfaces that don't stain easily, or use an old cutting board. You can use small amounts of beets as a natural red food coloring for things like frosting and dough batter.

1. Add 1 tablespoon olive oil to a large skillet over medium heat. Add beets and onions and cook 5 minutes until onions are tender. Add garlic and cook another 1 minute. Remove from heat.

2. Pour wine and almonds in a food processor. Pulse, then push ingredients down with a spatula. Pulse again 1 minute to turn mixture into a paste. Add cooked beets and onions and pulse 30 seconds to combine. Add chickpeas, basil, and salt and pulse again until smooth. Pulse in water, 1 tablespoon at a time, to reach a spreadable consistency.

3. Transfer to a medium lidded container and refrigerate up to 5 days.

4. Transfer cooked pasta to a separate large lidded container and refrigerate up to 5 days. To serve, spoon hummus over portioned-out pasta and cook in microwave in 30-second intervals until heated through. Top with vegan Parmesan.

PER SERVING Calories: 302 | Fat: 7.0 g | Protein: 9.8 g | Sodium: 280 mg | Fiber: 4.6 g | Carbohydrates: 47.1 g | Sugar: 4.0 g

Easy Vegan Lasagna

This recipe uses no-bake lasagna noodles to make an easy dish with layers of pasta, red sauce, and a cheesy beet filling. Enjoy this colorful, savory, and healthy vegetable lasagna all week with a side of fresh salad.

INGREDIENTS | SERVES 12

1 (15-ounce) package extra-firm tofu
1 (15-ounce) jar beets, including juice
¼ cup nutritional yeast flakes
¼ cup walnuts
2 teaspoons mild miso paste
1 teaspoon garlic powder
1 teaspoon dried basil
3 cups vegan mozzarella shreds, divided
5 cups pasta sauce
2 cups vegan crumbles
1 (8-ounce) box no-boil lasagna noodles

1. Preheat oven to 350°F. Spray a 9" × 13" baking dish with vegetable cooking spray.

2. Add tofu, beets (reserving juice), nutritional yeast, walnuts, miso paste, garlic powder, and basil to a food processor. Pulse until smooth. Add 3 tablespoons reserved beet juice and pulse until a spreadable consistency is achieved. Add 1 cup vegan mozzarella shreds and pulse again to combine. Set aside.

3. In a large bowl add pasta sauce and vegan crumbles. Stir to combine.

4. Pour 1 cup sauce mixture into bottom of prepared pan. Arrange 4 lasagna noodles on top of sauce. Pour 1 cup sauce mixture over noodles. Spread ½ beet filling over sauce. Repeat another layer of lasagna noodles, sauce, and filling. Finish with one more layer lasagna noodles, topped with remaining sauce. Sprinkle remaining mozzarella over top.

5. Tear off a piece of aluminum foil large enough to cover baking dish. Spray bottom side of foil with vegetable cooking spray. Cover baking dish with foil, crimping edges around sides of pan. Bake covered pan 45 minutes.

6. Use tongs to carefully remove foil and bake another 15 minutes uncovered. Remove from oven and let cool 10 minutes.

7. Refrigerate covered up to 5 days or freeze up to 2 months. To serve, place individual slices on a large plate and cook in microwave in 30-second intervals until heated through.

PER SERVING Calories: 292 | Fat: 11.5 g | Protein: 12.6 g | Sodium: 728 mg | Fiber: 5.2 g | Carbohydrates: 34.0 g | Sugar: 8.8 g

Simple Spaghetti Squash Casserole

This Simple Spaghetti Squash Casserole offers a healthy, low-carb alternative to traditional pasta. Savor one delicious bite after another!

INGREDIENTS | SERVES 6

1 teaspoon olive oil

1 large spaghetti squash, halved and seeded

1 (20-ounce) jar dairy-free marinara sauce

1 (8-ounce) package vegan mozzarella shreds

1 medium Roma tomato, thinly sliced

Cooking with Spaghetti Squash

Spaghetti squash is usually harvested in the fall but can be found in the produce section of most grocery stores year-round. When cooking this squash, you'll discover that the flesh turns into spaghetti-like strands. Use cooked spaghetti squash as a low-carb pasta and top with your favorite noodle sauces.

1. Preheat oven to 375°F. Line a baking sheet with parchment paper.

2. Brush olive oil on cut sides of each squash half. Place squash cut-side down on prepared pan.

3. Bake 40 minutes until tender. Leave oven on but remove squash from oven and cool 3 minutes.

4. Use a large spoon to scrape out squash innards into a 2-quart casserole dish. Distribute strands evenly across bottom of dish.

5. Pour marinara sauce over spaghetti squash. Sprinkle vegan cheese over top. Arrange tomato slices on top of cheese.

6. Bake 20 minutes until cheese is fully melted. Remove from oven and let cool 10 minutes before covering.

7. Refrigerate up to 5 days. To serve, cook in microwave in 30-second intervals until heated through.

PER SERVING Calories: 246 | Fat: 10.4 g | Protein: 4.5 g | Sodium: 820 mg | Fiber: 6.9 g | Carbohydrates: 33.8 g | Sugar: 12.1 g

Spaghetti Squash with Chickpea Meatballs

This easy, low-carb Spaghetti Squash with Chickpea Meatballs recipe is perfect for weekday lunches or dinners!

INGREDIENTS | SERVES 4

1 large spaghetti squash, halved and seeded

1 (15-ounce) can great northern beans, drained

1 tablespoon dried minced onions

1 teaspoon garlic powder

¼ cup ground flaxseed

2 tablespoons nutritional yeast flakes

1 teaspoon Italian seasoning

1 teaspoon dried rubbed sage

1 tablespoon chia seeds

1½ cups pasta sauce

1 cup vegan mozzarella shreds

1. Preheat oven to 375°F. Line two baking sheets with parchment paper.

2. Place squash halves face down on one prepared pan. Bake 40 minutes until tender. Remove from oven and let cool 3 minutes.

3. Place beans in a food processor with onions, garlic powder, flaxseed, nutritional yeast flakes, Italian seasoning, and sage. Pulse 3 seconds until combined.

4. Use an ice cream scoop to scoop bean mixture from food processor and place meatballs onto second prepared pan. Bake 30 minutes. Remove and set aside.

5. Use a large spoon to scrape spaghetti squash onto paper towels. Squeeze spaghetti squash to remove excess fluids. Place into a 2-quart casserole dish. Add chia seeds and stir gently to distribute. Pour pasta sauce on top.

6. Use tongs to transfer meatballs onto spaghetti sauce. Top with mozzarella shreds. Return to oven and bake another 10 minutes until cheese has melted. Remove from heat and let cool 10 minutes before covering.

7. Refrigerate up to 5 days. To serve, cook in microwave in 30-second intervals until heated through.

PER SERVING Calories: 456 | Fat: 13.2 g | Protein: 17.0 g | Sodium: 1,021 mg | Fiber: 18.2 g | Carbohydrates: 70.2 g | Sugar: 17.5 g

Spaghetti with Seared Cauliflower and Walnuts

Learn how to make spaghetti topped with delicious seared cauliflower and walnuts with this easy, healthy recipe.

INGREDIENTS | SERVES 2

1 (4-ounce) box spaghetti
1 tablespoon olive oil
1 tablespoon dairy-free margarine
3 cups cauliflower florets
2 cloves garlic, peeled and chopped
¼ cup walnuts, chopped
½ cup sliced cherry tomatoes
4 fresh basil leaves, chopped
⅛ teaspoon salt
⅛ teaspoon ground black pepper

Walnuts for Your Health

Walnuts are packed with many of the nutrients you need for a healthy life, including omega-3s, a healthy fat that can lower blood pressure, improve mental health, and reduce inflammation as well as the risk of certain types of cancer. Studies also show that daily consumption of a small amount of walnuts decreases appetite, which can lead to weight loss.

1. Cook pasta in a medium saucepan of boiling water 8 minutes. Drain, reserving ⅓ cup cooking liquid. Set aside.

2. Heat olive oil and margarine in a large skillet over medium-high heat. Add cauliflower, stirring to coat evenly. Cook until cauliflower is slightly tender and golden brown, about 10 minutes.

3. Remove from heat and add reserved cooking liquid, garlic, walnuts, and tomatoes. Stir so everything is evenly coated.

4. Stir basil, salt, and pepper into cauliflower mixture. Toss in pasta.

5. Let cool 10 minutes, then transfer to a large lidded container (or individual serving containers) and refrigerate up to 5 days. To serve, cook in microwave in 30-second intervals until heated through.

PER SERVING Calories: 441 | Fat: 19.2 g | Protein: 13.3 g | Sodium: 238 mg | Fiber: 6.6 g | Carbohydrates: 55.1 g | Sugar: 6.0 g

Easy Macaroni Casserole

This Easy Macaroni Casserole is a baked pasta dish that delivers vegan, cheesy deliciousness in every bite.

INGREDIENTS | SERVES 8

2 teaspoons olive oil

1 medium yellow onion, peeled and chopped

1 medium red bell pepper, seeded and chopped

3 cloves garlic, peeled and finely chopped

1 (15-ounce) can diced tomatoes, drained

2 cups dairy-free marinara sauce

2 cups water

1 cup vegan crumbles

1 (12-ounce) box whole-wheat macaroni noodles

2 cups vegan mozzarella shreds

1. Preheat oven to 375°F and prepare a 9" × 13" baking dish with a light coating of vegetable spray.

2. In a large skillet over medium heat add olive oil, onions, and red pepper. Cook until vegetables are tender, about 5 minutes. Turn heat to low and add chopped garlic. Stir.

3. Add tomatoes, marinara, and water and bring mixture to a boil over high heat. Reduce heat to medium and add vegan crumbles. Stir to combine.

4. Spoon out just enough marinara sauce mixture to cover bottom of prepared pan. Pour box of uncooked pasta over sauce, spreading evenly across pan. Pour remaining marinara mixture over macaroni. Top with mozzarella.

5. Cover casserole with aluminum foil, crimping edges just slightly to keep heat inside. Bake 50 minutes. Remove from oven and keep foil on pan 15 minutes.

6. Let cool about 15 minutes, then refrigerate up to 7 days. To serve, cook individual servings in microwave in 30-second intervals until heated through.

PER SERVING Calories: 324 | Fat: 8.8 g | Protein: 11.4 g | Sodium: 716 mg | Fiber: 7.8 g | Carbohydrates: 50.2 g | Sugar: 6.3 g

Vegan Baked Parmesan Chick'n

This Vegan Baked Parmesan Chick'n takes a simple chickpea burger and transforms it into a delicious twist on an Italian classic. Breaded chickpea patties are baked and smothered in marinara and vegan cheese. Serve with your favorite pasta and steamed vegetables on the side.

INGREDIENTS | SERVES 6

1 medium sweet potato, perforated with a fork

1 cup rolled oats

¼ cup chopped walnuts

1 (15-ounce) can chickpeas, rinsed and drained

1 tablespoon dried minced onions

1 teaspoon garlic powder

1 tablespoon poultry seasoning

1 tablespoon nutritional yeast flakes

2 tablespoons ground flaxseed, divided

¼ teaspoon salt

¼ teaspoon ground black pepper

¾ cup seasoned bread crumbs

¼ cup vegan Parmesan

2 tablespoons vegan butter, melted

2 tablespoons plain soy milk

1 cup dairy-free marinara sauce

1 cup vegan mozzarella shreds

1. Preheat oven to 400°F. Spray a large baking sheet and a large skillet with vegetable cooking spray.

2. Place potato in microwave and cook 2 minutes. Use oven mitts to remove from microwave and allow to cool about 5 minutes. Once cooled, chop into large cubes.

3. Place oats and walnuts in a food processor and pulse until a coarse flour is formed. Add potato, chickpeas, onions, garlic powder, poultry seasoning, nutritional yeast, and 1 tablespoon ground flaxseed. Pulse 3 seconds, then use a spatula to push ingredients back down. Pulse again 3 seconds.

4. Form mixture into 6 patties and place in prepared skillet over medium heat. Cook 5 minutes on one side. Sprinkle salt and pepper on uncooked sides, flip, and cook another 5 minutes until patties have firmed up slightly and are brown on both sides. Transfer from skillet to a large plate and set aside to cool about 5 minutes.

5. In a small bowl stir together bread crumbs and vegan Parmesan. Pour melted butter, milk, and remaining 1 tablespoon flaxseed into a separate small bowl. Dip each patty in butter mixture, then dip in bread crumbs and place on prepared baking sheet. Spray patties lightly with vegetable cooking spray.

6. Bake 25 minutes until bread crumbs are golden brown. Remove from oven.

7. Spoon equal amounts marinara sauce over each patty. Top with equal amounts mozzarella shreds. Return pan to oven and bake another 10 more minutes until cheese is melted.

8. Let cool 10 minutes, then transfer patties to a large lidded container and refrigerate up to 10 days or freeze up to 2 months. To serve, cook in microwave in 30-second intervals until heated through.

PER SERVING Calories: 365 | Fat: 13.3 g | Protein: 10.8 g | Sodium: 897 mg | Fiber: 8.3 g | Carbohydrates: 48.4 g | Sugar: 6.8 g

Meatless Baked Ziti

This Meatless Baked Ziti is layered almost like a lasagna, which makes every bite full of flavor, from the sauce to the creamy vegan ricotta. It's easy to make on the weekends and enjoy for the rest of the week, or serve to company.

INGREDIENTS | SERVES 12

2 tablespoons olive oil

1 small yellow onion, peeled and roughly chopped

2 cloves garlic, peeled and roughly chopped

1 (15-ounce) package extra-firm tofu, cut into 1" cubes

1 tablespoon mild miso paste

10 slices vegan provolone cheese, divided

¼ cup fresh basil leaves, chopped

⅛ teaspoon salt

⅛ teaspoon ground black pepper

3 cups dairy-free marinara sauce

1 (10-ounce) package vegan Italian sausages, chopped into ½" cubes

1 (16-ounce) box ziti pasta, cooked according to package instructions

1 cup vegan mozzarella shreds

Pasta Shapes

The different shapes of pasta mean they are best used in certain types of recipes. For example, rotini and farfalle are perfect for pasta salad because they have lots of edges to hold the dressing. Ziti and penne pastas are great with flavorful sauces, as the center holds lots of the sauce. These pastas are very similar in shape, except ziti has flat edges, whereas penne has tips that come to a point.

1. Preheat oven to 375°F. Spray bottom of a 9" × 13" baking dish with vegetable cooking spray.

2. Add olive oil, onion, garlic, tofu, and miso paste to a food processor. Pulse until smooth. Add 4 provolone slices and basil and pulse again. Sprinkle with salt and pepper. Set aside.

3. In a medium bowl combine marina sauce and vegan sausage slices. Set aside.

4. Add tofu mixture to pan with cooked pasta. Stir gently until pasta is coated.

5. Pour ½ pasta into prepared baking dish. Top with ½ marinara sauce mixture. Top with remaining slices provolone, followed by remaining pasta, then remaining sauce, then mozzarella shreds.

6. Cover dish with aluminum foil and bake 20 minutes until cheese is melted. Use tongs to remove foil and bake another 10 minutes until browned at edges. Remove from oven and let cool about 15 minutes.

7. Cover dish and refrigerate up to 7 days or freeze up to 2 months. To serve, cook in microwave in 30-second intervals until heated through.

PER SERVING Calories: 387 | Fat: 15.6 g | Protein: 17.1 g | Sodium: 784 mg | Fiber: 3.4 g | Carbohydrates: 43.5 g | Sugar: 6.1 g

Stuffed Pasta Shells

These pasta shells are stuffed with savory vegan crumbles and vegan ricotta, and topped with marinara sauce and vegan mozzarella cheese. If you love cheesy Italian dishes, this recipe will be right up your alley.

INGREDIENTS | SERVES 8

1 (15-ounce) package firm tofu, pressed

2 tablespoons olive oil

½ cup nutritional yeast flakes

1 tablespoon mild miso paste

2 teaspoons dried basil

3 cloves garlic, peeled and roughly chopped

1 (10-ounce) package frozen chopped spinach, thawed and squeezed

3½ cups spaghetti sauce, divided

24 jumbo pasta shells, cooked according to package instructions

1 cup vegan mozzarella shreds

1. Preheat oven to 350°F.

2. Place tofu in a food processor along with olive oil, yeast flakes, miso paste, basil, and garlic. Pulse until smooth. Add spinach and pulse 2 seconds to combine, leaving a creamy mixture with chopped spinach throughout.

3. Spread 1 cup marinara sauce evenly over bottom of an ungreased 9" × 13" baking dish. Use a spoon to fill cooked pasta shells with spinach mixture, placing shells in prepared baking dish as you fill them. Drizzle rest of marinara sauce over top of filled shells, followed by vegan mozzarella shreds.

4. Cover dish with aluminum foil. Bake until cheese melts, about 15 minutes. Use tongs to remove foil and bake another 15 minutes until edges are golden brown. Remove from oven and let cool about 15 minutes.

5. Cover dish and refrigerate up to 7 days or freeze up to 2 months. To serve, cook in microwave in 30-second intervals until heated through.

PER SERVING Calories: 354 | Fat: 11.4 g | Protein: 16.6 g | Sodium: 749 mg | Fiber: 6.4 g | Carbohydrates: 46.5 g | Sugar: 8.7 g

Spinach Pesto Flatbreads

Make these tasty Spinach Pesto Flatbreads in a few easy steps. Enjoy the health benefits of the spinach, pecans, fresh basil, and more.

INGREDIENTS | SERVES 8

⅓ cup pecans

1⅓ cups fresh spinach, divided

⅓ cup olive oil

2 teaspoons nutritional yeast flakes

½ teaspoon garlic powder

5 fresh basil leaves

½ teaspoon salt

4 (4-ounce) flatbreads

1 cup vegan mozzarella shreds

What Is Flatbread?

Flatbread, such as pita and naan, is made with a simple list of ingredients, usually flour, water, and a little salt. You can find flavored flatbreads with herbs such as basil and oregano, as well as gluten-free flatbreads. Serve alongside saucy dishes or as a base for delicious toppings.

1. Preheat oven to 425°F. Line a baking sheet with parchment paper.

2. Place pecans, 1 cup spinach, olive oil, nutritional yeast, garlic powder, and basil leaves in a food processor. Pulse 3 seconds, then use a spatula to push down ingredients. Pulse again until combined and spinach is broken down, but some texture remains.

3. Spread pesto evenly across each piece of flatbread. Sprinkle evenly with mozzarella shreds and remaining spinach leaves.

4. Bake 13 minutes until crust is golden brown and cheese has melted. Remove from oven and let cool about 5 minutes.

5. Slice flatbread, then place slices in a large sealed container and refrigerate up to 10 days or freeze up to 2 months.

6. To serve, place individual slices in a toaster oven and toast 5 minutes.

PER SERVING Calories: 311 | Fat: 15.1 g | Protein: 6.4 g | Sodium: 448 mg | Fiber: 2.3 g | Carbohydrates: 36.1 g | Sugar: 0.9 g

Vegan Pasta Primavera

This Vegan Pasta Primavera is full of garden-fresh vegetables, resulting in a light and fresh recipe. The sauce is infused with lemon and garlic, and the dish is topped with vegan Parmesan.

INGREDIENTS | SERVES 8

2 cloves garlic, peeled and mashed

½ teaspoon salt

3 tablespoons olive oil, divided

1 tablespoon lemon zest

½ cup chopped peeled red onion

1 small zucchini, ends removed and diced

1 medium carrot, peeled and cut into thin strips

1 medium red bell pepper, seeded and diced

1 cup small broccoli florets

½ cup halved sugar snap peas

½ cup frozen peas

1 cup cherry tomatoes, halved

1 (12-ounce) box penne pasta, cooked according to package instructions (reserving ½ liquid)

½ cup vegan Parmesan cheese

1 tablespoon chopped fresh basil leaves

1. Combine garlic with salt, 1 tablespoon olive oil, and lemon zest in a small bowl. Set aside.

2. Add remaining oil to a large skillet over medium-high heat. Add onions and cook until tender, about 5 minutes. Add remaining vegetables and reserved pasta cooking liquid. Stir until vegetables are coated and cook 7 minutes.

3. Reduce heat to medium and add pasta and lemon garlic mixture. Cook another 2 minutes. Remove from heat and let cool about 5 minutes.

4. Cover dish and refrigerate up to 7 days. Store Parmesan and basil in lidded container up to 7 days. To serve, cook in microwave in 30-second intervals until heated through. Top with Parmesan and basil.

PER SERVING Calories: 262 | Fat: 7.0 g | Protein: 7.1 g | Sodium: 310 mg | Fiber: 3.4 g | Carbohydrates: 41.3 g | Sugar: 4.1 g

Appetizers and Snacks

Fresh Black Bean Dip

Make up a batch of this simple Fresh Black Bean Dip with fewer than a dozen ingredients and you'll be rewarded with a healthy and flavorful new favorite. This dip is infused with fresh onions, jalapeños, and delicious spices.

INGREDIENTS | MAKES 5 CUPS

1 small yellow onion, peeled and chopped

2 jalapeño peppers, seeded and chopped

1 clove garlic, peeled and chopped

¼ cup chopped seeded red bell pepper

2 (15-ounce) cans black beans, drained

3 tablespoons water

1 teaspoon ground cumin

2 teaspoons cocoa powder

3 tablespoons fresh lime juice

2 tablespoons fresh chopped cilantro

4 cherry tomatoes, sliced

1. Add onion, jalapeño, garlic, bell pepper, black beans, and water to a food processor bowl. Pulse three times, pushing down contents that go up sides of bowl. Add cumin and cocoa powder and pulse again until smooth.

2. Pour into a medium microwave-safe container and cook 60 seconds. Stir and repeat. Remove from microwave and let cool 1 minute.

3. Stir in lime juice and cilantro. Cover and refrigerate up to 5 days or freeze up to 2 months. To serve, cook in microwave in 30-second intervals until heated through, then garnish with sliced cherry tomatoes.

PER SERVING (½ cup) Calories: 88 | Fat: 0.3 g | Protein: 5.5 g | Sodium: 191 mg | Fiber: 6.5 g | Carbohydrates: 18.9 g | Sugar: 1.4 g

Easy Vegan Queso Dip

Make this creamy, cheesy Easy Vegan Queso Dip with only six ingredients. It also takes less than 10 minutes to make, and it is perfect served over baked potatoes or burritos or with nachos or tortilla chips.

INGREDIENTS | SERVES 6

1 (8-ounce) package vegan cream cheese

1 (10-ounce) can mild green chili enchilada sauce

3 tablespoons nutritional yeast flakes

1 teaspoon garlic powder

½ teaspoon salt

¼ teaspoon black pepper

1. Scoop vegan cream cheese into a small microwave-safe bowl and microwave about 20 seconds. Remove, stir, and repeat until sauce is smooth and stirs easily.

2. Pour green chili enchilada sauce over cream cheese. Stir to combine. Stir in nutritional yeast flakes, garlic powder, salt, and pepper. Let cool about 5 minutes before covering and refrigerating up to 7 days.

3. To serve, remove from refrigerator and cook in microwave in 30-second intervals until heated through.

PER SERVING Calories: 142 | Fat: 11.3 g | Protein: 2.4 g | Sodium: 703 mg | Fiber: 0.5 g | Carbohydrates: 10.5 g | Sugar: 0.8 g

Vegan Spinach Artichoke Dip

This savory Vegan Spinach Artichoke Dip is easy to make and delivers a tasty, creamy appetizer perfect with chips or crackers. Best served hot, this cheesy dip is ready to go in just 30 minutes with a few ingredients!

INGREDIENTS | SERVES 6

¼ cup vegan butter

1 small yellow onion, peeled and chopped

½ cup all-purpose flour

2 cups water

1 tablespoon soy sauce

1 teaspoon garlic powder

¼ cup nutritional yeast flakes

½ teaspoon salt

2 cups vegan mozzarella shreds

2 cups chopped fresh spinach

1 (7.5-ounce) can artichoke hearts, drained

What Are Nutritional Yeast Flakes?

Nutritional yeast flakes, sometimes referred to as "nooch," are bright yellow flakes that can be found in the bulk section of many health food stores. They are a dried form of yeast that add a savory, cheesy flavor to recipes. You can also use these flakes in place of Parmesan cheese to sprinkle over things like popcorn and chips.

1. In a small saucepan add vegan butter and cook onions over medium heat about 5 minutes, until onions are translucent. Add flour and stir until a paste forms.

2. Place water in a small microwave-safe bowl and heat 2 minutes until hot. Pour hot water 1 cup at a time into saucepan, stirring in between until all ingredients are incorporated. Stir in soy sauce, garlic powder, nutritional yeast flakes, and salt.

3. Add vegan mozzarella. Stir mixture and then turn up heat to medium-high. Cook 10 minutes until cheese melts.

4. Once cheese has melted add spinach and artichoke hearts. Stir to combine and place lid on saucepan until spinach has wilted, about 5 minutes. Remove from heat and allow to cool about 10 minutes.

5. Transfer to a large lidded container. Store in refrigerator up to 7 days or freezer up to 2 months. To serve, cook in microwave in 30-second intervals until heated through.

PER SERVING Calories: 217 | Fat: 11.3 g | Protein: 4.7 g | Sodium: 929 mg | Fiber: 3.2 g | Carbohydrates: 21.4 g | Sugar: 0.9 g

Vegan Seven-Layer Dip

Nothing beats the presentation of this Vegan Seven-Layer Dip, with layers of black beans, seasoned "meat" crumbles, vegan Cheddar shreds, and more. It's easy to make and full of flavor!

INGREDIENTS | SERVES 10

1 (12-ounce) package vegan meat crumbles

1 tablespoon olive oil

3 tablespoons taco seasoning

1 (15-ounce) can black beans, rinsed and drained

1½ cups mild chunky salsa, divided

2 cups vegan Cheddar shreds

1 cup vegan sour cream

1 cup guacamole

1 (2.25-ounce) can black olives, chopped

½ cup chopped tomatoes

½ cup chopped green onion

DIY Taco Seasoning

It's very easy to make your own taco seasoning! Simply combine 1 tablespoon chili powder with ¼ teaspoon each of garlic powder, dehydrated onions, crushed red pepper flakes, dried oregano, and ground turmeric. Then add 1 teaspoon each of paprika and ground cumin, followed by salt and pepper to taste.

1. In a large skillet, brown vegan meat crumbles in olive oil over medium heat about 5 minutes. Add taco seasoning. Set aside to cool to room temperature, about 5 minutes.

2. Place beans in a blender or food processor with ½ cup salsa. Blend about 20 seconds until beans are consistency of refried beans.

3. Spread beans into bottom of a large serving tray that is about 1½" deep. Sprinkle shredded cheese on top of beans. Sprinkle vegan meat crumbles on top of cheese. Carefully spread sour cream on top of vegan crumbles, then spread guacamole on top of sour cream. Pour remaining salsa over guacamole and spread evenly. Sprinkle with olives. Garnish with tomatoes and green onions. Cover and refrigerate up to 3 days.

PER SERVING Calories: 325 | Fat: 19.8 g | Protein: 11.9 g | Sodium: 1,275 mg | Fiber: 9.9 g | Carbohydrates: 27.0 g | Sugar: 4.0 g

Chocolate Chip Peanut Butter Dip

This easy Chocolate Chip Peanut Butter Dip is made with wholesome ingredients, and is also flavorful thanks to the delicious combination of peanut butter and chocolate chips. Serve with vanilla wafers for dipping.

INGREDIENTS | MAKES 3 CUPS

1 (15-ounce) can chickpeas, rinsed and drained
¾ cup creamy peanut butter
½ cup agave nectar
1 teaspoon vanilla extract
3 tablespoons filtered water
1 cup dairy-free chocolate chips

1. Pour all ingredients except chocolate chips into bowl of a food processor.

2. Pulse 3 seconds. Use a spatula to push down ingredients from sides of bowl. Pulse an additional 40 seconds.

3. Transfer to a small lidded container and stir in chocolate chips. Store in refrigerator up to 5 days.

PER SERVING (2 tbsp) Calories: 310 | Fat: 17.8 g | Protein: 6.6 g | Sodium: 51 mg | Fiber: 4.0 g | Carbohydrates: 30.8 g | Sugar: 20.1 g

Air-Fried Tofu

Crispy, fried tofu is a protein-rich, delicious addition to many of your favorite meals. Serve with rice or steamed vegetables and a simple sauce, add it to salads, or even enjoy it plain with a favorite dipping sauce.

INGREDIENTS | SERVES 4

1 (15-ounce) package extra-firm tofu, pressed and cut into ½" cubes
2 teaspoons olive oil
¼ teaspoon salt

1. Preheat air fryer to 375°F and set timer for 18 minutes. Allow air fryer to heat up 30 seconds. Remove fryer basket and spray with vegetable cooking spray. Add tofu cubes and olive oil. Toss to coat, then place basket back in air fryer.

2. Every 5 minutes, remove basket and stir tofu by shaking basket carefully. Cook until timer goes off and tofu is crispy. Remove from basket and sprinkle with salt.

3. Let cool 10 minutes, then transfer tofu to a large sealed container and refrigerate up to 5 days.

4. To serve, reheat tofu in the air fryer heated at 350°F for 5 minutes.

PER SERVING Calories: 155 | Fat: 8.0 g | Protein: 10.8 g | Sodium: 238 mg | Fiber: 0.6 g | Carbohydrates: 11.4 g | Sugar: 1.8 g

Green Chili Hummus with Salsa

Enjoy this tasty twist on the classic hummus recipe. The savory hummus combines perfectly with the fresh salsa poured over the top! Serve with chips, crackers, or vegetables.

INGREDIENTS | SERVES 12

1 (15-ounce) can chickpeas, rinsed and drained

2 tablespoons tahini

2 tablespoons nutritional yeast flakes

2 teaspoons garlic powder

1 (4-ounce) can green chilies

½ cup fresh spinach

1 (8-ounce) jar mild chunky salsa

1. Combine chickpeas, tahini, nutritional yeast flakes, garlic powder, green chilies, and spinach in a food processor. Pulse 3 seconds until coarse and crumbly.

2. Place a colander over a bowl and pour salsa into colander to strain liquid.

3. Add liquid 1 tablespoon at a time to food processor and pulse until a spreadable consistency is reached.

4. Spoon hummus into a small serving dish and top with strained salsa.

5. Cover and keep refrigerated until ready to serve (up to 4 days). Alternatively, it can be frozen up to 1 month.

6. To serve, allow to sit at room temperature until spreadable, about 30 minutes.

PER SERVING Calories: 67 | Fat: 1.9 g | Protein: 3.4 g | Sodium: 265 mg | Fiber: 2.8 g | Carbohydrates: 9.7 g | Sugar: 2.0 g

Crostini with Pecan Basil Pesto

This savory Crostini with Pecan Basil Pesto makes a perfect appetizer to share with guests, take to parties, or even serve at home. It's an easy, tasty addition to your vegan kitchen.

INGREDIENTS | MAKES 24 CROSTINI

⅓ cup pecans

1 cup fresh spinach

⅓ cup olive oil

2 teaspoons vegan Parmesan

1 teaspoon garlic powder

5 fresh basil leaves

1 baguette, sliced into 24 (½"-thick) slices

Leaving the Dairy Out of Pesto

You may think dairy is required to make a good pesto. However, you can buy vegan Parmesan to replace the dairy in pesto and other Italian dishes. Alternatively, you can sub nutritional yeast flakes for the Parmesan.

1. Preheat oven to 350°F with rack in middle. Place pecans on an ungreased baking sheet and toast in oven about 5 minutes. Remove and cool about 2 minutes.

2. Place cooled pecans, spinach, olive oil, vegan Parmesan, garlic powder, and basil leaves in a food processor. Pulse 3 seconds to combine. Transfer to a small lidded container and refrigerate up to 5 days.

3. Arrange bread slices in one layer on a large ungreased baking sheet. Place in oven and toast about 5 minutes. Remove from oven and cool about 5 minutes, then transfer to a medium sealed container and refrigerate up to 3 days.

4. To serve, wrap toast with foil and heat in toaster oven at 350°F for 5 minutes, until heated through. Top with Pecan Basil Pesto.

PER SERVING (1 crostini) Calories: 65 | Fat: 4.1 g | Protein: 1.3 g | Sodium: 67 mg | Fiber: 0.4 g | Carbohydrates: 5.8 g | Sugar: 0.5 g

Baked Cauliflower Wings

These savory vegan Baked Cauliflower Wings are a delicious, satisfying snack for game day—or any day!

INGREDIENTS | SERVES 6

½ cup unsweetened almond milk
½ cup water
½ cup all-purpose flour
1 teaspoon garlic powder
1 teaspoon paprika
4 cups small cauliflower florets
1 cup store-bought wing sauce
1 tablespoon refined coconut oil

1. Preheat oven to 425°F. Line two baking sheets with parchment paper.

2. Mix almond milk, water, flour, garlic powder, and paprika in a medium bowl. Batter should be thick. Dip cauliflower florets into batter, letting excess drip off over bowl, then place on prepared baking sheets. Repeat until all cauliflower is coated and in a single layer on baking sheets.

3. Bake 20 minutes, using tongs to flip each piece halfway through baking.

4. In a small microwave-safe bowl combine wing sauce and coconut oil. Microwave 30 seconds until coconut oil begins to melt. Stir.

5. Once cauliflower is done, remove from oven and set aside until cooled enough to handle, about 5 minutes. Dip cauliflower pieces in prepared hot sauce, then place back on baking sheets and return to oven.

6. Bake another 10 minutes. Remove from oven and cool 10 minutes. Place in a large sealed container and refrigerate up to 3 days.

7. To serve, preheat oven to 300°F and cook on an ungreased baking sheet 10 minutes until heated through.

PER SERVING Calories: 147 | Fat: 8.0 g | Protein: 2.7 g | Sodium: 783 mg | Fiber: 2.0 g | Carbohydrates: 14.9 g | Sugar: 1.5 g

Black-Eyed Pea Dip

Some people believe that eating this dip on New Year's Day will bring a prosperous new year.

INGREDIENTS | SERVES 6

1 (15-ounce) can blackeye peas, drained

3 tablespoons finely chopped peeled yellow onion

¼ cup vegan sour cream

½ (8-ounce) jar mild chunky salsa

1 cup vegan Cheddar shreds

1. Preheat oven to 350°F.

2. Place blackeye peas in an ungreased 8" × 8" casserole dish and use a fork to mash up most of beans.

3. Add in onions, sour cream, salsa, and ½ vegan Cheddar shreds. Stir to combine. Top mixture with remaining vegan Cheddar shreds.

4. Bake 25 minutes until top cheese layer melts. Remove from oven and allow to cool 15 minutes.

5. Transfer dip to a large sealable container and refrigerate up to 5 days. To serve, cook in microwave in 30-second intervals until heated through.

PER SERVING Calories: 85 | Fat: 2.0 g | Protein: 3.4 g | Sodium: 280 mg | Fiber: 3.3 g | Carbohydrates: 12.9 g | Sugar: 1.5 g

Caramelized Onion Hummus

Onions sautéed in olive oil add a sweet, tender flavor to this creamy Caramelized Onion Hummus. It's a tasty dip made with minimal ingredients!

INGREDIENTS | SERVES 10

1 small yellow onion, peeled and thinly sliced

3 tablespoons olive oil, divided

1 teaspoon agave nectar

1 (15-ounce) can chickpeas, rinsed and drained

¼ cup pine nuts

3 tablespoons lime juice

½ teaspoon dried basil

1 tablespoon nutritional yeast flakes

1 clove garlic, peeled

1. Place a medium skillet over medium heat and add onions. Drizzle with 1 tablespoon olive oil. Cook until tender, about 5 minutes. Then add agave nectar and continue cooking about 10 minutes, until caramelized. Remove from heat and set aside.

2. Add chickpeas into a food processor with pine nuts and pulse 5 seconds. Add remaining tablespoons olive oil, lime juice, basil, nutritional yeast flakes, garlic, and ½ caramelized onions. Pulse 3 seconds until smooth. Top with remaining caramelized onions. Transfer to a medium lidded container and refrigerate up to 5 days.

PER SERVING Calories: 103 | Fat: 6.4 g | Protein: 2.7 g | Sodium: 57 mg | Fiber: 2.0 g | Carbohydrates: 8.3 g | Sugar: 2.0 g

Spicy Roasted Chickpeas

These seasoned, crispy roasted chickpeas make for a satisfying treat to enjoy over salads, in lunches, and even as a snack on their own.

INGREDIENTS | SERVES 4

1 (15-ounce) can chickpeas, drained and patted dry

1½ teaspoons olive oil

1 tablespoon Southwest Chipotle seasoning

½ teaspoon salt

⅛ teaspoon ground black pepper

1. Preheat oven to 400°F. Line a 9" × 13" baking pan with parchment paper.

2. Add chickpeas and olive oil to a medium bowl and stir until each chickpea is coated with oil. Place chickpeas on prepared pan.

3. Bake 25 minutes until chickpeas are crispy on outside.

4. Remove from oven and sprinkle seasoning over top. Stir until thoroughly coated. Sprinkle with salt and pepper. Let cool 10 minutes, then transfer to a small sealed container and refrigerate up to 5 days.

PER SERVING Calories: 106 | Fat: 2.7 g | Protein: 4.7 g | Sodium: 551 mg | Fiber: 4.2 g | Carbohydrates: 15.3 g | Sugar: 2.7 g

Southwestern Hummus

Southwestern Hummus is a gluten-free appetizer that's easy to throw together and will be enjoyed by everyone, even picky, non-vegan dieters!

INGREDIENTS | SERVES 10

1 (15-ounce) can chickpeas, rinsed and drained

¼ cup tahini

¼ cup lime juice

1 cup mild chunky salsa

1 tablespoon Southwest Chipotle seasoning

1. Pour all ingredients in bowl of food processor and pulse 3 seconds. Use a spatula to scrape down any ingredients on side of bowl. Pulse again until consistency is smooth.

2. Transfer to a small sealed container and refrigerate up to 5 days.

PER SERVING Calories: 88 | Fat: 3.2 g | Protein: 3.0 g | Sodium: 292 mg | Fiber: 2.6 g | Carbohydrates: 10.6 g | Sugar: 2.8 g

Vegan Bacon Ricotta Crostini

Vegan Bacon Ricotta Crostini is a savory experience of toasted bread, creamy cashew ricotta, crispy vegan bacon, and drizzles of maple syrup.

INGREDIENTS | MAKES 24 CROSTINI

1 baguette, cut into 24 slices
1 tablespoon olive oil
1 clove garlic, peeled and chopped
8 slices vegan bacon
1 cup cashews, soaked overnight in water, and drained
½ cup unsweetened almond milk
1 tablespoon nutritional yeast flakes
1 teaspoon dried basil
1 tablespoon mild miso paste
¼ cup maple syrup

1. Preheat oven to 375°F. Line a baking sheet with parchment paper.

2. Place baguette slices on prepared baking sheet and bake 10 minutes until toasted. Transfer to a large sealable bag and refrigerate up to 5 days.

3. Place a medium skillet over medium heat. Add olive oil and garlic. Cook 1 minute, then transfer to bowl of a food processor. Set aside.

4. In same skillet, cook vegan bacon 3 minutes per side. Color will become a darker red and may even have some dark brown or black edges. Remove from skillet and set aside to cool about 5 minutes, then break into pieces.

5. Add soaked cashews, almond milk, nutritional yeast flakes, basil, and miso paste to bowl of food processor. Pulse 3 seconds. Use a spatula to scrape sides of bowl. Repeat process until mixture is smooth and leaves no large pieces of cashews.

6. Transfer to a medium sealable container and refrigerate up to 5 days. To serve, top each piece of toasted crostini with one dollop cashew ricotta, followed by divided-out vegan bacon pieces and maple syrup. Toast in toaster oven at 300°F for 5 minutes until crispy.

PER SERVING (1 crostini) Calories: 86 | Fat: 4.1 g | Protein: 2.5 g | Sodium: 136 mg | Fiber: 0.6 g | Carbohydrates: 10.2 g | Sugar: 2.9 g

Vegan Beer Brats in a Blanket

These savory Vegan Beer Brats in a Blanket are the perfect comfort food. Vegan brats are simmered in beer, then cooked in a delicious crescent roll stuffed with sauerkraut and vegan cheese.

INGREDIENTS | MAKES 8 ROLLS

¼ cup yellow mustard

1 tablespoon agave nectar

1 (12-ounce) bottle pale lager beer

4 vegan brats

8 dairy-free crescent rolls

1 cup dill and garlic sauerkraut

1 cup vegan mozzarella cheese

4 slices vegan bacon, halved

1. Preheat oven to 350°F and line a baking sheet with parchment paper.

2. Combine mustard and agave nectar in a small lidded bowl. Cover and refrigerate up to 7 days.

3. Pour beer into a medium saucepan and bring to a boil over medium heat. Add brats and cook 7 minutes. Once done, transfer to a cutting board and cut each brat in half. Set aside.

4. Arrange dough pieces on prepared baking sheet, adding sauerkraut and vegan cheese evenly over each.

5. Wrap each brat piece in ½ slice vegan bacon. Place on piece of dough. Wrap dough tightly around each brat and pinch to seal dough. Bake 15 minutes.

6. Let rolls cool 10 minutes, then transfer to a large lidded container and refrigerate up to 5 days. To serve, remove from refrigerator and heat in microwave in 30-second intervals until heated through. Pour mustard sauce over each roll.

PER SERVING (1 roll) Calories: 297 | Fat: 17.8 g | Protein: 15.0 g | Sodium: 911 mg | Fiber: 1.5 g | Carbohydrates: 22.1 g | Sugar: 5.1 g

Baked Jalapeño Poppers

Transform a favorite sports bar appetizer into a vegan delight. You'll love these vegan Baked Jalapeño Poppers because they're easy to make and oh-so-tasty to eat.

INGREDIENTS | MAKES 20 POPPERS

½ (8-ounce) container dairy-free cream cheese, softened

½ (14.2-ounce) container Daiya Jalapeño Garlic Havarti Style Wedge, shredded

¾ cup + 1 tablespoon plain soy milk, divided

⅛ teaspoon garlic powder

½ teaspoon salt

10 jalapeños, halved and seeded

2 tablespoons ground flaxseed

½ cup all-purpose flour

½ cup bread crumbs

Cooking with Jalapeños

Jalapeños, like most peppers, add lots of flavor to your dishes. But there are some tricks to working with them. Be sure not to touch cut jalapeños with your bare hands or else you'll be feeling the burn later if you accidentally touch sensitive areas of your body. Most professionals recommend wearing gloves when cutting jalapeños and removing the seeds to reduce the heat in your recipe.

1. Preheat oven to 350°F. Spray a baking sheet with vegetable cooking spray.

2. Place vegan cream cheese, shredded vegan cheese, 1 tablespoon soy milk, garlic powder, and salt in a medium bowl and stir until well combined. Stuff each halved jalapeño with an even amount cream cheese mixture.

3. In a separate medium bowl combine flaxseed and remaining soy milk. Set aside.

4. Pour flour into a small dish and bread crumbs into another. Set aside.

5. Roll a stuffed jalapeño in flour, then dip in flaxseed mixture, followed by a final dip in bread crumbs. Place breaded popper on prepared pan and repeat dipping process with remaining stuffed jalapeños. Bake 30 minutes until crumbs are golden brown.

6. Remove from oven and let cool about 5 minutes. Transfer to a large sealed container and refrigerate up to 5 days. To serve, heat in a toaster oven at 350°F for about 5 minutes.

PER SERVING (1 popper) Calories: 52 | Fat: 3.1 g | Protein: 1.2 g | Sodium: 149 mg | Fiber: 0.7 g | Carbohydrates: 5.2 g | Sugar: 0.4 g

Vegan Spinach Cheese Pinwheels

This flaky puff pastry appetizer is made with a vegan cheesy spinach filling.
Believe it or not, this is an easy dish to make—and fun to eat!

INGREDIENTS | MAKES 24 PINWHEELS

½ cup shredded vegan jack cheese

¼ cup vegan Parmesan cheese

2 tablespoons chopped green onion

¼ teaspoon garlic powder

½ teaspoon salt

¼ cup all-purpose flour

1 Pepperidge Farm Puff Pastry Sheet

1 tablespoon vegan butter, melted

1 tablespoon plain soy milk

1 (10-ounce) package frozen chopped spinach, thawed and drained

1. In a medium bowl stir together vegan cheeses, green onions, garlic powder, and salt.

2. Prepare a work area by sprinkling with flour. Lay out pastry sheet on floured surface. Stir together melted vegan butter and soy milk in a small bowl and brush over top of pastry sheet, reserving remaining mixture.

3. Spread cheese mixture over buttered pastry sheet, then spread drained spinach over cheese mixture.

4. Begin with side closest to you and roll pastry sheet, wrapping ingredients in as you roll. Wrap pastry roll in aluminum foil and freeze about 30 minutes.

5. Preheat oven to 400°F. Grease a baking sheet with vegetable cooking spray.

6. Use a serrated knife to cut pastry roll into ½" slices. Place slices on prepared pan and brush with reserved butter mixture.

7. Bake 20 minutes until pinwheels are a golden color.

8. Remove from oven and let cool about 5 minutes before transferring to a large sealed container. Refrigerate up to 5 days. To serve, cook in a toaster oven at 350°F until heated through, about 5 minutes.

PER SERVING (1 pinwheel) Calories: 33 | Fat: 1.7 g | Protein: 0.8 g | Sodium: 112 mg | Fiber: 0.5 g | Carbohydrates: 3.5 g | Sugar: 0.1 g

Cocktail Lentil Meatballs

These baked lentil meatballs are served with lots of savory sweet sauce. Serve this recipe at your next party or family dinner. They're sure to be a hit!

INGREDIENTS | MAKES 36 MEATBALLS

1 cup chopped peeled yellow onion
1 cup dried brown lentils
3 cups water
1 cup extra-firm tofu, pressed
2 tablespoons ground flaxseed, divided
1¼ cups rolled oats, divided
1 tablespoon cashews
2 teaspoons Better Than Bouillon Seasoned Vegetable Base
1 tablespoon nutritional yeast flakes
1 teaspoon rubbed sage
¼ teaspoon ground turmeric
1 teaspoon paprika
¾ cup grape jelly
1½ cups ketchup
1 teaspoon sriracha

1. Add onions, lentils, and water to a small saucepan. Bring to a boil over high heat, then reduce heat to low, cover, and cook 25 minutes. Strain excess liquid and set aside.

2. In a food processor add tofu, 1 tablespoon flaxseed, ½ cup rolled oats, cashews, Better Than Bouillon, nutritional yeast flakes, sage, turmeric, and paprika. Pulse until combined.

3. Add 2 cups strained lentil mixture to tofu mixture. Pulse to combine. Add remaining lentil mixture and use a spatula to stir. Add remaining flaxseed and oats and stir to combine. Set aside about 5 minutes to allow mixture to thicken.

4. Preheat oven to 375°F. Line two baking sheets with parchment paper.

5. Use a cookie dough scoop to measure consistent portions from mixture. Form into balls.

6. Place lentil meatballs on prepared pans, allowing some space between them.

7. Bake 25 minutes, turning over once, halfway through bake. When lentil meatballs are done, remove from oven and let cool about 10 minutes.

8. To prepare sauce, combine grape jelly, ketchup, and sriracha in a large microwave-safe bowl. Heat in microwave 30 seconds then stir. Repeat heating until jelly has melted and a sauce forms. Add meatballs to sauce, stirring gently to coat.

9. Transfer meatballs to a large lidded container and refrigerate up to 5 days, or freeze up to 2 months.

PER SERVING (1 meatball) Calories: 35 | Fat: 1.1 g | Protein: 2.4 g | Sodium: 43 mg | Fiber: 1.2 g | Carbohydrates: 4.4 g | Sugar: 0.4 g

Carrot Hummus

A savory dip made of carrots, spices, and chickpeas, this Carrot Hummus is perfect served with chips or used as a condiment on your favorite sandwiches and wraps.

INGREDIENTS | SERVES 10

1 (15-ounce) can chickpeas, rinsed and drained

1 cup roughly chopped peeled carrots

1 tablespoon balsamic vinegar

2 teaspoons garlic powder

½ teaspoon ground cumin

½ teaspoon ground turmeric

1 teaspoon dried basil

1 tablespoon tamari

2 tablespoons all-natural peanut butter

4 tablespoons water

2 tablespoons olive oil

1. Place all ingredients except water and olive oil in a food processor and pulse until combined. Remove lid and stir ingredients, adding water 1 tablespoon at a time until desired consistency is reached.

2. Transfer to a medium lidded container and refrigerate up to 7 days. To serve, drizzle olive oil on top of hummus.

PER SERVING Calories: 89 | Fat: 4.7 g | Protein: 2.9 g | Sodium: 66 mg | Fiber: 2.3 g | Carbohydrates: 8.9 g | Sugar: 2.3 g

Vegan Cheesy Popcorn

This is the best microwave popcorn with a vegan twist. It's butter-free, healthy, and oh-so-delicious! Make extra and store up to 3 days at room temperature.

INGREDIENTS | SERVES 2

⅓ cup popcorn kernels

2 teaspoons nutritional yeast flakes

1 teaspoon paprika

½ teaspoon ground turmeric

⅛ teaspoon salt

1. Place popcorn kernels in a microwave popcorn popper. Place lid on container and microwave about 3 minutes.

2. Place nutritional yeast flakes, paprika, and turmeric in a small bowl. Stir to combine.

3. Use oven mitts to remove popcorn popper from microwave, then carefully remove lid.

4. Pour popcorn into a large sealable container, removing unpopped kernels. Spray popcorn generously with vegetable cooking spray. Sprinkle nutritional yeast mixture and salt over top and use your hands or a spoon to distribute seasonings evenly throughout popcorn.

PER SERVING Calories: 134 | Fat: 1.5 g | Protein: 4.5 g | Sodium: 147 mg | Fiber: 4.4 g | Carbohydrates: 24.7 g | Sugar: 0.1 g

Easy Vegan Rangoon Dip

Rich and creamy, this Rangoon dip tastes just like the crab Rangoon from your favorite Asian restaurant, but is vegan! It's ready in around 20 minutes. Serve this dip with chips.

INGREDIENTS | SERVES 10

1 cup Frank's RedHot Sweet Chili Sauce

1 (15-ounce) container extra-firm tofu, pressed and cut into ½" cubes

1 (8-ounce) container vegan cream cheese, divided

1 green onion, chopped

About 10 tortilla chips, crushed

1. Preheat oven to 350°F.

2. Pour sauce in a medium skillet over medium heat. Add tofu and allow to simmer in sauce 3 minutes. Be sure to stir tofu well while cooking. Use a spatula to break up tofu more.

3. Add 2 tablespoons cream cheese to tofu mixture and stir to incorporate. Remove from heat and set aside.

4. Spread remaining cream cheese in bottom of a 1.5-quart casserole dish. Top with green onions. Pour tofu and sauce over cream cheese and top with crushed tortilla chip pieces.

5. Bake 25 minutes, then remove from oven and let cool about 10 minutes.

6. Cover and refrigerate up to 7 days. To serve, let sit until room temperature or heat in microwave in 30-second intervals until heated through.

PER SERVING Calories: 177 | Fat: 8.9 g | Protein: 5.2 g | Sodium: 554 mg | Fiber: 0.3 g | Carbohydrates: 20.3 g | Sugar: 11.5 g

CHAPTER 15

Bars, Bites, and Cookies

Healthy Blueberry Crumble Bars

These Healthy Blueberry Crumble Bars are made with healthy oats, a gluten-free crumble, and a generous layer of blueberry filling. Enjoy for breakfast or dessert!

INGREDIENTS | MAKES 9 BARS

For Blueberry Filling
3 cups fresh blueberries
½ cup water
¼ cup cornstarch
1 teaspoon lemon juice
⅓ cup agave nectar
2 tablespoons chia seeds

For Bars
1½ cups rolled oats
2 cups almond meal
1 tablespoon ground flax meal
½ teaspoon baking powder
¼ teaspoon salt
⅓ cup agave nectar
¼ cup almond butter
½ cup unsweetened almond milk
1 teaspoon vanilla extract

1. Preheat oven to 350°F. Spray a 9" square baking dish with vegetable cooking spray.

2. **To make Blueberry Filling:** place blueberries in a small saucepan over medium-high heat. Stir together water and cornstarch in a small bowl, then add to blueberries. Stir gently to combine. Bring to a boil, then reduce heat to medium and simmer 5 minutes, stirring occasionally. Remove from heat and stir in lemon juice and ⅓ cup agave nectar and chia seeds. Transfer to a small covered bowl and refrigerate during next steps.

3. **To make Bars:** combine oats, almond meal, flax meal, baking powder, and salt in a medium bowl. Move ingredients to one side of bowl. In other half of bowl combine remaining ⅓ cup agave nectar, almond butter, almond milk, and vanilla. Stir wet and dry ingredients together.

4. Press ¾ oats mixture evenly across bottom of prepared pan. Set rest of batter aside.

Place crust in oven and bake 15 minutes. Remove from oven.

5. Spread thickened blueberry sauce over baked crust. Place dollops of remaining crust batter over blueberry filling and spread evenly. Return to oven and bake 15 minutes until top crust turns golden brown.

6. Remove from oven and set aside to cool about 15 minutes before covering and refrigerating at least one hour to allow filling to set completely.

7. Cut into bars and refrigerate in a large sealable container up to 7 days or freeze up to two months. Serve cold, or cook in microwave in 30-second intervals until heated through.

PER SERVING (1 bar) Calories: 358 | Fat: 18.3 g | Protein: 10.1 g | Sodium: 103 mg | Fiber: 7.4 g | Carbohydrates: 41.6 g | Sugar: 17.6 g

Chocolate Peanut Butter Rice Crispy Bars

These vegan Chocolate Peanut Butter Rice Crispy Bars combine the ultimate indulgent flavors (chocolate and peanut butter) in a delightful crispy treat. They are perfect for any occasion.

INGREDIENTS | MAKES 12 BARS

½ cup corn syrup

¼ cup granulated sugar

¼ cup packed light brown sugar

1½ cups creamy peanut butter, divided

½ cup cocoa powder

3 cups crispy rice cereal

1 (8-ounce) container vegan cream cheese

½ cup powdered sugar

2 cups dairy-free chocolate chips

2 tablespoons vegan butter

3 tablespoons unsweetened almond milk

1. Prepare a 9" square cake pan by greasing with vegetable cooking spray.

2. Combine corn syrup, granulated sugar, and brown sugar in a large saucepan over low heat and cover 3 minutes until mixture melts. Stir until smooth. Remove from heat and add ½ cup peanut butter and cocoa powder and stir until combined. Pour in rice cereal and stir until evenly coated.

3. Spread coated rice mixture into prepared pan. Set aside.

4. In a small microwave-safe bowl combine vegan cream cheese and remaining 1 cup peanut butter. Heat about 30 seconds, then stir to combine. Add powdered sugar and stir until combined. Spread cream cheese mixture over rice crispy layer in baking pan.

5. Combine chocolate chips and vegan butter in a small microwave-safe bowl. Cook in 30-second increments, stirring after each cook time, until chocolate chips are melted. Add almond milk, 1 tablespoon at a time, stirring in between each tablespoon. Spread over peanut butter layer in prepared pan.

6. Cover pan and set aside at room temperature 1 hour to set.

7. Slice into bars, then re-cover and store at room temperature up to 5 days or freeze up to 2 months.

PER SERVING (1 bar) Calories: 447 | Fat: 26.6 g | Protein: 7.6 g | Sodium: 161 mg | Fiber: 4.2 g | Carbohydrates: 47.8 g | Sugar: 32.8 g

Sugar Cookie Bars

These Sugar Cookie Bars boast a moist cookie crust with a sweet raspberry-infused frosting. Sprinkles are not required, but are encouraged.

INGREDIENTS | MAKES 30 BARS

1½ cups vegan butter, softened to room temperature, divided
1½ cups granulated sugar
1 (8-ounce) package vegan cream cheese, divided
1 tablespoon ground flaxseed
2 tablespoons cornstarch
6 tablespoons plain soy milk, divided
1 teaspoon apple cider vinegar
2 teaspoons raspberry extract, divided
½ teaspoon almond extract
½ cup fresh raspberries, smashed, divided
2½ cups all-purpose flour
½ teaspoon salt
1 teaspoon baking powder
½ teaspoon baking soda
3½ cups powdered sugar

1. Preheat oven to 350°F. Lightly grease a 9" × 13" cake pan with vegetable cooking spray.

2. Beat together 1 cup vegan butter and sugar in a large bowl until creamy, approximately 2 minutes. Add all but 2 tablespoons vegan cream cheese, ground flaxseed, cornstarch, 4 tablespoons soy milk, vinegar, 1 teaspoon raspberry extract, and almond extract. Mix again until all ingredients are combined and batter is light and fluffy. Add smashed raspberries, reserving 1 tablespoon. Stir to combine. Set aside.

3. In a separate large bowl stir together flour, salt, baking powder, and baking soda. Using electric mixer on low speed, gradually blend flour mixture into butter mixture until well combined. Press batter into prepared pan.

4. Bake 25 minutes until top is golden brown and a toothpick inserted in center comes out clean. When done, remove pan from oven and set aside to cool about 20 minutes.

5. Add ½ cup vegan butter and remaining 2 tablespoons cream cheese to a large bowl. Using mixer, beat on medium-high until smooth and fluffy, about 1 minute.

6. Add powdered sugar, reserved raspberries, and remaining raspberry extract. Beat again until combined. Mix in remaining 2 tablespoons soy milk, 1 tablespoon at a time, until a spreadable consistency is reached.

7. Top cooled cookie bars with raspberry cream frosting, then cut into bars. Cover and refrigerate up to 10 days or freeze up to 2 months.

PER SERVING (1 bar) Calories: 191 | Fat: 6.2 g | Protein: 1.5 g | Sodium: 208 mg | Fiber: 0.5 g | Carbohydrates: 21.2 g | Sugar: 21.6 g

Luscious Lemon Bars

Enjoy these Luscious Lemon Bars as a light and delicious treat. You'll love the classic lemon flavor served up in a vegan recipe!

INGREDIENTS | MAKES 9 BARS

½ cup vegan butter, softened
1 cup lightly packed light brown sugar
¾ cup all-purpose flour
¾ cup whole-wheat flour
½ teaspoon salt
1 teaspoon baking powder
1 cup rolled oats
1¼ cups vegan sweetened condensed milk
½ cup lemon juice
1 tablespoon lemon zest

Homemade Sweetened Condensed Milk

You can make your own nondairy sweetened condensed milk by combining 1 cup almond milk with ½ cup sugar and 1 tablespoon cornstarch in a large microwave-safe bowl. Microwave mixture in 30-second intervals, stirring in between each cook time, until thickened.

1. Preheat oven to 350°F. Line bottom of a 9" × 13" cake pan with parchment paper.

2. In a large bowl mix together vegan butter and brown sugar until well combined.

3. In a medium bowl stir together both flours, salt, and baking powder. Add to butter mixture, along with oats, and mix to combine. Press ½ mixture into bottom of prepared pan.

4. Mix together condensed milk, lemon juice, and lemon zest in a medium bowl. Spread onto crumb mixture in pan. Top with remaining crumb mixture, but don't press down.

5. Bake 25 minutes until crumble is golden brown.

6. Allow pan to sit on counter 30 minutes, then cover and refrigerate 1 hour.

7. Cut into bars and refrigerate up to 7 days, or freeze up to 2 months.

PER SERVING (1 bar) Calories: 377 | Fat: 9.4 g | Protein: 4.0 g | Sodium: 287 mg | Fiber: 2.6 g | Carbohydrates: 69.3 g | Sugar: 44.4 g

Strawberry Chocolate Dessert Bars

Enjoy heavenly layers of strawberry and chocolate with these deliciously simple Strawberry Chocolate Dessert Bars. This is a rich recipe perfect for sharing.

INGREDIENTS | MAKES 24 BARS

1 cup + 2 tablespoons unsweetened almond milk, divided

1 tablespoon cornstarch

1 tablespoon ground flaxseed

1 (15-ounce) can chickpeas, rinsed and drained

½ cup vegetable oil

1 box Duncan Hines Classic Dark Chocolate Fudge Cake Mix

1 cup dairy-free chocolate chips, divided

1 box Duncan Hines Signature Strawberry Supreme Cake Mix

4 tablespoons multicolored sprinkles, divided

1 cup pecans, chopped

1 cup powdered sugar

¼ teaspoon raspberry extract

1. Preheat oven to 350°F and grease a 9" × 13" cake pan with vegetable cooking spray.

2. Add 1 cup almond milk, cornstarch, flaxseed, chickpeas, and oil in bowl of a food processor. Pulse until smooth, up to 1 minute.

3. Pour chocolate cake mix into a large bowl. Add ½ chickpea mixture to bowl and stir to combine. Press mixture into bottom of prepared pan and sprinkle ½ chocolate chips over top.

4. Rinse out bowl and dry, then pour in strawberry cake mix and remaining ½ chickpea mixture. Stir to combine. Gently press over top of chocolate layer. Sprinkle with two tablespoons sprinkles, pecans, and remaining chocolate chips.

5. Bake 50 minutes. Remove from oven and set aside to cool.

6. Place powdered sugar in a small bowl. Add 2 tablespoons almond milk, 1 tablespoon at a time, until mixture has reached desired drizzling consistency. Add raspberry extract. Stir to combine. Drizzle over cooled dessert bar mixture and top with remaining sprinkles.

7. Cover and refrigerate up to 7 days or freeze up to 2 months. To serve, cut into bars and allow time to come to room temperature.

PER SERVING (1 bar) Calories: 311 | Fat: 14.7 g | Protein: 2.8 g | Sodium: 395 mg | Fiber: 1.9 g | Carbohydrates: 43.0 g | Sugar: 26.1 g

Caramel Chocolate Chip Cookie Bars

These ooey gooey Caramel Chocolate Chip Cookie Bars boast a flavorful base topped with a delightfully creamy vegan caramel sauce.

INGREDIENTS | MAKES 12 BARS

½ cup + 1 tablespoon vegan butter, softened, divided

½ cup creamy peanut butter

1 cup light brown sugar, divided

½ cup granulated sugar

1 tablespoon vanilla extract

1 tablespoon ground flaxseed

1 tablespoon cornstarch

4 tablespoons water

½ cup + 3 tablespoons unsweetened almond milk, divided

2¼ cups all-purpose flour

1 teaspoon baking soda

1½ teaspoons baking powder

½ teaspoon salt

1 cup dairy-free chocolate chips

Baking with Peanut Butter

When it comes to baking, the kind of peanut butter you use makes a difference. Ground peanut butter, oftentimes referred to as "all-natural," has to be stirred before use because it easily separates from the oil on top of the container. This peanut butter does not work as well in baked goods like cookies and bars because it's oily consistency changes the texture of the recipe. Stick to creamy peanut butter unless otherwise specified.

1. Preheat oven to 375°F. Spray a 9" square baking pan with vegetable cooking spray.

2. In a large bowl use an electric mixer to combine ½ cup vegan butter, peanut butter, ½ cup brown sugar, and granulated sugar until fluffy. Add vanilla, flaxseed, cornstarch, water, and 3 tablespoons almond milk. Mix to combine.

3. Push wet ingredients to one side of bowl. In other side, add flour, baking soda, baking powder, and salt. Stir dry ingredients together, then incorporate wet ingredients into dry mixture. Stir in chocolate chips.

4. Pour mixture into prepared baking pan and bake 25 minutes until crust is lightly golden on top. When done, remove from oven and let cool about 15 minutes.

5. Cover, and refrigerate up to 10 days or freeze up to 2 months.

6. To make caramel sauce, add ½ cup brown sugar and ½ cup almond milk to a small saucepan over medium-high heat. Bring to a boil while stirring, then reduce heat to medium and cook 5 minutes, stirring occasionally. Remove from heat.

7. Stir in 1 tablespoon vegan butter, then let cool about 10 minutes. Cover and refrigerate up to 10 days.

8. To serve, cut into bars and let come to room temperature. Heat caramel sauce by cooking in microwave in 15-second intervals until heated through. Drizzle bars with warmed caramel sauce.

PER SERVING (1 bar) Calories: 403 | Fat: 16.0 g | Protein: 5.5 g | Sodium: 289 mg | Fiber: 2.7 g | Carbohydrates: 58.5 g | Sugar: 35.5 g

Chocolate Brownie Magic Bars

Everyone will love these Chocolate Brownie Magic Bars made with a chocolate brownie base, sweetened almond milk middle, and chocolate chip and coconut topping.

INGREDIENTS | MAKES 9 BARS

½ cup vegan butter

1⅓ cups dairy-free chocolate chips, divided

1 tablespoon ground flaxseed

3 tablespoons water

2 tablespoons cornstarch, divided

1 tablespoon + 1 teaspoon vanilla extract, divided

1½ cups unsweetened almond milk, divided

1 cup packed light brown sugar

½ cup cocoa powder

1¼ cups all-purpose flour

¼ teaspoon salt

½ cup granulated sugar

1 cup unsweetened coconut flakes

½ cup walnuts, chopped

1. Preheat oven to 350°F and grease bottom of a 9" square baking pan with vegetable cooking spray.

2. In a large microwave-safe bowl combine vegan butter with ⅓ cup chocolate chips. Heat 30 seconds until chocolate begins to melt. Stir and return to microwave another 15 seconds. Stir and repeat until chocolate is melted.

3. Add ground flaxseed, water, 1 tablespoon cornstarch, 1 tablespoon vanilla, ½ cup almond milk, brown sugar, and cocoa powder to melted chocolate. Stir until well combined.

4. In a medium bowl stir together flour and salt. Pour flour mixture into chocolate mixture and stir until just combined. Spread into prepared baking pan. Bake 20 minutes.

5. While brownies are baking, combine remaining 1 cup almond milk and cornstarch, along with granulated sugar, in a large, microwave-safe bowl. Microwave 1 minute and stir. Repeat until mixture is thick, about 3 minutes. Add remaining vanilla and stir again to combine.

6. Remove brownies from oven and top with sweetened almond milk mixture, followed by 1 cup chocolate chips, and walnuts. Return to oven and bake another 20 minutes, then set aside to cool about 20 minutes.

7. Cover and refrigerate up to 10 days or freeze up to 2 months. To serve, cut into bars and allow time to come to room temperature.

PER SERVING (1 bar) Calories: 563 | Fat: 26.9 g | Protein: 5.6 g | Sodium: 175 mg | Fiber: 7.2 g | Carbohydrates: 75.9 g | Sugar: 50.2 g

Pineapple Red Velvet Dessert Bars

Two different flavors combine to create ultimately rich and delicious Pineapple Red Velvet Dessert Bars. Everything's better with a little red velvet involved, and these cake bars are a perfect example.

INGREDIENTS | MAKES 24 BARS

1 cup unsweetened almond milk

1 tablespoon cornstarch

1 tablespoon ground flaxseed

1 (15-ounce) can chickpeas, rinsed and drained

½ cup vegetable oil

1 box Duncan Hines Signature Red Velvet Cake Mix

1 box Duncan Hines Signature Pineapple Supreme Cake Mix

1. Preheat oven to 350°F and grease a 9" × 13" cake pan with vegetable spray.

2. Add almond milk, cornstarch, ground flaxseed, chickpeas, and oil to a food processor. Pulse until smooth, about 1 minute. Set aside.

3. Pour red velvet cake mix into a large bowl and stir in ½ chickpea mixture. Press mixture into bottom of prepared pan.

4. Rinse out bowl and dry, then pour pineapple cake mix and remaining ½ chickpea mixture. Stir to combine. Gently press mixture over top of red velvet layer.

5. Bake 45 minutes. Remove from oven and set aside to cool about 15 minutes.

6. Cover and refrigerate up to 10 days or freeze up to 2 months. To serve, cut into bars and allow time to come to room temperature.

PER SERVING (1 bar) Calories: 210 | Fat: 8.3 g | Protein: 2.1 g | Sodium: 310 mg | Fiber: 1.2 g | Carbohydrates: 30.9 g | Sugar: 15.9 g

Pumpkin Magic Bars

These Pumpkin Magic Bars are a vegan twist on the original seven-layer recipe. They are ooey, gooey, and full of magical pumpkin flavor!

INGREDIENTS | **MAKES 18 BARS**

20 dairy-free chocolate sandwich cookies
4 tablespoons coconut oil
1 (8-ounce) container vegan cream cheese
1 cup unsweetened vanilla almond milk
½ cup granulated sugar
1 tablespoon cornstarch
1 (15-ounce) can pumpkin purée
1 teaspoon pumpkin pie spice
1 cup dried cranberries
1 cup unsweetened coconut flakes
1 cup dairy-free chocolate chips
1 cup chopped walnuts

1. Preheat oven to 350°F. Lightly grease a 9" × 13" baking dish with vegetable cooking spray.

2. Place sandwich cookies in a food processor. Pulse until coarse crumbs form. Add coconut oil and pulse again until a coarse crust is achieved. Press mixture into bottom of prepared baking dish.

3. In same food processor bowl add vegan cream cheese, almond milk, sugar, cornstarch, pumpkin, and spice. Pulse until smooth.

4. Pour pumpkin mixture over crust. Sprinkle top with 1 layer each of dried cranberries, coconut flakes, chocolate chips, and nuts.

5. Bake 45 minutes. Remove from oven and cool about 20 minutes.

6. Cover and refrigerate up to 10 days or freeze up to 2 months. To serve, slice and allow to come to room temperature.

PER SERVING (1 bar) Calories: 301 | Fat: 19.5 g | Protein: 2.9 g | Sodium: 159 mg | Fiber: 3.6 g | Carbohydrates: 29.8 g | Sugar: 18.1 g

Blueberry Lemon Pie Bars

You're in for a special treat with these Blueberry Lemon Pie Bars—made with plenty of fresh ingredients. It's a dessert everyone will love!

INGREDIENTS | MAKES 9 BARS

For Crust and Topping
1 cup all-purpose flour
½ cup vegan butter
¼ cup powdered sugar
½ cup rolled oats

For Lemon Filling
1 (12-ounce) package firm silken tofu, pressed
½ cup granulated sugar
2 teaspoons vanilla extract
Zest of 1 lemon
Juice of 1 lemon

For Blueberry Filling
2 cups frozen blueberries
½ cup granulated sugar
1 tablespoon cornstarch
2 tablespoons lemon juice

Reducing Refined Sugars

It's a good idea to limit the amount of refined sugars in your diet. One way you can do this is by using alternatives like coconut sugar or dates in place of the refined sugar in your recipes.

1. Preheat oven to 350°F. Line a 9" square baking pan with foil and spray with a light coating of vegetable spray.

2. **To make Crust and Topping:** in a food processor add flour, vegan butter, powdered sugar, and oats. Pulse until combined. Use a spatula to press down any ingredients on sides of container, then pulse again until smooth. Reserve 1 cup mixture and press remaining mixture into prepared pan.

3. **To make Lemon Filling:** to processor bowl (do not clean out) add silken tofu, sugar, vanilla, lemon zest, and lemon juice. Pulse until smooth. Pour mixture over crust.

4. **To make Blueberry Filling:** in a medium bowl add frozen blueberries. Sprinkle sugar and cornstarch over blueberries. Add lemon juice and gently stir to distribute equally over blueberries. Gently spoon blueberry mixture over lemon filling. Spoon dollops of reserved topping evenly over top.

5. Bake 60 minutes until crust becomes a golden brown. When done, remove pan and let cool completely, about 30 minutes.

6. Cover and refrigerate up to 10 days or freeze up to 2 months. To serve, cut into bars and allow to come to room temperature.

PER SERVING (1 bar) Calories: 258 | Fat: 5.7 g | Protein: 5.0 g | Sodium: 86 mg | Fiber: 2.0 g | Carbohydrates: 45.8 g | Sugar: 28.7 g

Chocolate Wafer Bars

Imagine a crispy wafer cookie dipped in chocolate. It's sort of like your favorite candy bar, except vegan!

INGREDIENTS | MAKES 16 BARS

1 cup dairy-free chocolate chips
1 tablespoon coconut oil
16 dairy-free vanilla sugar wafers

1. Line a baking sheet with wax paper.

2. Place chocolate chips in a small microwave-safe container and stir in coconut oil, making sure chips are coated. Microwave 15 seconds, then stir. Repeat until chocolate is melted.

3. Place wafers on waxed paper. Use a spoon to drizzle chocolate over each wafer, until it is thoroughly coated. Set tray in refrigerator until chocolate has firmed up, about 15 minutes.

4. Refrigerate in a large sealable container up to 10 days or freeze up to 2 months. To serve, either eat cold, or allow to come to room temperature.

PER SERVING (1 bar) Calories: 104 | Fat: 6.4 g | Protein: 0.6 g | Sodium: 15 mg | Fiber: 1.1 g | Carbohydrates: 10.9 g | Sugar: 7.5 g

Gooey Neapolitan Brownie Bars

You'll enjoy the classic chocolate, strawberry, and vanilla layers in these Gooey Neapolitan Brownie Bars.

INGREDIENTS | **MAKES 24 BARS**

1 (15-ounce) can sweetened coconut milk

1 tablespoon cornstarch

1 cup granulated sugar

1 teaspoon vanilla extract

1½ cups vegan butter, melted, divided

1 box Duncan Hines Classic Dark Chocolate Fudge Cake Mix

1 box Duncan Hines Signature French Vanilla Cake Mix

1 box Duncan Hines Signature Strawberry Supreme Cake Mix

1. Combine 2 tablespoons coconut milk with cornstarch in a small microwave-safe bowl. Add in remaining coconut milk and sugar. Stir, then heat in microwave 45 seconds. Stir and repeat until mixture has thickened. Stir in vanilla and set aside to cool about 10 minutes.

2. Preheat oven to 350°F. Line bottom and sides of a 9" × 13" cake pan with aluminum foil sheet. Spray foil with vegetable cooking spray.

3. In a large bowl stir together ½ cup vegan butter, ¼ cup coconut milk mixture, and chocolate cake mix. Spread chocolate dough in bottom of prepared pan.

4. Rinse and dry bowl, then add in ½ cup vegan butter, ¼ cup coconut milk mixture, and vanilla cake mix. Mix, then gently spread out over chocolate dough layer in pan.

5. Add remaining ½ cup vegan butter, ¼ cup coconut milk mixture, and strawberry cake mix to same bowl. Mix, then spread over vanilla layer in pan.

6. Pour remaining coconut milk mixture over top of strawberry layer. Be sure that foil is standing tall on each side of pan to prevent spills.

7. Bake 45 minutes until a toothpick inserted in center comes out clean. Remove from oven and set aside to cool about 20 minutes.

8. Cover and refrigerate up to 10 days or freeze up to 2 months. To serve, cut into bars and allow to come to room temperature.

PER SERVING Calories: 351 | Fat: 11.3 g | Protein: 1.7 g | Sodium: 599 mg | Fiber: 0.0 g | Carbohydrates: 59.7 g | Sugar: 39.6 g

Almond Surprise Cookies

The flavors of a favorite candy bar come together in this vegan recipe.
These homemade cookies are healthier and just as tasty!

INGREDIENTS | MAKES 32 COOKIES

½ cup coconut oil

½ cup almond butter

1 cup packed light brown sugar

1 tablespoon ground flaxseed

1 tablespoon cornstarch

3 tablespoons unsweetened almond milk

½ cup water

1 teaspoon coconut extract

1¼ cups all-purpose flour

3 cups quick-cooking oats

½ cup cocoa powder

1 teaspoon baking soda

1 teaspoon baking powder

½ teaspoon salt

1 cup unsweetened coconut flakes

1 cup dairy-free chocolate chips

1 cup almonds, roughly chopped

Keeping Cookies Fresh Longer

No one likes stale cookies. One trick to keep cookies fresh longer is to add a piece of sliced bread to the storage container with your cookies. You'll notice that the bread becomes stale after a few days. This is because the cookies absorb all the moisture from the bread, keeping them soft for a longer period of time.

1. Preheat oven to 350°F. Line two baking sheets with parchment paper.

2. In a large bowl add coconut oil, almond butter, and sugar. Use an electric mixer on medium speed to beat until light and fluffy. Add flaxseed, cornstarch, almond milk, water, and coconut extract. Mix again until combined. Set aside.

3. In a separate large bowl combine flour, oats, cocoa powder, baking soda, baking powder, and salt. Stir into butter mixture, along with coconut, chocolate chips, and almonds.

4. Use a cookie dough dispenser or a large tablespoon to drop cookie dough onto prepared sheets, roughly 2" apart.

5. For soft cookies, bake 9 minutes. For crispier cookies, bake up to 12 minutes. When done, remove cookies from oven and allow to cool 2 minutes, then transfer to a rack to cool completely. Repeat with rest of dough.

6. Transfer cooled cookies to a large lidded container and store at room temperature up to 3 days, refrigerate up to 10 days, or freeze up to 2 months.

PER SERVING (1 cookie) Calories: 213 | Fat: 12.0 g | Protein: 4.0 g | Sodium: 94 mg | Fiber: 3.4 g | Carbohydrates: 23.1 g | Sugar: 10.4 g

Chocolate Chip Cookies

Delicious Chocolate Chip Cookies are soft and chewy, with lots of melted chocolate chips throughout. Perfect for dipping in vanilla almond milk!

INGREDIENTS | MAKES 36 COOKIES

1 cup vegan butter, softened

¾ cup packed light brown sugar

¾ cup granulated sugar

1 tablespoon vanilla extract

1 tablespoon chia seeds

3 tablespoons water

2¼ cups all-purpose flour

1½ teaspoons baking soda

1½ teaspoons baking powder

1 teaspoon salt

2 cups dairy-free chocolate chips

Baking Without Eggs

It can be tricky to bake without eggs, which are a binding agent, so use chia seeds or flaxseeds in their place. Both seeds create a gel-like substance when exposed to moisture, binding your recipe and also adding moisture to the finished product.

1. Preheat oven to 350°F. Line two baking sheets with parchment paper.

2. Place vegan butter and sugars in a large bowl. Use an electric mixer on medium speed to beat until light and fluffy. Add vanilla, chia seeds, and water and mix again to combine.

3. In a separate large bowl combine flour, baking soda, baking powder, and salt. Pour flour mixture into butter mixture. Stir to combine. Add chocolate chips and stir until combined.

4. Drop rounded spoonfuls of dough, about 2" apart, onto prepared baking sheets. Bake 10 minutes. Batter will yield approximately 36 cookies.

5. Once cookies are done, allow them to cool 2 minutes before transferring to a wire rack to cool completely about 10 minutes.

6. Store either at room temperature or in refrigerator in a large sealed container up to 7 days, or freeze up to 2 months.

PER SERVING (1 cookie) Calories: 156 | Fat: 6.7 g | Protein: 1.2 g | Sodium: 174 mg | Fiber: 1.2 g | Carbohydrates: 22.1 g | Sugar: 14.0 g

Peanut Butter Cookies

*These tender Peanut Butter Cookies are melt-in-your-mouth delicious.
Share with friends, or enjoy as a treat for yourself all week.*

INGREDIENTS | MAKES 24 COOKIES

½ cup vegan butter
½ cup creamy peanut butter
¾ cup granulated sugar, divided
½ cup packed light brown sugar
1 tablespoon chia seeds
1 teaspoon vanilla extract
1¼ cups all-purpose flour
½ teaspoon baking soda
1 teaspoon baking powder
½ teaspoon salt
2 tablespoons unsweetened almond milk

1. Use an electric mixer to combine vegan butter and peanut butter in a medium bowl, beating on medium-high speed 30 seconds. Add ½ cup granulated sugar and brown sugar and beat until combined, scraping sides of bowl occasionally. Beat in chia seeds and vanilla until combined.

2. In a large bowl combine flour, baking soda, baking powder, and salt. Pour flour mixture into peanut butter mixture and stir until ingredients are combined. Add almond milk, 1 tablespoon at a time, stirring between each addition. Cover and refrigerate 30 minutes.

3. When cookie dough is chilled, heat oven to 375°F. Cover two baking sheets with parchment paper.

4. Shape dough into 24 1" balls. Roll balls in small bowl with remaining granulated sugar to coat, then place 2" apart on prepared sheets. Use a fork to create crisscross marks on top of each dough ball, slightly flattening each ball.

5. Bake 8 minutes until light brown. Let cool 1 minute on baking sheets before transferring to a wire rack to cool about 10 minutes.

6. Store in a large sealed container at room temperature or in refrigerator up to 7 days, or freeze up to 2 months.

PER SERVING (1 cookie) Calories: 113 | Fat: 4.4 g | Protein: 2.1 g | Sodium: 125 mg | Fiber: 1.1 g | Carbohydrates: 16.8 g | Sugar: 11.3 g

Red Velvet Chocolate Cookies

If you love chocolate chips and red velvet, this recipe is for you. These vegan Red Velvet Chocolate Cookies are easy to make and full of rich, gooey chocolate chips!

INGREDIENTS | MAKES 32 COOKIES

1 box Duncan Hines Signature Red Velvet Cake Mix
½ cup vegan butter, softened
2 tablespoons ground flaxseed
2 tablespoons cornstarch
½ cup water
1½ cups dairy-free chocolate chips
1 cup powdered sugar

Frozen Cookie Dough Balls

Running low on time, or only need a small amount of cookies? Rather than baking a whole batch at one time, try freezing some of the cookie dough balls. Place dough balls on a tray in the freezer. Once the dough balls are frozen, about 30 minutes, transfer to a freezer bag and keep them frozen until you're ready to bake. Be sure to bake frozen cookie dough balls a few minutes longer than just-made cookie dough.

1. Pour cake mix in a large bowl and add vegan butter. Stir to combine. Create a well in center and set aside.

2. In a small bowl stir together flaxseed, cornstarch, and water. Pour into well in cake mixture. Stir together. Add chocolate chips and stir again. Cover and refrigerate 20 minutes.

3. When ready to bake, preheat oven to 350°F.

4. Use a cookie dough scoop to create 32 cookie dough balls. Roll cookie dough balls in a small bowl with powdered sugar and place on ungreased baking sheets, about 1½" apart.

5. Bake 10 minutes, then remove from oven and let sit on pan 2 minutes before transferring to a rack to cool about 10 minutes.

6. Store in a large sealed container at room temperature or in refrigerator up to 7 days, or freeze up to 2 months.

PER SERVING (1 cookie) Calories: 144 | Fat: 6.5 g | Protein: 1.0 g | Sodium: 123 mg | Fiber: 1.2 g | Carbohydrates: 20.1 g | Sugar: 13.2 g

Lemon Thumbprint Cookies

*These Lemon Thumbprint Cookies have a buttery vegan cookie
shell with a creamy, zesty lemon curd in the middle.*

INGREDIENTS | MAKES 36 COOKIES

For Cookie Crust
¾ cup vegan butter, softened
¾ cup granulated sugar
1 tablespoon ground flaxseed
1 tablespoon cornstarch
Juice of 1 lemon
3 tablespoons unsweetened almond milk
1 teaspoon lemon extract
2 cups all-purpose flour
½ teaspoon baking powder
½ teaspoon baking soda
½ teaspoon salt

For Lemon Sugar
¼ cup granulated sugar
Zest of 1 lemon

For Lemon Curd
1 tablespoon cashews
2 tablespoons coconut oil, melted
1 cup powdered sugar
Juice of 1 lemon
Zest of 1 lemon
⅛ teaspoon ground turmeric

1. **To make Cookie Crust:** in a large bowl combine vegan butter, sugar, flaxseed, cornstarch, lemon juice, almond milk, and lemon extract. Use an electric mixer on medium-high speed to beat until light and fluffy, about 1 minute.

2. In a medium bowl combine flour, baking powder, baking soda, and salt. Pour dry ingredients over lemon butter mixture and stir to combine. Cover and place bowl in refrigerator to chill 1 hour.

3. **To make Lemon Sugar:** combine sugar with lemon zest in a small bowl. Set aside.

4. **To make Lemon Curd:** place cashews in a coffee grinder or food processor. Pulse until consistency is a sticky flour.

5. Place cashew flour in a small bowl. Stir in coconut oil, powdered sugar, lemon juice, lemon zest, and turmeric. Set aside.

6. When dough is chilled, preheat oven to 325°F and line two baking sheets with parchment paper.

7. Use a tablespoon to measure out 36 balls of dough. Roll balls in Lemon Sugar and place on prepared sheets 1½" apart. Use a teaspoon to create an indentation in each cookie dough ball and pour Lemon Curd into each indent.

8. Bake 13 minutes, then remove from oven and allow cookies to cool completely on baking sheets about 10 minutes.

9. Store in a large sealed container at room temperature or in refrigerator up to 7 days, or freeze up to 2 months.

PER SERVING (1 cookie) Calories: 89 | Fat: 2.5 g | Protein: 0.8 g | Sodium: 84 mg | Fiber: 0.3 g | Carbohydrates: 15.7 g | Sugar: 9.8 g

Chocolate Chip Sprinkle Cookies

Sugar cookie meets chocolate chips and sprinkles in these delicious Chocolate Chip Sprinkle Cookies. Add color and fun to a simple vegan chocolate chip cookie recipe.

INGREDIENTS | MAKES 32 COOKIES

½ cup vegan butter

½ cup creamy peanut butter

1½ cups granulated sugar

2 tablespoons ground flaxseed

2 tablespoons cornstarch

½ cup unsweetened almond milk

1 teaspoon apple cider vinegar

1 teaspoon vanilla extract

1 teaspoon almond extract

2½ cups all-purpose flour

1 teaspoon baking soda

1 teaspoon baking powder

¼ teaspoon salt

1 cup dairy-free chocolate chips

1 cup multicolored sprinkles

Measuring Flour

How you measure flour makes a difference in a recipe. This is why some people weigh their flour to get more exact measurements. However, you can get a better measurement by using your measuring cup to "fluff" up the flour in its container. Then, lightly fill the measuring cup and use a butter knife to scrape along the top, creating a level surface.

1. Place vegan butter, peanut butter, and sugar in a large bowl and using an electric mixer, mix on medium-high speed until light and fluffy, about 1 minute. Push mixture to one side of bowl. In other side combine flaxseed, cornstarch, almond milk, vinegar, vanilla, and almond extract. Use mixer to slowly incorporate flaxseed mixture into butter mixture until light and fluffy.

2. In a separate large bowl combine flour, baking soda, baking powder, and salt. Pour flour mixture over butter mixture and use mixer to combine. Add chocolate chips and sprinkles and hand mix until incorporated throughout dough.

3. Cover bowl and freeze about 20 minutes or refrigerate 1 hour.

4. When ready to bake, preheat oven to 350°F. Use a cookie dough dispenser to drop cookie dough balls roughly 1½" apart onto ungreased baking sheet.

5. Place cookies in oven and bake 9 minutes. Remove pan from oven and allow cookies to cool 2 minutes before placing on a wire rack to cool about 10 minutes. Repeat with remaining dough.

6. Store in a large sealed container at room temperature or in refrigerator up to 7 days, or freeze up to 2 months.

PER SERVING (1 cookie) Calories: 175 | Fat: 7.2 g | Protein: 2.2 g | Sodium: 96 mg | Fiber: 1.1 g | Carbohydrates: 28.5 g | Sugar: 18.9 g

Confetti Cookies

These colorful Confetti Cookies boast a tender cookie flavor with added fun. It's a party for your taste buds!

1 cup granulated sugar

½ cup vegan butter, softened

¼ cup coconut oil, softened

1 teaspoon vanilla extract

½ cup unsweetened applesauce

2½ cups all-purpose flour

2 tablespoons cornstarch

¾ teaspoon salt

1 teaspoon baking powder

⅓ cup multicolored sprinkles

1. Add sugar, vegan butter, and coconut oil into a large bowl. Using an electric mixer, beat until smooth and fluffy. Add vanilla and applesauce and beat again to combine. Set aside.

2. Combine flour, cornstarch, salt, baking powder, and sprinkles in a separate large bowl. Pour flour mixture into bowl with sugar mixture and stir to combine.

3. Form dough into a ball and cover with plastic wrap. Refrigerate at least 1 hour.

4. When ready to bake, preheat oven to 350°F and line two baking sheets with parchment paper.

5. Use a cookie dough dispenser to drop cookie dough balls roughly 1½" apart onto baking sheet. Bake 8 minutes. Remove from oven and allow to cool 2 minutes before placing on a wire rack to cool an additional 10 minutes. Repeat with remaining dough.

6. Store cookies in a large sealed container at room temperature or in refrigerator up to 7 days, or freeze up to 2 months.

PER SERVING (1 cookie) Calories: 130 | Fat: 4.3 g | Protein: 1.4 g | Sodium: 120 mg | Fiber: 0.4 g | Carbohydrates: 22.3 g | Sugar: 11.5 g

Double Chocolate Chip Cookies

These vegan Double Chocolate Chip Cookies are like mini brownies because of their crispy outer crust and gooey chocolatey center. Made from a simple list of ingredients, you'll love making these cookies almost as much as everyone will love eating them.

INGREDIENTS | MAKES 32 COOKIES

2 cups dairy-free chocolate chips, divided
1 cup vegan butter, softened
¾ cup granulated sugar
½ cup packed light brown sugar
1 teaspoon vanilla extract
½ cup unsweetened almond milk
2 cups whole-wheat pastry flour
1 tablespoon ground flaxseed
1 tablespoon cornstarch
½ cup cocoa powder
1½ teaspoons baking powder
½ teaspoon salt
½ cup chopped walnuts

Making Gorgeous Homemade Cookies

Make your homemade cookies look as good as they taste with this simple tip: Always reserve a little of one or two of the ingredients, like chocolate chips, to distribute across the top of the cookie dough balls before baking. This way, the finished cookie will be dotted with melty chocolate chips (or raisins, etc.).

1. Preheat oven to 350°F.

2. Place 1 cup chocolate chips in a small microwave-safe bowl and heat in microwave 30 seconds. Place a lid over bowl and let sit 1 minute until chocolate is melted. Set aside to cool about 5 minutes.

3. In a large bowl use an electric mixer to beat together vegan butter and sugars until light and fluffy. Add vanilla and almond milk and mix until combined. Pour cooled melted chocolate into mixture. Beat until chocolate is incorporated.

4. In a separate large bowl combine flour, ground flaxseed, cornstarch, cocoa powder, baking powder, and salt. Add remaining chocolate chips and walnuts to flour mixture and stir before adding to chocolate butter mixture. Stir until combined.

5. Drop dough by rounded spoonfuls onto two ungreased baking sheets and bake 10 minutes. Then remove from oven and let sit on baking sheets 1 minute before transferring to wire racks to cool about 10 minutes.

6. Store in a large sealed container at room temperature or in refrigerator up to 7 days, or freeze up to 2 months.

PER SERVING (1 cookie) Calories: 180 | Fat: 8.8 g | Protein: 1.8 g | Sodium: 103 mg | Fiber: 2.7 g | Carbohydrates: 23.4 g | Sugar: 14.1 g

Chocolate No-Bake Cookies

Every time you bite into these tender Chocolate No-Bake Cookies you'll experience peanut butter, chocolate, and hints of coconut in every bite. It's no wonder this recipe has stood the test of time!

INGREDIENTS | MAKES 26 COOKIES

½ cup coconut sugar
½ cup Swerve granulated sugar
½ cup unsweetened vanilla almond milk
⅓ cup coconut oil
¼ cup cocoa powder
¾ cup creamy peanut butter
2 teaspoons vanilla extract
3 cups quick-cooking oats
1 tablespoon ground flaxseed
¼ cup unsweetened coconut flakes

1. Line two baking sheets with wax paper.

2. In a medium saucepan over medium heat, combine sugar, sweetener, almond milk, coconut oil, and cocoa powder. Stir over heat until everything has melted, about 2 minutes. Bring mixture to a boil 1 minute, then remove from heat.

3. Stir in peanut butter and vanilla. Continue stirring until peanut butter is melted and combined with rest of ingredients. Pour in oats, flaxseed, and coconut flakes. Stir to combine.

4. Use a cookie scoop to drop rounded cookie balls onto prepared baking sheets. Use scoop or bottom of a small drinking glass to press cookie balls and flatten them slightly. Set aside to let set at room temperature 1 hour, or in refrigerator 30 minutes.

5. Store in a large sealed container at room temperature or in refrigerator up to 7 days, or freeze up to 2 months.

PER SERVING (1 cookie) Calories: 98 | Fat: 5.1 g | Protein: 2.1 g | Sodium: 4 mg | Fiber: 1.6 g | Carbohydrates: 16.0 g | Sugar: 4.2 g

Chunky Monkey Cookies

The flavors of chocolate, peanut butter, and banana combine in these veganized Chunky Monkey Cookies. Deliciousness in every bite!

INGREDIENTS | MAKES 36 COOKIES

1¼ cups all-purpose flour
1 cup whole-wheat pastry flour
1 teaspoon baking soda
½ teaspoon salt
½ cup vegan butter, softened
½ cup creamy peanut butter
½ cup packed light brown sugar
1 teaspoon vanilla extract
2 medium ripe bananas, mashed
¼ cup unsweetened almond milk
1 teaspoon apple cider vinegar
1 cup dairy-free chocolate chips
½ cup chopped walnuts

Where to Buy Dairy-Free Chocolate Chips

You can find dairy-free chocolate chips at many big-name grocery stores and online. Great brands include Enjoy Life, Simply Delicious By Nestlé Toll House, and Guittard (certain products). It's important to always read labels because sometimes manufacturers may change their formulas.

1. Preheat oven to 375°F. Line two baking sheets with parchment paper.

2. In a large bowl combine flours, baking soda, and salt. Set aside.

3. In a separate large bowl stir together vegan butter and peanut butter. Add brown sugar and vanilla and stir vigorously until creamy. Add bananas, almond milk, and vinegar and stir until combined. Set aside.

4. Pour chocolate chips and walnuts into flour mixture. Stir. Pour peanut butter mixture into flour mixture and stir until combined. Drop dough by rounded spoonfuls onto prepared baking sheets.

5. Bake 10 minutes until golden brown. Remove and let cool on baking sheets 2 minutes before transferring to wire racks to cool about 10 minutes.

6. Store in a large sealed container at room temperature or in refrigerator up to 7 days, or freeze up to 2 months.

PER SERVING (1 cookie) Calories: 124 | Fat: 6.1 g | Protein: 2.1 g | Sodium: 88 mg | Fiber: 1.5 g | Carbohydrates: 15.0 g | Sugar: 6.9 g

Orange-Pumpkin Chocolate Chip Cookies

These sweet Orange-Pumpkin Chocolate Chip Cookies are packed with chocolate chips, orange and pumpkin flavors, and oats.

INGREDIENTS | MAKES 32 COOKIES

½ cup vegan butter, softened

½ cup creamy peanut butter

½ cup granulated sugar

½ cup packed dark brown sugar

1 (15-ounce) can plain pumpkin purée

1 teaspoon vanilla extract

Zest of 1 orange

1 tablespoon ground flaxseed

2 cups all-purpose flour

¼ cup cornstarch

½ cup rolled oats

1 teaspoon baking soda

1 teaspoon baking powder

½ teaspoon salt

1 cup chopped walnuts

2 cups dairy-free chocolate chips

1. Preheat oven to 350°F.

2. In a large bowl use an electric mixer to blend together vegan butter, peanut butter, and sugars until light and fluffy. Add pumpkin purée, vanilla, orange zest, and flaxseed and mix again until well combined. Set aside.

3. In a separate large bowl combine flour, cornstarch, oats, baking soda, baking powder, and salt. Pour into butter mixture and mix until combined. Add walnuts and chocolate chips and stir until distributed throughout. Use a cookie dough dispenser to drop cookie dough onto ungreased baking sheets, approximately 1" apart.

4. Bake 12 minutes. Remove from oven and cool on a wire rack about 10 minutes.

5. Store in a large sealed container at room temperature or in refrigerator up to 7 days, or freeze up to 2 months.

PER SERVING (1 cookie) Calories: 210 | Fat: 10.7 g | Protein: 3.0 g | Sodium: 113 mg | Fiber: 2.3 g | Carbohydrates: 25.1 g | Sugar: 13.6 g

Raspberry Coconut Thumbprint Cookies

You'll love this crispy, pastry-like cookie with a tender, sweet filling. These Raspberry Coconut Thumbprint Cookies also include a coconut cream icing that make them even more delightful.

INGREDIENTS | MAKES 32 COOKIES

For Cookies

½ cup vegan butter

5 tablespoons coconut oil

1 teaspoon coconut extract

½ cup powdered sugar

½ cup cornstarch

1½ cups all-purpose flour

½ cup unsweetened coconut flakes

For Raspberry Filling

½ cup unsweetened coconut flakes

½ cup raspberry jam

For Coconut Drizzle

1 tablespoon coconut oil

1 cup powdered sugar

2 teaspoons unsweetened vanilla almond milk

1. Preheat oven to 350°F and line two baking sheets with parchment paper.

2. **To make Cookies:** in a food processor add vegan butter, coconut oil, coconut extract, and powdered sugar. Pulse until well combined. Add cornstarch and flour and pulse until combined.

3. Place coconut in a small bowl. Roll dough into balls and roll each ball through coconut, then place on prepared baking sheets, about 1" apart.

4. **To make Raspberry Filling:** in same bowl used for coconut, add another ½ cup shredded coconut and raspberry jam. Stir to combine.

5. Use your thumb or a spoon to create an indentation in center of each cookie dough ball. Add a bit of Raspberry Filling to each.

6. Place baking sheets in oven and bake 10 minutes until outside of cookies are slightly golden. Remove from oven and let cool 1 minute before transferring to a rack to cool about 10 minutes.

7. **To make Coconut Drizzle:** place coconut oil and powdered sugar in a small bowl. Stir to combine. Add almond milk, 1 teaspoon at a time, until desired consistency is reached. Drizzle onto cooled cookies.

8. Store cookies in a large sealed container at room temperature or in refrigerator up to 7 days, or freeze up to 2 months.

PER SERVING (1 cookie) Calories: 103 | Fat: 4.4 g | Protein: 0.7 g | Sodium: 22 mg | Fiber: 0.5 g | Carbohydrates: 14.8 g | Sugar: 7.1 g

Chocolate Mint Cookies

Make these homemade vegan Chocolate Mint Cookies! Crunchy chocolate cookies dipped in melted chocolate make a treat perfect for dunking in vanilla almond milk.

INGREDIENTS | MAKES 24 COOKIES

½ cup vegan butter, softened
¾ cup granulated sugar
⅓ cup plain soy milk
2 tablespoons unflavored vodka
1 teaspoon peppermint extract
2 cups all-purpose flour
¼ cup cornstarch
½ cup cocoa powder
1 teaspoon salt
1½ cups dairy-free chocolate chips
3 tablespoons coconut oil

Baking with Vodka

Using vodka in your baking is a great trick, especially when it comes to pastry-type baking. Recipes need moisture to help them come together, and yet too much moisture can be detrimental to things like pie crust, as it can keep them from rising properly. To create flaky crusts and cookies, baking with vodka is the perfect solution because the alcohol bakes off in the heat of the oven.

1. In a large bowl use an electric mixer to cream together butter and sugar until light and fluffy. Add soy milk, vodka, and peppermint. Blend until well mixed. Set aside.

2. In a medium bowl mix together flour, cornstarch, cocoa powder, and salt. Add mixture to wet ingredients in large bowl and stir.

3. Divide cookie dough into two balls, wrap each in plastic wrap, and refrigerate at least 1 hour.

4. When dough is ready, preheat oven to 350°F.

5. Lay one dough ball on counter and smooth out plastic on counter so it extends well beyond dough. Tear off another sheet of plastic and cover top of dough. Use a rolling pin to roll dough to ¼" thickness. Use a round or scalloped cookie cutter to cut rolled dough and transfer cookies to ungreased baking sheets.

6. Bake 7 minutes. Allow baked cookies to sit on pan 2 minutes before transferring to a wire rack to cool about 5 minutes.

7. Line another baking sheet with wax paper. Combine chocolate chips and coconut oil in a small microwave-safe bowl and microwave 30 seconds. Stir and repeat until chocolate is melted. Dip each cookie in chocolate, then transfer to wax paper. Place tray in refrigerator to set about 15 minutes.

8. Store cookies in a large sealed container in refrigerator up to 7 days, or freeze up to 2 months.

PER SERVING (1 cookie) Calories: 184 | Fat: 8.5 g | Protein: 1.9 g | Sodium: 125 mg | Fiber: 2.0 g | Carbohydrates: 24.6 g | Sugar: 12.3 g

Chocolate-Dipped Macaroons

Chocolate-Dipped Macaroons are delicious and easy cookies your whole family will enjoy!

INGREDIENTS | MAKES 40 MACAROONS

For Cookies

1½ cups almond meal

3 cups unsweetened shredded coconut flakes

½ cup agave nectar

⅓ cup coconut oil, melted

1 tablespoon vanilla extract

½ teaspoon salt

For Chocolate Coating

1 cup dairy-free chocolate chips

1 tablespoon coconut oil

Make Your Own Almond Meal

Almond meal is a great addition to baked goods, as it adds more moisture to the finished product. To make your own almond meal, simply place almonds in a food processor and pulse until a coarse meal forms. Store the meal in the refrigerator up to 10 days or freezer up to 2 months.

1. Line two baking sheets with wax paper.

2. **To make Cookies:** in a large bowl combine almond meal, coconut, agave nectar, coconut oil, vanilla, and salt. Use a cookie dough dispenser to dispense rounded balls of mixture onto prepared pans. Place in refrigerator 1 hour to firm up.

3. **To make Chocolate Coating:** mix chocolate chips and 1 tablespoon coconut oil in a small microwave-safe bowl. Cook in microwave 30 seconds and stir. Repeat until chocolate is melted.

4. Dip bottom of refrigerated macaroons in chocolate and place back on wax paper until chocolate hardens about 10 minutes.

5. Once chocolate is firm, store macaroons in a large sealed container in refrigerator up to 10 days, or freeze up to 2 months.

PER SERVING (1 macaroon) Calories: 124 | Fat: 9.7 g | Protein: 1.5 g | Sodium: 29 mg | Fiber: 2.1 g | Carbohydrates: 7.8 g | Sugar: 4.9 g

Chocolate Chip Peanut Butter Energy Bites

These Chocolate Chip Peanut Butter Energy Bites are packed with lots of good-for-you ingredients such as flaxseed, oats, and coconut.

INGREDIENTS | MAKES 20 BITES

½ cup all-natural peanut butter

¼ cup agave nectar

1 teaspoon vanilla extract

1 cup rolled oats

½ cup unsweetened coconut flakes

½ cup ground golden flaxseed

¼ cup dairy-free chocolate chips

1. Place everything except chocolate chips in a food processor. Pulse 3 seconds, then push down ingredients and pulse again until combined. Add chocolate chips and pulse three more times to break down chocolate chips.

2. Roll dough into bite-sized balls and transfer to a large sealed container. Store at room temperature or in refrigerator up to 7 days, or freeze up to 2 months.

PER SERVING (1 bite) Calories: 118 | Fat: 7.4 g | Protein: 3.1 g | Sodium: 2 mg | Fiber: 2.6 g | Carbohydrates: 10.1 g | Sugar: 4.1 g

Brownie Energy Bites

These energy bites may taste like brownies, but they deliver a punch with healthy ingredients like dates, walnuts, and flaxseed.

INGREDIENTS | MAKES 20 BITES

1 cup medjool dates, pitted and softened

½ cup rolled oats

1 cup walnuts

4 tablespoons cocoa powder

1 teaspoon vanilla extract

¼ cup unsweetened coconut flakes

¼ cup ground flaxseed

¼ cup dairy-free chocolate chips

1. Place all ingredients except chocolate chips in a food processor. Pulse 3 seconds, then push down ingredients and pulse again until combined.

2. Add chocolate chips and pulse two times to combine. Roll dough into bite-sized balls.

3. Store bites in a large sealed container at room temperature or in refrigerator up to 7 days, or freeze up to 2 months.

PER SERVING (1 bite) Calories: 105 | Fat: 5.9 g | Protein: 2.0 g | Sodium: 0 mg | Fiber: 2.6 g | Carbohydrates: 12.6 g | Sugar: 7.9 g

Frosted Banana Cookies

Frosted Banana Cookies are like little cakes bursting with so much flavor that you won't be able to stop at one, or two, or maybe even three! Top with granola, sliced almonds, coconut slivers, or coconut whipped cream.

INGREDIENTS | MAKES 32 COOKIES

1 cup vegan butter, divided

¾ cup + 2 tablespoons packed dark brown sugar, divided

2 medium ripe bananas, peeled and mashed

2 tablespoons plain soy milk

1 tablespoon ground flaxseed

2 cups all-purpose flour

1 tablespoon cornstarch

1 teaspoon baking powder

½ teaspoon baking soda

½ teaspoon salt

2 tablespoons plain soy milk

1½ cups powdered sugar

1. Preheat oven to 350°F. Line two baking sheets with parchment paper.

2. Combine vegan butter (reserving 1 tablespoon) and ¾ cup brown sugar in a large bowl and beat with an electric mixer on high speed 2 minutes until light and fluffy. Add banana, soy milk, and flaxseed. Beat another 1 minute. Set aside.

3. In a separate large bowl combine flour, cornstarch, baking powder, baking soda, and salt. Pour into wet mixture and beat until combined. Use a cookie dough scoop to drop cookie dough onto prepared sheets, 1½" apart.

4. Bake 11 minutes until edges are a light golden color. Remove from oven and let cool 2 minutes before transferring to a wire rack to cool about 10 minutes.

5. Prepare frosting by combing reserved vegan butter, 2 tablespoons brown sugar, and soy milk in a small saucepan. Cook and stir over medium heat until it comes to a boil, then remove from heat and add powdered sugar. Stir until smooth.

6. Spread frosting over cooled cookies, then store cookies in a large sealed container at room temperature or in refrigerator up to 7 days, or freeze up to 2 months.

PER SERVING (1 cookie) Calories: 102 | Fat: 2.5 g | Protein: 1.0 g | Sodium: 114 mg | Fiber: 0.5 g | Carbohydrates: 18.7 g | Sugar: 11.4 g

CHAPTER 16

Desserts

Chocolate Chia Pudding

This Chocolate Chia Pudding is a rich, chocolate-infused dessert that tantalizes your sweet tooth while meeting your health goals too.

INGREDIENTS | SERVES 2

2 tablespoons cocoa powder

1 cup unsweetened almond milk

⅓ cup chia seeds

1 tablespoon vanilla extract

½ cup pitted medjool dates, softened

2 teaspoons dairy-free dark chocolate chips, chopped

1. Add all ingredients except chocolate chips to a food processor bowl. Pulse until dates are smooth.

2. Cover and refrigerate at least 1 hour or up to 8 hours.

3. Sprinkle top with chopped chocolate chips. Cover and refrigerate individual servings up to 4 days.

PER SERVING Calories: 33 | Fat: 1.2 g | Protein: 0.7 g | Sodium: 9 mg | Fiber: 1.5 g | Carbohydrates: 5.5 g | Sugar: 3.5 g

Easy Chocolate Peanut Butter Pie

This is a supersimple chocolate and peanut butter pie that you can make in no time with a few ingredients. A perfect combination of flavors, this pie will have you coming back time and time again!

INGREDIENTS | SERVES 8

1 (5.1-ounce) box Jell-O Cook & Serve Chocolate Pudding & Pie Filling

2 cups unsweetened vanilla almond milk

½ cup creamy peanut butter

1 teaspoon vanilla extract

1 Oreo Pie Crust (see Chapter 17 for recipe)

1 cup vegan whipped topping

1. Pour pudding mix into a medium saucepan. Add almond milk and stir to combine. Turn heat to medium and bring mixture to a light boil, stirring frequently. Reduce heat to medium-low and continue cooking and stirring until pudding becomes thick, about 3 minutes.

2. Remove from heat and immediately add peanut butter and vanilla and stir until combined.

3. Allow pudding to cool about 3 minutes, then pour into pie crust, using a spatula to spread pudding equally across crust. Refrigerate at least 1 hour up to 7 days. Serve with dollops of vegan whipped topping.

PER SERVING Calories: 313 | Fat: 15.7 g | Protein: 5.6 g | Sodium: 482 mg | Fiber: 2.3 g | Carbohydrates: 37.7 g | Sugar: 23.1 g

Frozen Chocolate Drumsticks

These Frozen Chocolate Drumsticks are made with vegan chocolate ice cream, chocolate toppings, and roasted almonds. They're the perfect warm-weather dessert!

INGREDIENTS | SERVES 4

4 cups vegan chocolate ice cream

1 cup dairy-free dark chocolate chips

2 tablespoons coconut oil

4 sugar cones

¼ cup finely chopped almonds

1. Place vegan ice cream on counter to allow to soften, about 5 minutes.

2. Combine chocolate chips and coconut oil in a small microwave-safe container. Place in microwave and heat 30 seconds. Stir and repeat heating until chocolate chips and coconut oil have melted. Stir well to combine.

3. Pour 1 tablespoon melted chocolate into bottom of each sugar cone. Turn cones on their sides and roll to help spread melted chocolate inside. Place cones in four tall glasses and put in freezer 5 minutes.

4. Use an ice cream scoop or a large spoon to ladle softened ice cream into prepared sugar cones (still in glasses). Place glasses back in freezer to allow ice cream to firm up, about 10 minutes.

5. Spread a generous amount melted chocolate mixture over one drumstick and roll in chopped nuts while chocolate is still soft. Place in freezer. Repeat with remaining cones.

6. Allow all drumsticks to firm up in freezer once more, about 30 minutes. Once frozen, place in a large freezer bag and freeze up to 1 month. To serve, remove from freezer and let soften 5 minutes before eating.

PER SERVING Calories: 800 | Fat: 49.6 g | Protein: 5.8 g | Sodium: 52 mg | Fiber: 9.0 g | Carbohydrates: 79.4 g | Sugar: 55.7 g

Strawberry Shortcake

Hot-weather fun begins with this vegan Strawberry Shortcake, made with vegan shortcakes, sweet strawberries, and a delicious vegan whipped cream.

INGREDIENTS | SERVES 12

3 cups all-purpose flour

2 tablespoons baking powder

3 tablespoons granulated sugar

½ teaspoon salt

¾ cup chilled vegan butter, chopped

1¼ cups unsweetened vanilla almond milk

1 teaspoon apple cider vinegar

6 cups fresh strawberries, cored and sliced

⅓ cup coconut sugar

1 cup vegan whipped topping

Vegan Whipped Topping

You can make your own whipped topping with just a few ingredients. Chill 1 (15-ounce) can full-fat coconut milk for 2 hours in the refrigerator. Meanwhile, add a whisk attachment to a mixing bowl and place bowl in freezer 2 hours. Scoop fat into the chilled mixing bowl and whip 7 minutes, adding 3 tablespoons granulated sugar and 1 teaspoon vanilla extract to bowl as you whip. Peaks should form.

1. Preheat oven to 400°F and line a baking sheet with parchment paper.

2. In a food processor pulse together flour, baking powder, sugar, and salt. Add vegan butter and pulse until coarse crumbs form.

3. In a small bowl combine almond milk and vinegar. Stir to combine, then pour it over flour mixture. Pulse until just combined and a sticky dough is formed.

4. Drop dough by large, rounded spoonfuls onto prepared baking sheet.

5. Bake 20 minutes until golden brown.

6. Add sliced strawberries into a medium bowl with coconut sugar. Use a fork to mash strawberries a little to help release their juices. Place in a small sealed container and refrigerate up to 3 days.

7. Once shortcakes are done, remove from oven and set aside to cool about 10 minutes. Place in a large plastic bag and refrigerate up to 7 days or freeze up to 2 months.

8. To serve, slice shortcakes in half and cook in a toaster oven about 5 minutes until heated through. Fill and top with strawberries and vegan whipped topping.

PER SERVING Calories: 240 | Fat: 6.7 g | Protein: 3.8 g | Sodium: 441 mg | Fiber: 2.4 g | Carbohydrates: 41.0 g | Sugar: 14.1 g

Walnut Blondies with Peanut Butter Glaze

This recipe is rich and elegant, but not so pretentious that you wouldn't have it on a Tuesday afternoon at home. No sharing required!

INGREDIENTS | MAKES 12 BLONDIES

For Blondies
¾ cup almond flour

2 cups all-purpose flour

1 teaspoon baking powder

½ teaspoon baking soda

1 teaspoon salt

10 tablespoons vegan butter, softened

1½ cups light brown sugar

1 tablespoon ground flaxseed

3 tablespoons cornstarch

6 tablespoons plain soy milk

1 teaspoon apple cider vinegar

1 teaspoon vanilla extract

2 tablespoons light rum

½ cup chopped walnuts

For Peanut Butter Coconut Topping
¼ cup coconut oil

1 tablespoon PB2 Powdered Peanut Butter

4 tablespoons powdered sugar

3 cups vegan vanilla ice cream

1. Preheat oven to 350°F. Spray a 9" × 13" baking pan with vegetable cooking spray.

2. **To make Blondies:** add flours, baking powder, baking soda, and salt to a large bowl and stir. Set aside.

3. In a medium bowl combine vegan butter, brown sugar, flaxseed, cornstarch, soy milk, vinegar, vanilla, and rum. Pour into flour mixture along with walnuts and combine.

4. Pour batter into prepared pan and bake 35 minutes until lightly brown. Let cool about 20 minutes, then cut into bars and refrigerate in a large sealable bag up to 10 days.

5. **To make Peanut Butter Coconut Topping:** place coconut oil in a medium microwave-safe bowl. Microwave in 8-second intervals until melted. Stir in peanut butter powder and powdered sugar. Cover and refrigerate up to 7 days.

6. To serve, cook individual servings in microwave in 30-second intervals until heated through. Top with a scoop of vegan vanilla ice cream drizzled with Peanut Butter Coconut Topping.

PER SERVING (1 blondie) Calories: 430 | Fat: 18.3 g | Protein: 5.9 g | Sodium: 344 mg | Fiber: 1.9 g | Carbohydrates: 59.7 g | Sugar: 37.4 g

Cherry Parfaits

Busy days mean easy desserts are necessary! Enjoy these easy and delicious vegan Cherry Parfaits with creamy vanilla pudding.

INGREDIENTS | SERVES 3

1 (4.6-ounce) box Jell-O Cook & Serve Vanilla Pudding & Pie Filling

3 cups unsweetened almond milk

20 graham crackers

2 tablespoons coconut oil

1 (15-ounce) can lite cherry pie filling

¾ cup vegan whipped topping

Vegan Pudding

It may be surprising to learn that Jell-O pudding is dairy-free. This has not always been the case. And who knows, companies change their recipes, so someday Jell-O pudding may no longer be dairy-free. That's why it's important to read the labels. Mix with a plant-based milk and enjoy a simple, affordable dessert any day of the week!

1. Combine pudding and almond milk in a medium saucepan over medium heat. Stir until mixture comes to a boil. Cook another 2 minutes until pudding thickens. Remove from heat.

2. Place graham crackers in a food processor. Pulse until a sand-like texture develops. Add coconut oil. Pulse until combined.

3. Press graham cracker mix into bottom of three medium serving dishes, reserving some to crumble on top of each. Use a spoon to press graham cracker mixture into bottom of dishes.

4. Pour pudding over graham cracker crust. Fill each dish until ¾ of the way full. Refrigerate until pudding thickens, about 10 minutes.

5. Top each dish with cherry pie filling. Cover and refrigerate up to 5 days. To serve, top with vegan whipped cream and reserved graham cracker crumbs.

PER SERVING Calories: 808 | Fat: 24.7 g | Protein: 8.4 g | Sodium: 1,251 mg | Fiber: 5.9 g | Carbohydrates: 137.8 g | Sugar: 82.9 g

Chocolate Banana Brownies

You're going to love these rich, moist Chocolate Banana Brownies, filled with ripe bananas and chocolate. Thanks to whole-wheat flour, these bars boast fiber, potassium, and other tasty nutrients, making it both delicious and a healthier dessert alternative!

INGREDIENTS | SERVES 12

1 cup dairy-free chocolate chips

3 tablespoons vegan butter

1 tablespoon chia seeds

1 tablespoon vanilla extract

2 medium ripe bananas, peeled and mashed

½ cup unsweetened applesauce

¼ cup water

1 cup whole-wheat pastry flour

1 teaspoon baking powder

½ teaspoon salt

¾ cup coconut sugar

1. Preheat oven to 350°F. Spray a 9" × 9" square baking pan with vegetable cooking spray.

2. Place chocolate chips and vegan butter in microwave in a large microwave-safe bowl and heat 1 minute. Stir to combine. Add chia seeds and vanilla and stir to combine. Add bananas, applesauce, and water and stir. Set aside.

3. In a medium bowl combine flour, baking powder, salt, and sugar. Pour into chocolate mixture. Stir to combine. Pour into prepared baking dish.

4. Bake 35 minutes until a butter knife or toothpick inserted in center comes out clean. Remove from oven and let cool about 15 minutes.

5. Slice and store brownies in a large sealed container in refrigerator up to 7 days, or freeze up to 2 months.

PER SERVING Calories: 184 | Fat: 8.1 g | Protein: 1.9 g | Sodium: 158 mg | Fiber: 3.6 g | Carbohydrates: 24.6 g | Sugar: 11.5 g

Pumpkin Pie

Here's an easy, delicious vegan Pumpkin Pie recipe with a gingersnap cookie crust for the pumpkin lovers out there!

INGREDIENTS | SERVES 8

For Gingersnap Cookie Crust

40 gingersnap cookies
3 tablespoons vegan butter
2 tablespoons coconut oil
1 teaspoon ground ginger

For Pie Filling

1 (15-ounce) can pumpkin purée
1 (12-ounce) container firm silken tofu
¾ cup dairy-free hazelnut creamer
½ cup packed light brown sugar
3 tablespoons cornstarch
2 teaspoons pumpkin pie spice
1 cup vegan whipped topping

1. **To make Gingersnap Cookie Crust:** place gingersnap cookies in a food processor and pulse until a coarse meal is formed. Add vegan butter, coconut oil, and ginger and pulse 3 more seconds until combined. Press into an ungreased 9" pie pan. Set aside.

2. Preheat oven to 350°F.

3. **To make Pie Filling:** place pumpkin purée, tofu, dairy-free creamer, brown sugar, cornstarch, and pumpkin pie spice in a food processor. Pulse until smooth, pushing down ingredients as needed. Pour into prepared pie crust and use a spatula to smooth top.

4. Bake 50 minutes until filling is firm and crust is a dark golden brown. Remove from oven and let cool about 30 minutes.

5. Cover and refrigerate up to 7 days or slice and freeze in freezer bags up to 2 months. To serve, slice and heat individual servings in microwave in 30-second intervals until heated through. Top with vegan whipped topping.

PER SERVING Calories: 358 | Fat: 11.5 g | Protein: 5.4 g | Sodium: 242 mg | Fiber: 2.2 g | Carbohydrates: 53.6 g | Sugar: 26.1 g

Banana Blondies with Peanut Butter Frosting

Superdelicious and easy to make, these Banana Blondies with Peanut Butter Frosting require just a few ingredients and take 30 minutes to prepare!

INGREDIENTS | MAKES 12 BLONDIES

For Banana Blondies

½ cup vegan butter
1 tablespoon ground flaxseed
1 tablespoon cornstarch
1 cup light brown sugar
½ cup mashed peeled banana
1 tablespoon vanilla extract
1¼ cups all-purpose flour
¼ teaspoon salt

For Peanut Butter Frosting

¼ cup creamy peanut butter
2 tablespoons coconut oil
1 cup powdered sugar
4 tablespoons unsweetened vanilla almond milk

1. Preheat oven to 350°F and line bottom of an 8" × 8" baking pan with parchment paper. Spray paper with a light coating of vegetable cooking spray.

2. **To make Banana Blondies:** place vegan butter in a large microwave-safe bowl and heat in microwave 1 minute until melted. Add flaxseed, cornstarch, brown sugar, banana, and vanilla and stir until well incorporated.

3. In a medium bowl combine flour and salt. Pour into banana batter. Stir to combine. Pour batter into prepared pan.

4. Bake 25 minutes until a toothpick inserted into center comes out clean.

5. **To make Peanut Butter Frosting:** stir together peanut butter and coconut oil in a medium microwave-safe bowl. Heat in microwave 15 seconds to thin. Add powdered sugar and stir until crumbly. Add milk, 1 tablespoon at a time, until a spreadable consistency is achieved.

6. Let blondies cool about 15 minutes, then remove from pan, cut into bars, and top with Peanut Butter Frosting.

7. Transfer to a large lidded container and refrigerate up to 7 days or freeze up to 2 months. To serve, cook blondies in microwave in 30-second intervals until heated through.

PER SERVING (1 blondie) Calories: 250 | Fat: 8.3 g | Protein: 2.8 g | Sodium: 112 mg | Fiber: 1.1 g | Carbohydrates: 40.7 g | Sugar: 27.8 g

Banana Cream Pie

A light and fluffy vegan Banana Cream Pie will make your nights extra special.
Enjoy the golden cookie crust with a silky filling loaded with bananas.

INGREDIENTS | SERVES 16

For Crust

24 Golden Oreo Sandwich Cookies
4 tablespoons vegan butter, sliced

For Banana Cream Filling

½ cup granulated sugar
⅓ cup cornstarch
¼ teaspoon salt
1½ cups Ripple Original Plant-Based Half & Half
1 cup unsweetened vanilla almond milk
1 (12-ounce) container firm silken tofu, pressed
2 tablespoons vegan butter
1 teaspoon nutritional yeast flakes
3 medium bananas, peeled and sliced
1 cup vegan whipped topping

1. **To make Crust:** place cookies in a food processor. Pulse 3 seconds until broken up into smaller pieces. Add vegan butter. Pulse again until a coarse consistency resembling large sand grains develops. Press crust into an ungreased 9" pie pan. Refrigerate about 15 minutes.

2. **To make Banana Cream Filling:** mix sugar, cornstarch, and salt in a medium saucepan. Add milks and stir until combined. Place saucepan over medium heat and bring to a boil, stirring occasionally. Continue cooking until mixture thickens, about 7 minutes.

3. Place tofu, vegan butter, and nutritional yeast flakes in food processor. Pulse 3 seconds until mixture becomes very smooth. Remove lid and push contents down to bottom and pulse again.

4. Add pudding mixture to food processor and pulse again until all ingredients are combined and any lumps are gone. Set aside and allow to cool about 20 minutes.

5. Once pie filling is cooled, remove pie crust from refrigerator and pour ½ pie filling onto pie crust. Top with a layer of sliced bananas. Pour remaining pie filling over sliced bananas. Cover and place in refrigerator to set at least 1 hour.

6. To serve, remove from refrigerator, cut individual slices, and add a dollop of vegan whipped topping. Pie will keep in refrigerator up to 5 days.

PER SERVING Calories: 216 | Fat: 10.6 g | Protein: 3.0 g | Sodium: 141 mg | Fiber: 1.0 g | Carbohydrates: 27.5 g | Sugar: 16.6 g

Chocolate Sheet Cake

This delicious vegan Chocolate Sheet Cake recipe is easy and delivers a supermoist cake topped with silky smooth chocolate frosting. It's the ultimate chocolate lover's dream come true!

1. Preheat oven to 350°F. Prepare a 12" × 16" pan by spraying with vegetable cooking spray.

2. **To make Cake:** in a small bowl combine almond milk and vinegar. Set aside.

3. Combine vegan butter, peanut butter, water, and cocoa powder in a large microwave-safe bowl. Place in microwave and heat in 20-second intervals until butters melt.

4. In a medium bowl add sugar, flours, salt, and baking soda. Stir to combine. Add to vegan butter mixture and stir to combine. Stir in milk mixture, apple sauce, vegan sour cream, and vanilla. Pour batter into prepared pan.

5. Bake 25 minutes until a toothpick inserted in center of cake comes out clean.

6. **To make Frosting:** stir together vegan butter, cocoa powder, and soy milk in a small microwave-safe bowl. Heat in 30-second intervals until mixture begins to boil. Stir in powdered sugar and vanilla, then add chopped pecans.

7. Spread frosting over cake while cake is still hot. Place ½ whole pecan in center of where each slice will be. Let cool about 20 minutes before covering.

8. Store at room temperature up to 5 days, or refrigerate up to 10 days. To serve, heat individual slices in microwave 5 seconds.

PER SERVING Calories: 335 | Fat: 12.0 g | Protein: 4.7 g | Sodium: 212 mg | Fiber: 3.7 g | Carbohydrates: 55.3 g | Sugar: 39.0 g

Banana Chia Pudding with Blackberry Topping

Enjoy this creamy, delicious, and gorgeous Banana Chia Pudding with Blackberry Topping. It's made with only a few ingredients but lots of flavor.

INGREDIENTS | SERVES 2

For Blackberry Topping
½ cup fresh blackberries
1 teaspoon stevia sweetener
½ teaspoon chia seeds

For Banana Pudding
1½ cups unsweetened vanilla almond milk
1 medium banana, peeled
2 teaspoons stevia
⅓ cup chia seeds
½ teaspoon vanilla extract
¼ cup granola

1. **To make Blackberry Topping:** place blackberries in a small bowl and mash with a fork. Add 1 teaspoon stevia and ½ teaspoon chia seeds. Stir to combine. Cover and refrigerate at least 45 minutes up to 3 days.

2. **To make Banana Pudding:** in a food processor add almond milk, banana, 2 teaspoons stevia, ⅓ cup chia seeds, and vanilla. Pulse until smooth. Let sit 2 minutes to allow chia seeds to soften, then pulse again. Pour into a small lidded container. Refrigerate at least 45 minutes up to 5 days.

3. When ready to serve, pour equal amounts pudding into small serving dishes. Top with equal amounts Blackberry Topping. Add granola for garnish.

PER SERVING Calories: 296 | Fat: 14.4 g | Protein: 8.8 g | Sodium: 136 mg | Fiber: 15.2 g | Carbohydrates: 38.4 g | Sugar: 12.8 g

Vegan Frosting

Serve this easy, delicious frosting on your favorite vegan cake recipes.

INGREDIENTS | MAKES 1 CUP

6 tablespoons vegan butter
1½ cups powdered sugar
3 tablespoons vanilla almond milk

Make It Chocolate!
Craving chocolate frosting? Simply add ¼ cup cocoa powder to this recipe and then follow instructions as usual.

1. Combine vegan butter and powdered sugar in a small sealable container.

2. Add 1 teaspoon almond milk at a time, stirring as you add, until a spreadable consistency is achieved.

3. Refrigerate up to 14 days.

PER SERVING (1 cup) Calories: 694 | Fat: 9.7 g | Protein: 0.2 g | Sodium: 193 mg | Fiber: 0.2 g | Carbohydrates: 153.2 g | Sugar: 149.5 g

Easy Chocolate Cake

This rich, moist Easy Chocolate Cake will become your go-to favorite cake recipe. Serve as an elegant dessert for guests, or as a weekday after-dinner treat. For a pop of color, top individual slices with sprinkles before serving!

INGREDIENTS | SERVES 16

1½ cups all-purpose flour
1 cup granulated sugar
⅓ cup cocoa powder
½ teaspoon salt
1 teaspoon baking soda
⅓ cup vegetable oil
1 cup cold water
1 tablespoon apple cider vinegar
1 teaspoon vanilla extract
1 batch Vegan Frosting (chocolate version; see this chapter for recipe)

1. Preheat oven to 350°F. Spray an 8" round cake pan with vegetable cooking spray.

2. Combine flour, sugar, cocoa powder, salt, and baking soda in a large bowl. Set aside.

3. In a small bowl stir together vegetable oil, water, vinegar, and vanilla. Pour water mixture into flour mixture. Stir until combined.

4. Pour batter into prepared pan and bake 35 minutes until a toothpick inserted in center comes out clean.

5. Let cool about 20 minutes before adding frosting. Cover and store at room temperature up to 5 days, or refrigerate up to 10 days. To serve, heat individual slices in microwave 5 seconds.

PER SERVING Calories: 141 | Fat: 4.7 g | Protein: 1.6 g | Sodium: 153 mg | Fiber: 1.0 g | Carbohydrates: 23.6 g | Sugar: 13.5 g

Blueberry Cake

Take a bite out of this moist vegan Blueberry Cake. Made with minimal ingredients, this flavorful cake with creamy frosting is ready in around 35 minutes!

INGREDIENTS | SERVES 16

3 cups all-purpose flour
1¾ cups granulated sugar
⅔ cup vanilla soy protein powder
½ teaspoon salt
2 teaspoons baking soda
1 cup fresh blueberries
⅔ cup vegetable oil
2 cups cold water
2 tablespoons apple cider vinegar
2 teaspoons vanilla extract
1 batch Vegan Frosting (see this chapter for recipe)

1. Preheat oven to 350°F. Spray two round 8" cake pans with vegetable cooking spray.

2. Combine flour, sugar, protein powder, salt, and baking soda in a large bowl. Add blueberries and gently stir to coat blueberries. Set aside.

3. In a small bowl stir together vegetable oil, water, vinegar, and vanilla. Pour into flour mixture. Stir until combined.

4. Pour batter into prepared pans and bake 35 minutes until a toothpick inserted in center comes out clean.

5. Allow cakes to cool about 15 minutes before inverting onto a large serving plate.

6. Spread ½ frosting on top of one cake. Place second cake on top of frosted cake. Spread remaining frosting on top cake.

7. Cover and store at room temperature up to 4 days, refrigerate up to 8 days, or slice and freeze in freezer bags up to 2 months. To serve, heat individual slices in microwave 5 seconds.

PER SERVING Calories: 317 | Fat: 9.5 g | Protein: 4.5 g | Sodium: 258 mg | Fiber: 0.9 g | Carbohydrates: 52.6 g | Sugar: 33.9 g

Banana Cake

Love tender, moist cake with cream cheese frosting? This vegan Banana Cake will be your new favorite! There's no shortage of banana in this cake recipe, which is spiced with ginger and cinnamon and topped with a dreamy, creamy vegan cream cheese frosting!

INGREDIENTS | SERVES 16

For Cake

3 cups all-purpose flour
1½ teaspoons baking soda
1½ teaspoons baking powder
½ teaspoon salt
1 teaspoon ground ginger
1 teaspoon ground cinnamon
⅔ cup vegetable oil
1½ cups granulated sugar
3 large bananas, peeled and sliced
1 cup unsweetened almond milk
1 teaspoon vanilla extract
1 tablespoon apple cider vinegar

For Frosting

½ cup vegan cream cheese, softened
¼ cup vegan butter, softened
1½ cups powdered sugar
2 tablespoons unsweetened almond milk

1. Preheat oven to 350°F. Spray a 9" × 13" cake pan with vegetable cooking spray.

2. **To make Cake:** combine flour, baking soda, baking powder, salt, and spices in a large bowl. Set aside.

3. In a food processor bowl add oil, sugar, bananas, almond milk, vanilla, and vinegar. Pulse until smooth.

4. Pour banana mixture into flour mixture and stir until well combined. Pour batter into prepared cake pan.

5. Bake 50 minutes until top is golden brown and a toothpick inserted in center comes out clean. Let cool about 20 minutes.

6. **To make Frosting:** cream together vegan cream cheese and vegan butter until smooth. Add powdered sugar a little at a time until well combined. Add almond milk 1 tablespoon at a time until a spreadable consistency is achieved.

7. Once cake has cooled, top with frosting. Cover and store at room temperature up to 5 days, refrigerate up to 10 days, or slice and freeze in freezer bags up to 2 months. To serve, heat individual slices in microwave 5 seconds.

PER SERVING Calories: 336 | Fat: 12.2 g | Protein: 3.0 g | Sodium: 327 mg | Fiber: 1.5 g | Carbohydrates: 53.6 g | Sugar: 31.1 g

Strawberry Cake

If you need a reason to celebrate, this vegan Strawberry Cake will help. It's loaded with tender strawberries in every bite. You'll love the rich and oh-so-delicious cake topped with strawberry frosting. More proof that you can be vegan and have your (strawberry) cake too!

INGREDIENTS | SERVES 16

For Cake

2 cups all-purpose flour

1 cup whole-wheat flour

1½ cups granulated sugar

1½ teaspoons baking soda

1½ teaspoons baking powder

1 teaspoon salt

1 (1.6-ounce) box vegan Strawberry Jel Dessert

1½ cups stemmed, chopped fresh strawberries

1 cup vegetable oil

2 tablespoons ground flaxseed

1½ cups unsweetened almond milk

1½ teaspoons vanilla extract

1 tablespoon apple cider vinegar

4 drops plant-based red food coloring

For Strawberry Frosting

½ cup vegan butter, softened

3½ cups powdered sugar

3 fresh strawberries, stems removed, mashed

1. Preheat oven to 350°F. Grease a 9" × 13" cake pan with vegetable cooking spray.

2. **To make Cake:** mix flours, sugar, baking soda, baking powder, and salt together in a large bowl. Add gelatin. Stir to combine. Add strawberries and stir once more to combine. Set aside.

3. In a medium bowl combine vegetable oil, flaxseed, almond milk, vanilla, vinegar, and food coloring.

4. Stir milk mixture into flour mixture. Pour batter into prepared pan.

5. Bake 55 minutes until a toothpick inserted in center of cake comes out clean. Remove cake from oven and let cool about 20 minutes.

6. **To make Strawberry Frosting:** mix vegan butter with powdered sugar in a small bowl until smooth. Add strawberries and stir until a smooth consistency is reached.

7. Once cake has cooled, spread frosting over top of cake. Cover and store at room temperature up to 5 days, refrigerate up to 10 days, or slice and freeze in freezer bags up to 2 months. To serve, heat individual slices in microwave 5 seconds.

PER SERVING Calories: 415 | Fat: 16.3 g | Protein: 3.2 g | Sodium: 373 mg | Fiber: 2.6 g | Carbohydrates: 62.3 g | Sugar: 42.6 g

Chunky Monkey Cake

This moist, rich Chunky Monkey Cake is made with bananas, peanut butter, and chocolate. Each slice of this surprisingly vegan recipe yields a buttery banana cake base, with melted chocolate chips and a generous layer of chocolate frosting!

INGREDIENTS | SERVES 16

½ cup all-natural peanut butter

¾ cup vegetable oil

2 cups granulated sugar

1 teaspoon vanilla extract

3 large bananas, peeled and mashed

1 cup unsweetened almond milk

1 tablespoon ground flaxseed

1 tablespoon cornstarch

1 teaspoon apple cider vinegar

2 cups all-purpose flour

1 cup whole-wheat flour

3 teaspoons baking powder

½ teaspoon baking soda

1 teaspoon salt

1½ cups dairy-free chocolate chips

1 batch Vegan Frosting (chocolate version; see this chapter for recipe)

1. Preheat oven to 375°F. Spray a 9" × 13" cake pan with vegetable cooking spray.

2. In a large bowl combine peanut butter, vegetable oil, sugar, vanilla, bananas, almond milk, flaxseed, cornstarch, and vinegar. Set aside.

3. In separate large bowl combine flours, baking powder, baking soda, and salt. Pour into bowl with wet ingredients. Stir vigorously until combined. Add chocolate chips and stir to incorporate.

4. Pour batter into prepared pan and bake 50 minutes until a toothpick inserted in center comes out clean.

5. Let cool completely, about 20 minutes, then top cake with chocolate version of Vegan Frosting.

6. Cover cake and store at room temperature up to 5 days, refrigerate up to 10 days, or slice and freeze in freezer bags up to 2 months. To serve, heat individual slices in microwave 5 seconds.

PER SERVING Calories: 432 | Fat: 22.4 g | Protein: 3.1 g | Sodium: 210 mg | Fiber: 3.3 g | Carbohydrates: 55.7 g | Sugar: 47.4 g

Pumpkin Swirl Brownies

A fudgy brownie batter combines with swirly, cream cheese–infused pumpkin mixture to transform this recipe into a decadent, delicious treat! A dollop of brownie here and a smidge of Pumpkin Swirl there makes each bite a surprise!

INGREDIENTS | SERVES 16

For Pumpkin Swirl

½ cup canned pumpkin purée

1 (8-ounce) package vegan cream cheese, softened

2 tablespoons coconut sugar

1 teaspoon vanilla extract

For Brownie Base

½ cup vegan butter

½ cup creamy peanut butter

½ cup dairy-free chocolate chips

2 cups granulated sugar

1 teaspoon vanilla extract

1 (15-ounce) canned pumpkin purée, minus ½ cup

1½ cups all-purpose flour

½ cup cocoa powder

1 tablespoon ground flaxseed

2 tablespoons cornstarch

2 cups dairy-free chocolate chips, divided

1 cup chopped walnuts, divided

1. Preheat oven to 350°F. Grease a 9" × 13" cake pan with a light coating of vegetable cooking spray.

2. **To make Pumpkin Swirl:** combine ½ cup pumpkin purée, vegan cream cheese, coconut sugar, and vanilla in a medium bowl. Set aside.

3. **To make Brownie Base:** combine vegan butter, peanut butter, and chocolate chips in a large microwave-safe bowl. Place in microwave and heat 30 seconds until chocolate chips are soft enough to stir. Stir in sugar, vanilla, and remaining pumpkin purée.

4. In a medium bowl combine flour, cocoa powder, ground flaxseed, and cornstarch. Add to chocolate mixture. Stir until just combined.

5. Pour ½ Brownie Base into prepared pan, using a spoon to spread across bottom of pan. Sprinkle 1 cup chocolate chips and ½ cup chopped walnuts over brownie batter.

6. Drop Pumpkin Swirl and remaining Brownie Base batters by rounded spoonfuls evenly across Brownie Base. Run a butter knife through batter using a back and forth motion to create a swirled look across top of batter. Top with remaining chocolate chips and walnuts.

7. Bake 40 minutes until a toothpick inserted in center comes out clean. Remove from oven and let cool about 20 minutes.

8. Cover and store at room temperature up to 5 days, refrigerate up to 10 days, or slice and freeze in freezer bags up to 2 months. To serve, heat individual slices in microwave 5 seconds.

PER SERVING Calories: 531 | Fat: 27.8 g | Protein: 6.4 g | Sodium: 152 mg | Fiber: 5.5 g | Carbohydrates: 65.6 g | Sugar: 43.7 g

Healthy No-Bake Fruit Crisp

Most fruit crisps require time in the oven, but this healthy fruit crisp is a no-bake vegan twist. Cherries, strawberries, blueberries, and raspberries combine with a crumbly nut topping, garnished with vegan whipped topping!

INGREDIENTS | SERVES 4

2 cups fresh sweet cherries, pitted and quartered

2 cups mixed sliced strawberries, blueberries, and raspberries

4 tablespoons maple syrup, divided

3 tablespoons chia seeds

½ cup almonds

½ cup rolled oats

1 teaspoon vanilla extract

1 cup vegan whipped topping

Berries: A Nutritional Superfood!

Not only are berries nutritionally dense—offering fiber, potassium, antioxidants, vitamin C, and more—but they are also low in calories. You can buy berries fresh or frozen all year-round!

1. Place cherries in a large bowl with mixed berries. Add 2 tablespoons maple syrup and stir to combine.

2. Place chia seeds in a coffee grinder or food processor and pulse until a powder forms. Pour into fruit mixture and stir until combined. Cover mixture and refrigerate up to 1 hour.

3. Place almonds and oats in food processor. Pulse 3 seconds until crumbly. Add remaining maple syrup and vanilla. Pulse again 3 seconds to create a thick, crumbly crust. Cover and refrigerate up to 5 days.

4. To serve, spoon cherry mixture into four serving bowls. Sprinkle almond crisp on top, then top with vegan whipped topping.

PER SERVING Calories: 383 | Fat: 15.9 g | Protein: 8.2 g | Sodium: 3 mg | Fiber: 10.1 g | Carbohydrates: 54.8 g | Sugar: 33.7 g

Vanilla Cake with Chocolate Frosting

This veganized Vanilla Cake with Chocolate Frosting is made with chocolate icing and vanilla protein powder—the best of both essential dessert flavors! It is beautiful, easy to make, and delicious!

INGREDIENTS | SERVES 9

1½ cups all-purpose flour

1 cup granulated sugar

⅓ cup vanilla soy protein powder

½ teaspoon salt

1 teaspoon baking soda

⅓ cup vegetable oil

1 cup cold water

1 tablespoon apple cider vinegar

1 teaspoon vanilla extract

1 batch Vegan Frosting (chocolate version; see this chapter for recipe)

1. Preheat oven to 350°F. Spray an 8" round cake pan with vegetable cooking spray.

2. Combine flour, sugar, protein powder, salt, and baking soda in a large bowl. Set aside.

3. In a small bowl combine vegetable oil, water, vinegar, and vanilla. Pour into flour mixture. Stir until combined.

4. Pour batter into prepared pan and bake 35 minutes until a toothpick inserted in center comes out clean.

5. Allow cake to cool about 10 minutes before inverting onto a large serving plate. Once cake cools, top with Vegan Frosting (chocolate version).

6. Cover and store at room temperature up to 5 days, refrigerate up to 10 days, or slice and freeze in large freezer bags up to 2 months. To serve, heat individual slices in microwave 5 seconds.

PER SERVING Calories: 331 | Fat: 9.3 g | Protein: 4.4 g | Sodium: 165 mg | Fiber: 1.5 g | Carbohydrates: 58.2 g | Sugar: 40.4 g

Simple Banana Ice Cream

This dreamy, delicious, and surprisingly vegan banana ice cream is sweetened naturally with ripe bananas. It's an unbelievably simple recipe that can be adapted to include your favorite flavors.

INGREDIENTS | SERVES 4

4 medium bananas, peeled and cut into 2" slices

1 tablespoon macadamia nuts

¼ cup vanilla soy milk

1 teaspoon vanilla extract

1. Place bananas in a large freezer bag and freeze up to 3 hours.

2. Once frozen, add bananas to a food processor or blender. Add macadamia nuts, soy milk, and vanilla. Let sit 3 minutes to allow bananas to soften slightly, then pulse until smooth. Place in a large sealed container and freeze up to 2 months.

3. When ready to serve, scoop ice cream into serving dishes.

PER SERVING Calories: 128 | Fat: 1.8 g | Protein: 1.8 g | Sodium: 6 mg | Fiber: 3.3 g | Carbohydrates: 28.0 g | Sugar: 15.1 g

Simple Caramel Sauce

This vegan Simple Caramel Sauce will be your new go-to sauce, not just because it's easy to make and delicious, but also because it's made from wholesome ingredients! Serve it over oatmeal, vegan ice cream, fresh fruits, and more!

INGREDIENTS | SERVES 4

1 cup medjool dates, pitted

½ cup + 2 tablespoons water, divided

1 tablespoon all-natural peanut butter

Focus On Whole Foods

Weekends are a perfect time for indulgences, while most people try to stay more disciplined on weekdays. One way to make it easy to stick with your goals is to find whole foods to satisfy your sweet tooth. Simple Banana Ice Cream and date-infused Simple Caramel Sauce are two treats that will satisfy your sweet tooth in a healthy way.

1. Place dates and ½ cup water in a small pot over medium heat and bring to a simmer. Cook 1 minute, then turn heat off and set aside.

2. Place dates and water in a food processor with peanut butter. Pulse until smooth. Add more water, 1 tablespoon at a time, until desired consistency is reached.

3. Spoon sauce into a small lidded container and refrigerate up to 7 days. To serve, remove from refrigerator and cook in microwave in 30-second intervals until heated through.

PER SERVING Calories: 156 | Fat: 2.0 g | Protein: 1.8 g | Sodium: 0 mg | Fiber: 3.4 g | Carbohydrates: 36.9 g | Sugar: 32.3 g

Key Lime Pie

Get ready to enjoy this creamy, tart—yet still sweet—vegan Key Lime Pie. You'll love the easy-to-follow, no-bake instructions!

INGREDIENTS | SERVES 8

1½ cups graham cracker crumbs

2 tablespoons coconut oil, softened

Zest from 7 key limes

½ cup key lime juice

½ cup water

1 tablespoon agar-agar flakes

¼ cup granulated sugar

1 (8-ounce) container vegan cream cheese

1 (5.3-ounce) container dairy-free vanilla yogurt

1 (10-ounce) container extra-firm silken tofu

5 fresh spinach leaves

1 cup vegan whipped topping

¼ cup fresh raspberries

Working with Agar-Agar Flakes

You may not have heard of agar-agar flakes before, but that shouldn't stop you from trying them. These flakes are made from sea vegetables and are used to create a gel. Most gelatins have been made from hooves, meaning they are not vegan. You can buy agar-agar flakes in the Asian section of most health food stores, or online.

1. Spray a 9" pie pan with vegetable cooking spray.

2. Combine graham cracker crumbs and coconut oil in a medium bowl. Press into prepared pie pan.

3. Combine lime zest, lime juice, water, agar-agar flakes, and sugar in a small saucepan. Bring to a low boil over medium-high heat, then reduce heat to a simmer and cook 5 minutes.

4. Let saucepan mixture cool 1 minute before placing in refrigerator to cool about 20 minutes.

5. Add vegan cream cheese, yogurt, tofu, and spinach to a food processor. Pulse until smooth and creamy. Fold in cooled lime mixture and whip until smooth.

6. Pour filling into prepared pie crust, cover, and refrigerate at least 1 hour up to 5 days. Serve topped with whipped topping and raspberries.

PER SERVING Calories: 600 | Fat: 21.6 g | Protein: 24.2 g | Sodium: 861 mg | Fiber: 7.3 g | Carbohydrates: 74.9 g | Sugar: 7.3 g

CHAPTER 17

Weekend Gourmet Meals

Vegan Taco Casserole

What should you do with the crumbs at the bottom of the bag of tortilla chips...that's the question. This Vegan Taco Casserole delivers the answer! The epitome of easy, this dish can be made in minutes. Store the leftovers for the rest of the week.

INGREDIENTS | SERVES 9

1 cup crushed corn tortilla chips, divided

1 (15-ounce) can fat-free refried beans

1 (10-ounce) can mild diced tomatoes and green chilies, including juice, divided

1¼ cups Mexican-flavored vegan crumbles, divided

½ cup diced peeled yellow onions, divided

½ cup diced black olives, divided

1 (15-ounce) can black beans, rinsed and drained, divided

1¼ cups vegan Cheddar shreds, divided

Make It Spicy!

Replace vegan Cheddar shreds with shredded Daiya Jalapeño Havarti Style Farmhouse Block cheese for extra spice and flavor in Mexican recipes. Want even more spice? Add pickled jalapeños as a condiment. Be sure to have hot sauce like sriracha or Tabasco on hand for an added kick as well.

1. Preheat oven to 350°F. Spread ½ chips on bottom of an ungreased 9" square baking dish.

2. In a medium bowl combine refried beans and juice from can diced tomatoes and chilies. Spoon ½ mixture over chips in baking dish. Gently spread mixture, but do not stir.

3. Sprinkle ½ vegan crumbles over beans, followed by ½ onions, ½ black olives, ½ black beans, ½ tomatoes and chilies, and ½ Cheddar shreds. Repeat layers once more, beginning with remaining tortilla chips and ending with Cheddar shreds.

4. Cover dish with aluminum foil and bake 20 minutes. Use tongs to remove foil and bake another 5 minutes until edges are crispy.

5. Remove from oven and let cool about 15 minutes. Cover and refrigerate dish up to 5 days, or slice into individual servings and freeze up to 1 month. To serve, cook in microwave in 30-second intervals until heated through.

PER SERVING Calories: 206 | Fat: 6.9 g | Protein: 10.2 g | Sodium: 753 mg | Fiber: 8.0 g | Carbohydrates: 27.4 g | Sugar: 1.7 g

Vegan Chili Corn-Bread Casserole

This quick and easy vegan casserole creates a healthy, delicious, and filling meal that also yields lots of leftovers. Enjoy layers of corn bread, meatless taco filling, and a creamy center, topped with crumbled corn chips.

INGREDIENTS | SERVES 8

2 cups vegan crumbles

1 (1.25-ounce) envelope salt-free taco seasoning

2 (15-ounce) cans diced tomatoes, including liquid

1 cup cooked brown rice

1 (4-ounce) can diced green chilies, including liquid

2 (8-ounce) packages vegan corn-bread mix

1 cup plain soy milk

1 tablespoon ground flaxseed

1 tablespoon cornstarch

1 teaspoon apple cider vinegar

1 (15-ounce) can corn kernels, including liquid

1 cup vegan sour cream

2 cups corn chips, crumbled and divided

2 cups shredded vegan Cheddar cheese, divided

1. Preheat oven to 400°F. Spray a 9" × 13" baking dish with a light coating of vegetable cooking spray.

2. In a large bowl combine vegan crumbles and taco seasoning. Add tomatoes, rice, and green chilies. Stir to combine. Set aside.

3. Pour packets of corn-bread mix into a separate large bowl. Create a well in middle and pour soy milk, flaxseed, cornstarch, and vinegar into well. Stir center, gradually incorporating corn-bread mixture. Add corn, stirring to combine.

4. Pour ½ corn-bread batter into bottom of prepared dish. Top with ½ vegan meat mixture, all sour cream, ½ corn chips, and ½ vegan Cheddar shreds. Then repeat layers with remaining ingredients except Cheddar shreds.

5. Place in oven and bake 50 minutes. Top with remaining shredded cheese and bake another 5 minutes until cheese has melted.

6. Remove from oven and let cool about 15 minutes. Refrigerate up to 7 days, or cut into individual slices, place on a tray and place in freezer. Once slices have frozen, transfer to individual freezer bags and freeze up to 3 months.

7. To serve, cook in microwave in 30-second intervals until heated through.

PER SERVING Calories: 601 | Fat: 23.6 g | Protein: 14.8 g | Sodium: 1,319 mg | Fiber: 12.9 g | Carbohydrates: 85.6 g | Sugar: 17.5 g

Vegan Shepherd's Pie

When you're craving a savory comfort-food classic, prepare this Vegan Shepherd's Pie made with vegan crumbles, carrots, and potatoes.

INGREDIENTS | **SERVES 10**

For Potato Topping

5 pounds russet potatoes, chopped into small cubes

½ cup vegan butter, sliced

1½ cups unsweetened almond milk

1½ teaspoons salt

For Vegetable Filling

1 teaspoon olive oil

1 medium yellow onion, peeled and chopped

2 cups chopped peeled carrots

2 cloves garlic, peeled and minced

2 tablespoons tomato paste

½ cup white wine

4 cups vegetable broth

2 teaspoons soy sauce

2 bay leaves

2 tablespoons cornstarch

2 tablespoons cold water

1 (13.7-ounce) package vegan crumbles

1 cup frozen corn kernels

1 cup frozen peas

1. **To make Potato Topping:** place potatoes in a large pot over medium-high heat and cover with water. Bring to a boil, then reduce to medium-low heat and simmer until potatoes are fork tender, about 20 minutes. Remove from heat and let cool about 5 minutes before draining.

2. Place cooked potatoes into a large bowl. Add vegan butter slices and use a mashing tool to mash potatoes. Slowly add almond milk. Continue mashing until a thick consistency is attained. Add salt and stir to combine. Set aside.

3. Preheat oven to 400°F.

4. **To make Vegetable Filling:** pour olive oil into a large pot over medium heat. Add onions and carrots. Cook until tender, about 15 minutes. Add garlic and cook another 1 minute. Add tomato paste, wine, vegetable broth, and soy sauce. Stir to combine.

5. Add bay leaves and bring to a simmer, then continue cooking about 10 minutes.

6. Add cornstarch and water to a small bowl. Stir to dissolve cornstarch. Add into pot with onions and continue to simmer until a thick sauce forms, about 5 minutes. Add vegan crumbles, corn, and peas. Stir to combine. Discard bay leaves.

7. Pour Vegetable Filling into bottom of a 9" × 13" casserole dish. Top with mashed potatoes.

8. Bake 30 minutes until potatoes are golden brown and edges are bubbly. When done, remove from oven and set aside to cool about 20 minutes.

9. Cover and refrigerate up to 10 days. To serve, dish out individual servings and cook in microwave in 30-second intervals until heated through.

PER SERVING Calories: 317 | Fat: 5.8 g | Protein: 14.3 g | Sodium: 916 mg | Fiber: 7.0 g | Carbohydrates: 52.8 g | Sugar: 5.8 g

Vegan Mac and Cheese with Smoky Chickpeas

This Vegan Mac and Cheese with Smoky Chickpeas is an easy, creamy recipe you'll want to make on repeat! It's perfect for weekend dinners with friends.

INGREDIENTS | SERVES 6

⅓ cup cashews

1 tablespoon vegan butter

1 teaspoon garlic powder

1 teaspoon onion powder

1 teaspoon Dijon mustard

1 tablespoon tomato paste

¼ cup nutritional yeast flakes

½ teaspoon salt

1 (12-ounce) box elbow pasta, cooked according to package instructions, 1 cup liquid reserved

1 teaspoon olive oil

1 (15-ounce) can chickpeas, drained

2 tablespoons agave nectar

1 tablespoon liquid smoke

1. Add cashews, vegan butter, garlic powder, onion powder, mustard, tomato paste, nutritional yeast flakes, and salt to a food processor. Pulse to combine. Add reserved liquid from pasta. Pulse again 1 minute until a smooth sauce forms. Set aside.

2. Pour cheese sauce over cooked macaroni in a large pot and stir to combine. Place over medium-low heat and cook 5 minutes. Transfer to a large serving dish.

3. In a medium skillet over medium heat add olive oil. Add chickpeas and stir to coat with oil. Add agave nectar and liquid smoke and stir until chickpeas are coated. Continue cooking 10 minutes until chickpeas have turned golden.

4. Top Mac and Cheese with Smoky Chickpeas. Let cool 10 minutes, then cover and refrigerate up to 10 days or freeze up to 2 months. To serve, dish out individual servings and cook in microwave in 30-second intervals until heated through.

PER SERVING Calories: 360 | Fat: 6.4 g | Protein: 13.3 g | Sodium: 332 mg | Fiber: 5.6 g | Carbohydrates: 60.1 g | Sugar: 7.2 g

Vegan Mac and Cheese Casserole

Warm and creamy, this Vegan Mac and Cheese Casserole will satisfy your comfort-food cravings with healthy, savory deliciousness!

INGREDIENTS | SERVES 12

6 cups cold + 3 cups boiling water, divided

3½ cups uncooked elbow pasta

½ cup vegan butter

1 small yellow onion, peeled and chopped

½ cup all-purpose flour

2 tablespoons soy sauce

½ teaspoon salt

1½ teaspoons garlic powder

⅛ teaspoon ground turmeric

¼ cup vegetable oil

1 cup nutritional yeast flakes

½ teaspoon paprika

1½ cups vegan crumbles

2 cups broccoli florets

Using Whole-Wheat Pasta

For an added boost of nutrition, look for either whole-wheat pasta or pasta made with increased fiber. There are also some pasta brands made with beans or non-wheat grains that include more protein and fewer carbohydrates and that are often-times gluten-free as well.

1. Preheat oven to 350°F.

2. In a large pot add 6 cups cold water and bring to a boil over high heat. Add pasta and cook 8 minutes, stirring occasionally. Drain well. Pour cooked pasta into an ungreased 9" × 13" baking pan and set aside.

3. In a medium saucepan melt vegan butter over medium heat 30 seconds. Add onions and sauté 5 minutes until translucent. Stir in flour and whisk until mixture is smooth and bubbly.

4. Stir in remaining hot water, soy sauce, salt, garlic powder, and turmeric to saucepan. Continue cooking until sauce thickens and bubbles. Stir in oil, nutritional yeast flakes, and paprika, then remove from heat.

5. Pour ⅔ sauce on top of pasta and stir. Add vegan crumbles and broccoli and stir to distribute. Top with remaining sauce.

6. Bake 20 minutes, until edges are golden brown. Remove from oven and let cool about 15 minutes.

7. Cover and refrigerate dish up to 10 days or freeze up to 2 months. To serve, dish out individual servings and cook in microwave in 30-second intervals until heated through.

PER SERVING Calories: 255 | Fat: 8.3 g | Protein: 11.0 g | Sodium: 371 mg | Fiber: 3.4 g | Carbohydrates: 32.1 g | Sugar: 1.7 g

Vegan Chicken and Rice Casserole

This Vegan Chicken and Rice Casserole is magical because it's so full of comfort-food goodness that it disappears like that!

INGREDIENTS | SERVES 6

1 tablespoon olive oil

1 small yellow onion, peeled and chopped

1 (10-ounce) package Gardein Chick'n Scallopini, thawed and chopped

2 cups sliced white mushrooms

3 cups small broccoli florets

3 tablespoons gluten-free flour

1 cup unsweetened almond milk

1 cup cooked brown rice

⅔ cup vegan sour cream

2 tablespoons Vegan Mayonnaise (see Chapter 7 for recipe)

2 tablespoons nutritional yeast flakes

¼ teaspoon dried thyme

1 cup vegan Cheddar shreds

1. Preheat oven to 350°F.

2. Pour olive oil into a large skillet with onions. Cook over medium heat 5 minutes until onions are tender. Add vegan chicken, mushrooms, and broccoli. Cook 7 minutes until mushrooms and broccoli are tender.

3. Sprinkle flour over mixture and stir to incorporate. Cook 2 minutes. Gradually add almond milk. Cook and stir another 2 minutes until a sauce forms. Stir in cooked brown rice, vegan sour cream, Vegan Mayonnaise, nutritional yeast, and thyme.

4. Transfer mixture to a 9" × 9" ungreased baking dish and sprinkle with vegan Cheddar cheese. Bake 20 minutes until cheese melts. Remove from oven and let cool about 15 minutes.

5. Cover and refrigerate up to 10 days or freeze up to 2 months. To serve, dish out individual servings and cook in microwave in 30-second intervals until heated through.

PER SERVING Calories: 276 | Fat:16.3 g | Protein: 10.5 g | Sodium: 503 mg | Fiber: 6.2 g | Carbohydrates: 25.6 g | Sugar: 2.7 g

Crispy Orange Tofu

Rather than calling for takeout, enjoy this delicious Crispy Orange Tofu with sticky orange sauce. You'll like the food—and how you feel too!

Stay Organized

Active meal preppers know there can be a lot going on in your kitchen at any given time. Being organized can help you stay on top of it all. Keep measuring cups and spoons in the same location, and clean out your refrigerator at regular intervals.

1. In a small bowl combine flaxseed, water, cornstarch, and flour. Add tofu and toss to thoroughly coat.

2. Place a large skillet over medium-high heat and add ½ sesame oil. Place three sheets of paper towels on a large plate nearby. Use tongs to place ½ tofu in heated oil, allowing space between each piece. Cook about 5 minutes on each side.

3. Once golden on each side, transfer to paper towel–lined plate. Repeat with remaining oil and tofu. Set aside.

4. **To make Coating:** in a small bowl combine ingredients. Set aside.

5. Return tofu to skillet and add Coating. Cook over medium heat until sauce thickens, about 5 minutes.

6. Let tofu cool about 5 minutes, then transfer to a large sealed container and refrigerate up to 10 days.

7. **To make Orange Sauce:** combine all ingredients (except rice) in a medium microwave-safe bowl. Heat in microwave 30 seconds, then stir. Repeat until sauce thickens. Let cool, 10 minutes, then cover and refrigerate up to 10 days.

8. To serve, heat rice in microwave in 30-second intervals until heated through. Place in bowls. Cook tofu in microwave in 30-second intervals until heated through. Place tofu over warmed rice. Cook Orange Sauce in microwave in 10-second intervals until heated through and drizzle over tofu.

PER SERVING Calories: 483 | Fat: 17.3 g | Protein: 17.1 g | Sodium: 1,018 mg | Fiber: 5.6 g | Carbohydrates: 66.1 g | Sugar: 7.2 g

Baked Nachos

These crispy vegan nachos are loaded with all your favorite toppings, making for a delicious, cheesy experience!

INGREDIENTS | SERVES 8

2 cups vegan crumbles

1 tablespoon taco seasoning

1 (15-ounce) can black beans, drained

1 cup frozen corn kernels

12 ounces tortilla chips

1 cup vegan Cheddar shreds

½ cup shredded Daiya Jalapeño Havarti Style Farmhouse Block

½ cup red cabbage, sliced into thin strips

1 cup cherry tomatoes, quartered

1 tablespoon diced green onion

¼ cup sliced pickled jalapeños

2 tablespoons vegan sour cream

1. Combine vegan crumbles with taco seasoning in a small bowl. If crumbles are frozen, heat in microwave 30 seconds, then stir to combine with seasoning. Transfer to a small lidded container and refrigerate up to 7 days.

2. Combine black beans and corn in a small lidded container. Refrigerate up to 10 days. Refrigerate remaining ingredients (except chips) in separate lidded containers up to 5 days.

3. To serve, preheat oven to 400°F. Line a baking sheet with parchment paper.

4. Arrange tortilla chips in a single layer on prepared baking sheet. Top with vegan crumble mixture, black beans and corn, and shredded cheeses. Bake 7 minutes until cheese is melted.

5. When nachos are done, remove from oven and serve immediately topped with cabbage, tomatoes, green onions, jalapeños, and vegan sour cream.

PER SERVING Calories: 408 | Fat: 16.4 g | Protein: 13.2 g | Sodium: 712 mg | Fiber: 9.1 g | Carbohydrates: 51.8 g | Sugar: 2.6 g

Vegan Meatloaf

Enjoy healthy comfort food with this homemade Vegan Meatloaf. It's made with black beans, quinoa, and lots of savory flavorings, with a sweet tomato topping.

INGREDIENTS | SERVES 10

For Vegan Meatloaf

1 tablespoon olive oil

1 large yellow onion, peeled and chopped

1 teaspoon dried thyme

1 teaspoon dried oregano

2 tablespoons soy sauce

1 teaspoon Better Than Bouillon Seasoned Vegetable Base

1 tablespoon tomato paste

1 (14-ounce) package Gimme Lean Vegan Sausage

1 (15-ounce) can black beans, drained and rinsed

1 cup cooked quinoa

½ cup shredded peeled carrots

2 tablespoons blackberry jam

½ cup bread crumbs

2 tablespoons ground flaxseed

2 tablespoons cornstarch

For Topping

½ cup ketchup

½ cup agave nectar

½ teaspoon ground nutmeg

1. Preheat oven to 350°F. Spray a 9" × 5" loaf pan with vegetable cooking spray.

2. **To make Vegan Meatloaf:** pour olive oil into a large skillet over medium heat. Add onions, thyme, and oregano and cook until onions are tender, about 5 minutes. Remove from heat and stir in soy sauce, Better Than Bouillon, and tomato paste. Set aside.

3. In a large bowl combine vegan sausage, black beans, quinoa, carrots, blackberry jam, bread crumbs, flaxseed, cornstarch, and onion mixture. Use a spatula to break up vegan sausage and beans.

4. Press meatloaf mixture into prepared loaf pan. Bake 45 minutes until edges separate from pan and look crispy.

5. **To make Topping:** combine ketchup, agave nectar, and nutmeg in a small bowl. Set aside.

6. When meatloaf is done, remove from oven and invert loaf pan onto an ungreased baking sheet. Turn oven up to 400°F.

7. Use a spatula to spread ketchup topping across top of meatloaf, allowing it to spill over sides. Place meatloaf back in oven and bake 15 minutes, then remove from oven and let cool 15 minutes.

8. Transfer to a large lidded container and refrigerate up to 10 days or slice and freeze up to 2 months. To serve, place slices in a toaster oven and cook about 5 minutes until heated through.

PER SERVING Calories: 251 | Fat: 5.2 g | Protein: 12.1 g | Sodium: 715 mg | Fiber: 5.6 g | Carbohydrates: 36.5 g | Sugar: 14.1 g

Vegan Fettuccine Alfredo

*Comfort food at its very best. Enjoy this Vegan Fettuccine Alfredo
for an easy dinner full of healthy ingredients!*

INGREDIENTS | SERVES 6

½ cup cashews

1 cup water

1 medium sweet potato, perforated with a fork

¼ cup nutritional yeast flakes

1 clove garlic, peeled and roughly chopped

¼ teaspoon salt

⅛ teaspoon ground black pepper

2 tablespoons vegan butter

2 tablespoons Ripple Original Plant-Based Half & Half

1 (16-ounce) package fettuccine noodles, cooked according to package instructions

1 teaspoon olive oil

1. Place cashews in a small saucepan with water over medium-high heat. Bring to a boil, then reduce to a simmer over medium heat and cook 5 minutes. Set aside.

2. Place potato in microwave and cook 3 minutes. Remove with oven mitts and let cool 3 minutes, then slice.

3. Pour cooked cashews (with water), nutritional yeast, garlic, salt, pepper, sweet potato slices, and vegan butter into a food processor. Pulse until smooth. Add half-and-half and pulse again until creamy.

4. Let cool 10 minutes, then transfer mixture to a medium lidded container and refrigerate up to 5 days.

5. Transfer fettuccine noodles to a large lidded serving bowl and drizzle with olive oil. Stir to combine. Refrigerate up to 5 days.

6. To serve, cook portioned pasta and sauce in microwave in 30-second intervals until heated through.

PER SERVING Calories: 403 | Fat: 8.8 g | Protein: 13.4 g | Sodium: 148 mg | Fiber: 3.9 g | Carbohydrates: 65.7 g | Sugar: 3.5 g

Vegan Beef Empanadas

A crispy crust combines with vegan beef and potatoes to make Vegan Beef Empanadas: a delicious dinner you'll want to serve time and time again!

INGREDIENTS | SERVES 20

For Dough

1 cup whole-wheat flour
3 cups all-purpose flour
2 teaspoons baking powder
1 teaspoon salt
½ cup cold vegan butter, sliced
¾ cup cold water
¼ cup chilled vodka

For Filling

1 teaspoon olive oil
1 cup chopped peeled yellow onion
1 large red potato, diced
1½ cups vegan crumbles, thawed
1 cup vegan chorizo
4 cloves garlic, peeled and minced
2 teaspoons dried thyme

1 teaspoon paprika
1 cup vegetable broth
1½ cups vegan Cheddar shreds
2 tablespoons Ripple Original Plant-Based Half & Half
1 cup dairy-free marinara sauce

1. **To make Dough:** add both flours, baking powder, and salt to a food processor. Pulse until combined. Add butter pieces and pulse until well incorporated. Add water and vodka and continue pulsing until dough comes together.

2. Transfer dough to a bowl. Cover in plastic wrap and refrigerate during next steps.

3. **To make Filling:** add olive oil, onions, and potatoes to a large skillet over medium heat. Cook 10 minutes until onions are tender. Add vegan crumbles and vegan chorizo. Stir, breaking any larger chorizo pieces apart. Add garlic, thyme, and paprika. Stir to combine. Add broth and bring to a simmer, then cook another 10 minutes until potatoes are tender and sauce thickens. Remove from heat and let cool about 5 minutes.

4. Preheat oven to 400°F. Line a baking sheet with parchment paper.

5. Create a ball out of dough. Cut in half. Wrap one half in plastic wrap and place back in refrigerator. Divide other half into 5 dough balls about the size of golf balls. Use a rolling pin to roll each ball into a 5" circle.

6. Run your spatula down center of skillet to divide contents in half. Spoon 2 tablespoons of filling into center of one dough round and top with a little bit of vegan Cheddar shreds.

7. Wet your finger with water, then run around edges of dough. Wrap dough around filling and use moisture on edges to press together. Fold edge back to create a crust and use your fingers to pinch pleats. Repeat process with remaining rounds, filling, and cheese, then repeat again with second half dough and skillet contents.

8. Brush tops of each empanada with half-and-half. Bake 15 minutes until golden brown. Once done, remove from oven and let cool about 10 minutes.

9. Store in a large sealed container in refrigerator up to 10 days or in freezer up to 2 months. To serve, cook in a toaster oven about 5 minutes until heated through. Serve with marinara sauce.

PER SERVING Calories: 185 | Fat: 6.0 g | Protein: 6.0 g | Sodium: 470 mg | Fiber: 290.0 g | Carbohydrates: 26.2 g | Sugar: 1.8 g

Vegan Enchilada Bowl with Brown Rice

Enjoy the flavors of classic enchiladas in this Vegan Enchilada Bowl with Brown Rice. Ready in less than 30 minutes, this simple, tasty recipe makes healthy meals a breeze.

INGREDIENTS | SERVES 3

1 tablespoon maple syrup

2 tablespoons soy sauce

2 tablespoons chili powder, divided

1 tablespoon almond butter

1 (10-ounce) package Gardein Chick'n Strips, thawed

2 teaspoons olive oil, divided

1 medium yellow onion, peeled and finely chopped

1 clove garlic, peeled and chopped

1 (8-ounce) can tomato sauce

¼ teaspoon ground cumin

4 tablespoons nutritional yeast flakes

1 cup cooked brown rice

1 (15-ounce) can black beans, including liquid

1 medium avocado, peeled, pitted, and sliced

1 cup mild chunky salsa

1. Make marinade by pouring maple syrup, soy sauce, 1 tablespoon chili powder, and almond butter into an 8" × 8" ungreased casserole dish. Stir to combine. Add vegan chicken pieces. Stir to coat. Set aside.

2. Place 1 teaspoon olive oil in a medium saucepan over medium heat. Add onion and cook until tender, about 5 minutes. Add garlic and cook another 1 minute.

3. Pour tomato sauce, remaining chili powder, cumin, and nutritional yeast into pan with onion. Stir until combined. Add brown rice and black beans. Stir to combine. Cook about 5 minutes.

4. Heat remaining teaspoon oil in a large skillet over medium heat. Place marinated vegan chicken pieces in skillet. Cook 5 minutes on each side. Add rest of marinade to skillet and cook until sauce thickens, about 5 minutes.

5. Add chicken mixture to rice mixture and stir together. Remove from heat and let cool about 5 minutes.

6. Transfer to a large lidded container and refrigerate up to 7 days or freeze up to 2 months. To serve, spoon individual servings into bowls and cook in microwave in 30-second intervals until heated through. Garnish with sliced avocado and salsa.

PER SERVING Calories: 618 | Fat: 20.7 g | Protein: 32.6 g | Sodium: 2,590 mg | Fiber: 20.4 g | Carbohydrates: 73.1 g | Sugar: 15.9 g

Vegan Beef Stroganoff

This easy Vegan Beef Stroganoff is ready in 30 minutes and is perfect for either lunch or dinner!

INGREDIENTS | SERVES 5

1 tablespoon vegetable oil, divided

1 (10-ounce) package Gardein Beefless Tips, thawed

¼ cup peeled minced yellow onion

2 cloves garlic, peeled and minced

1 tablespoon all-purpose flour

2 teaspoons Better Than Bouillon No Beef Base

1 tablespoon white wine

1 teaspoon vegan Worcestershire sauce

1 cup water

¼ cup vegan sour cream

10 ounces egg-free wide noodles, prepared according to package instructions

Is Vegan Worcestershire Sauce Different?

Standard Worcestershire sauce is made using anchovies, but the good news is that some brands offer vegan Worcestershire sauce that is anchovy-free. You can find vegan Worcestershire sauce at most health food stores and in the health food section of some grocery stores.

1. Pour ½ vegetable oil into a large skillet over medium-high heat. Add vegan beefless tips in a single layer and cook until browned on one side, about 5 minutes. Flip pieces and cook on other side another 5 minutes. Place cooked pieces on a paper towel and set aside.

2. Add remaining ½ vegetable oil to same skillet and add onions, cooking 1 minute. Add garlic and cook until fragrant, about 30 seconds. Sprinkle with flour and stir to coat.

3. In a small bowl combine Better Than Bouillon, white wine, and vegan Worcestershire sauce. Add water and stir to combine.

4. Add ½ mixture to skillet. Use a spatula to stir and scrape bits in skillet. Add remaining ½ mixture and stir to combine. Cook over medium heat another 5 minutes.

5. Stir in vegan sour cream and cook another 1 minute to allow sauce to thicken further. Add vegan beefless tips back into skillet. Add noodles and stir until tips and noodles are coated.

6. Remove from heat and let cool about 10 minutes. Then transfer to a large lidded container and refrigerate up to 10 days. To serve, dish out into individual bowls and cook in microwave in 30-second intervals until heated through.

PER SERVING Calories: 306 | Fat: 9.3 g | Protein: 17.5 g | Sodium: 753 mg | Fiber: 3.7 g | Carbohydrates: 38.2 g | Sugar: 1.5 g

Vegan Teriyaki Rice Bowls

Enjoy a tasty Vegan Teriyaki Rice Bowl this week. This recipe is made with fewer than 10 ingredients and is ready in 30 minutes. "Vegan, Vegan Chick'n Dinner!"

INGREDIENTS | SERVES 4

1 tablespoon olive oil

2 cups broccoli florets

1 cup chopped peeled yellow onion

1 cup sliced seeded red and yellow bell pepper

2 teaspoons dried ginger

1 teaspoon garlic powder

1 (10.5-ounce) package Gardein Teriyaki Chick'n Strips

1 cup frozen shelled edamame

3 cups cooked brown rice

1. In a large skillet over medium heat add olive oil, broccoli, onion, peppers, ginger, and garlic powder. Stir and cook until broccoli is tender, about 5 minutes.

2. Push vegetables to outer edges of pan, creating space in middle of skillet. Add vegan chicken pieces (not including sauce packet) to center of skillet. Cook until browned, about 7 minutes. Add edamame and cook 1 minute until heated through.

3. Pour in sauce packet and stir ingredients, including vegetables, around edges of pan. Add rice and stir until coated.

4. Let cool 10 minutes, then transfer mixture to a large lidded container (or individual serving containers) and refrigerate up to 7 days or freeze up to 2 months. To serve, spoon into individual serving bowls and cook in microwave in 30-second intervals until heated through.

PER SERVING Calories: 397 | Fat: 9.8 g | Protein: 23.5 g | Sodium: 275 mg | Fiber: 8.7 g | Carbohydrates: 50.5 g | Sugar: 4.2 g

Beefless Pot Pie Casserole

Ready for a hearty dish that yields lots of delicious leftovers? You'll want to dig into this Beefless Pot Pie Casserole with a cheesy biscuit topping.

INGREDIENTS | SERVES 9

⅓ cup all-purpose flour

1 teaspoon dried thyme

1 tablespoon nutritional yeast flakes

½ teaspoon salt

¼ teaspoon ground black pepper

1 package Gardein Beefless Tips, thawed

1 teaspoon vegetable oil

1 medium yellow onion, peeled and chopped

2 cups chopped peeled carrots

2 cups chopped russet potatoes

1 cup chopped celery

2 cups small cauliflower florets

3 cups vegetable broth

2 bay leaves

1 cup frozen corn kernels

1 cup frozen peas

For Biscuit Topping

2 cups all-purpose flour

1 cup whole-wheat flour

1 teaspoon baking powder

½ teaspoon baking soda

½ teaspoon salt

½ cup vegan butter

1 cup unsweetened almond milk

1 cup shredded vegan Cheddar cheese

1. Preheat oven to 350°F.

2. Place flour, thyme, nutritional yeast, salt, and pepper in a large sealable bag. Shake to mix together. Add beefless tips and shake to coat.

3. Add vegetable oil to a large skillet over medium heat. Place beefless tips in skillet, reserving leftover flour mixture. Cook until browned on both sides, about 5 minutes per side. Set aside on a large plate.

4. To same skillet add onions, carrots, potatoes, celery, cauliflower, and vegetable broth. Stir together and top with bay leaves. Cook and stir gently, until vegetables are slightly tender, about 15 minutes.

5. Pour in reserved flour mixture and stir to incorporate. Bring to a boil, then reduce to simmer over medium-low heat. Continue to simmer until liquid thickens, about 5 minutes.

6. Stir in corn and peas, then pour into an ungreased 9" × 13" casserole dish and top with cooked beefless tips. Discard bay leaves.

7. **To make Biscuit Topping:** add flours, baking powder, baking soda, and salt to a food processor. Pulse to combine. Add vegan butter. Pulse until mixture forms small pea-sized crumbles. Add almond milk. Pulse to combine. Add vegan cheese and pulse once more.

8. Spoon topping evenly across beefless stew in casserole dish and cook, uncovered, 40 minutes until topping is golden brown. Remove from oven and let cool about 20 minutes.

9. Cover and refrigerate up to 10 days or freeze up to 2 months. To serve, cook in microwave in 30-second intervals until heated through.

PER SERVING Calories: 378 | Fat: 10.8 g | Protein: 13.7 g | Sodium: 943 mg | Fiber: 7.3 g | Carbohydrates: 60.0 g | Sugar: 4.6 g

Vegan Sushi with Cauliflower Rice

You'll love this supereasy, superhealthy Vegan Sushi with Cauliflower Rice. If you haven't made sushi at home before, don't worry: the instructions are a snap, and the result is stunning and delicious!

INGREDIENTS | SERVES 8

4 sheets nori

1 batch Easy Cauliflower Rice (see Chapter 8 for recipe)

1 medium red bell pepper, seeded and thinly sliced

1 medium avocado, peeled, pitted, and sliced

¼ head medium red cabbage, thinly sliced

2 green onions, thinly sliced lengthwise

2 cups chopped field greens

For Dipping Sauce

¼ cup all-natural peanut butter

2 teaspoons agave nectar

2 teaspoons soy sauce

1 teaspoon sriracha

1 teaspoon water

2 teaspoons chopped peanuts

1. Place one nori sheet on a bamboo roller. Top ½ sheet with a thin layer of cauliflower rice. Top rice with a portion of red bell pepper, avocado, red cabbage, green onion, and field greens. Use bamboo roller to roll nori, using your fingers to press down on nori sheet as it rolls up. Roll tightly, then let roll sit 2 minutes, seam-side down. Slice into six pieces. Repeat with remaining nori and portioned-out ingredients.

2. Transfer sushi to a large lidded container and refrigerate up to 5 days.

3. **To make Dipping Sauce:** combine peanut butter, agave nectar, soy sauce, sriracha, and water in a small lidded container. Sprinkle top with chopped peanuts. Cover and refrigerate up to 10 days.

PER SERVING Calories: 107 | Fat: 6.7 g | Protein: 3.6 g | Sodium: 107 mg | Fiber: 3.2 g | Carbohydrates: 9.4 g | Sugar: 4.3 g

Vegan Bulgogi Jackfruit Street Tacos

Dig into these Vegan Bulgogi Jackfruit Street Tacos that are easy to make, fun to throw together, and so delicious to eat. You'll be coming back for more!

INGREDIENTS | SERVES 12

1 batch Slow Cooker Vegan Bulgogi Jackfruit (see Chapter 12 for recipe)

1 batch Brussels Sprouts Slaw (see Chapter 6 for recipe)

⅓ cup vegan sour cream

½ teaspoon fresh lime zest

2 tablespoons fresh lime juice

1 teaspoon garlic powder

12 (6") corn tortillas

4 fresh lime slices

1. Transfer Slow Cooker Vegan Bulgogi Jackfruit to a large lidded container and refrigerate up to 10 days. Transfer Brussels Sprouts Slaw to a medium lidded container and refrigerate up to 10 days.

2. In a small lidded bowl combine vegan sour cream, lime zest, lime juice, and garlic powder. Cover and refrigerate up to 7 days.

3. To serve, cook jackfruit in microwave in 30-second intervals until heated through. Let Brussels Sprouts Slaw and sour cream sauce come to room temperature while jackfruit is cooking.

4. Lay two corn tortillas flat on a large plate. Spoon a portion of jackfruit in middle of tortilla and spread it in a line. Top with a spoonful of slaw. Repeat with each taco. Drizzle each taco with sour cream sauce. Serve with lime slices.

PER SERVING Calories: 216 | Fat: 8.1 g | Protein: 5.2 g | Sodium: 1,189 mg | Fiber: 5.7 g | Carbohydrates: 31.6 g | Sugar: 10.1 g

Vegan Twice-Baked Potatoes

Enjoy these Vegan Twice-Baked Potatoes as a filling main dish. You'll love the cheesy flavors and delicious toppings that make this the perfect baked potato!

INGREDIENTS | SERVES 2

2 large russet potatoes, perforated with a fork

1 teaspoon olive oil

1 medium sweet potato, perforated with a fork

½ cup vegan sour cream

½ cup unsweetened almond milk

2 tablespoons vegan butter

½ cup nutritional yeast flakes

½ teaspoon salt

¼ cup chopped green onion

2 tablespoons chopped fresh chives

½ cup shredded vegan Cheddar cheese

1. Preheat oven to 400°F.

2. Rub russet potatoes with olive oil and place potatoes directly on middle rack in oven to cook 1½ hours, until fork tender. Leave oven on.

3. Place sweet potato in microwave and cook 3 minutes. Remove with an oven mitt and set aside to cool about 5 minutes before chopping into large cubes.

4. Once russet potatoes are done, use tongs to remove them from oven. Let cool about 7 minutes, then cut each potato in half lengthwise. Scoop out middle of potatoes, leaving about ⅛" thickness around skin so potatoes don't collapse.

5. Add scooped potatoes, vegan sour cream, almond milk, vegan butter, nutritional yeast, sweet potato cubes, and salt to a food processor. Pulse until smooth.

6. Spoon filling into scooped-out potatoes. Sprinkle with green onions, chives, and vegan Cheddar cheese.

7. Place potatoes back in heated oven 10 minutes to reheat. Remove from oven and set aside to cool about 15 minutes.

8. Transfer potatoes to a medium lidded container and refrigerate up to 7 days or freeze in freezer bags up to 3 months. To serve, cook in microwave in 30-second intervals until heated through.

PER SERVING Calories: 665 | Fat: 25.4 g | Protein: 17.5 g | Sodium: 1,107 mg | Fiber: 15.4 g | Carbohydrates: 95.6 g | Sugar: 5.5 g

Stuffed Peppers

Recipes take on a new meaning when vegan crumbles are used. That's because there's no cooking involved, so dishes like these delicious vegan Stuffed Peppers come together with ease.

INGREDIENTS | SERVES 6

6 large green bell peppers, tops removed, cored and seeded

1½ cups cooked brown rice

1 (13.7-ounce) package vegan crumbles

½ cup chopped peeled yellow onion

1 (8-ounce) can tomato sauce

1 teaspoon salt

½ teaspoon garlic powder

1 cup vegan Cheddar shreds, divided

1. Trim a little off bottom of each bell pepper to create a level surface. Place peppers hollow-side up in a 9" × 13" ungreased baking dish.

2. Preheat oven to 350°F. In a large bowl stir together rice, vegan crumbles, onions, tomato sauce, salt, garlic powder, and ½ vegan cheese.

3. Stuff each pepper with equal amounts filling. Top each with equal amounts remaining cheese. Cover dish with foil.

4. Bake 30 minutes. Once done, use tongs to remove foil and bake another 10 minutes until pepper filling is golden around edges. Let cool about 10 minutes.

5. Once cooled, transfer to a large lidded container and refrigerate up to 7 days or freeze up to 2 months. To serve, cook in microwave in 30-second intervals until heated through.

PER SERVING Calories: 184 | Fat: 6.2 g | Protein: 12.2 g | Sodium: 941 mg | Fiber: 6.7 g | Carbohydrates: 23.2 g | Sugar: 6.9 g

Vegan Mexican Lasagna

This Vegan Mexican Lasagna is made with layers of the best south-of-the-border flavors. It will yield lots of leftovers, so it's perfect for batch cooking meal plans!

INGREDIENTS | SERVES 9

1 medium yellow onion, peeled and chopped

1 tablespoon olive oil

2 cloves garlic, peeled and chopped

1 (13.7-ounce) package vegan crumbles

1 package fajita seasoning

½ cup water

½ cup cornmeal

1 (15-ounce) package extra-firm tofu

1 medium avocado, peeled and chopped

1 can chickpeas, drained

½ teaspoon ground turmeric

½ teaspoon onion powder

1 teaspoon garlic powder

½ teaspoon salt

2 cups mild chunky salsa

18 (6") corn tortillas

1 (7-ounce) package vegan Cheddar shreds

1. Preheat oven to 350°F.

2. In a medium skillet over medium heat, sauté onion in oil 5 minutes until onions are tender. Add garlic, soy crumbles, and fajita seasoning. Stir in water and cornmeal and cook over low heat 5 minutes. Set aside to cool during next step.

3. Add tofu, avocado, chickpeas, turmeric, onion powder, garlic powder, and salt to a food processor and pulse until well combined.

4. Spoon some of salsa into bottom of an ungreased 9" × 13" baking pan and top with 6 corn tortillas. Spoon ½ fajita-spiced vegan crumbles over tortillas, followed by ½ avocado mixture, then ½ Cheddar and additional salsa, and top with remaining Cheddar shreds.

5. Bake 30 minutes until cheese melts. Remove from oven and let cool about 20 minutes.

6. Cover and refrigerate up to 10 days or freeze up to 3 months. To serve, cook in microwave in 30-second intervals until heated through.

PER SERVING Calories: 435 | Fat: 14.5 g | Protein: 19.8 g | Sodium: 1,268 mg | Fiber: 10.7 g | Carbohydrates: 55.3 g | Sugar: 7.5 g

Vegan Carnitas Taco Bar

Nothing beats a taco bar for fun weekend entertainment. This vegan version is made with jackfruit and served with all the trimmings to make your taco bar a festive event!

INGREDIENTS | SERVES 6

1 tablespoon olive oil

1 cup thinly sliced peeled red onion

2 cloves garlic, peeled and minced

1 jalapeño pepper, seeded and finely diced

2 (15-ounce) cans young green jackfruit (not in syrup), drained

2 cups mild chunky salsa, divided

1 teaspoon ground cumin

½ teaspoon salt

⅛ teaspoon ground black pepper

Juice of 1 large navel orange

1 cup water

1 bay leaf

1 cup Fresh Corn Salsa (see Chapter 8 for recipe)

1 cup guacamole

10 green onions, chopped

1 cup canned black beans, drained

½ cup pickled jalapeños

1 cup vegan Cheddar shreds

¼ cup roughly chopped fresh cilantro

12 (6") soft taco corn tortillas

1. Place olive oil and onions in a large saucepan over medium-high heat. Cook 5 minutes until onions are tender. Reduce heat to medium and add garlic and jalapeño. Cook another 1 minute.

2. Stir in jackfruit, 1 cup salsa, cumin, salt, black pepper, orange juice, and water. Top with bay leaf and cook 30 minutes until jackfruit becomes tender. Use a spatula to break jackfruit into smaller pieces while cooking.

3. Remove bay leaf and let mixture cool about 10 minutes, then transfer to a large sealed container and refrigerate up to 5 days.

4. Transfer topping ingredients to separate sealed containers and refrigerate up to 5 days.

5. To serve, cook carnitas in microwave in 30-second intervals until heated through. Warm corn tortillas about 10 seconds in microwave to make them soft and pliable. Top each tortilla with portioned-out carnitas and toppings.

PER SERVING Calories: 429 | Fat: 16.5 g | Protein: 9.7 g | Sodium: 2,074 mg | Fiber: 13.2 g | Carbohydrates: 62.0 g | Sugar: 14.5 g

Multipurpose Recipes

In some recipes, the main ingredients can be used to make a sandwich, top a salad or baked potato, or more. For example, you can toss this taco "meat" into your favorite mac and cheese recipe. Try repurposing your ingredients for even more variety in your meal prepping.

Vegan Jalapeño Havarti Cheese Ball

This Vegan Jalapeño Havarti Cheese Ball is easy to make, requiring fewer than ten ingredients. You'll be surprised that it's vegan! Serve with your favorite crackers.

INGREDIENTS | SERVES 12

¼ cup whole + ⅓ cup chopped candied pecans, divided

2 tablespoons agave nectar

⅛ teaspoon + ½ teaspoon salt, divided

1 (7-ounce) package Daiya Jalapeño Havarti Style Farmhouse Block, chopped into ½" cubes

1 (8-ounce) container vegan cream cheese

1 teaspoon garlic powder

1 medium jalapeño, seeded and chopped

1. Preheat oven to 350°F and line a baking sheet with parchment paper.

2. Combine chopped pecans with agave nectar and sprinkle with ⅛ teaspoon salt. Pour onto prepared baking sheet and bake 8 minutes. Remove from oven to cool about 10 minutes.

3. Add Havarti cheese, vegan cream cheese, garlic powder, and remaining salt to a food processor and pulse 3 seconds. Push ingredients down and pulse again until combined and mostly smooth.

4. In a small skillet add jalapeño and spray tops with a bit of vegetable cooking spray. Cook over medium heat until jalapeños are tender, about 5 minutes.

5. Add whole candied pecans and cooked jalapeño to cream cheese mixture in food processor and pulse again 3 seconds. Leave bits of jalapeño throughout cheese ball.

6. Form mixture into a ball on a medium plate, cover with plastic wrap, and refrigerate 20 minutes.

7. Add chopped pecans to a small dish. Roll firmed cheese ball in pecans until mostly covered. Place back on a plate and serve immediately or refrigerate up to 10 days.

PER SERVING Calories: 142 | Fat: 10.3 g | Protein: 1.6 g | Sodium: 378 mg | Fiber: 0.9 g | Carbohydrates: 11.6 g | Sugar: 3.4 g

Chocolate-Covered Peanut Butter Balls

Say goodbye to cholesterol-laden peanut butter balls, and say hello to these veganized peanut butter balls covered in rich chocolate.

INGREDIENTS | MAKES 120 BALLS

3 cups creamy peanut butter, softened
1 cup dairy-free margarine, softened
5 cups powdered sugar
2 cups dairy-free chocolate chips
2 tablespoons coconut oil

1. Stir together peanut butter and margarine in a large bowl until well blended. Stir in powdered sugar.

2. Cover and refrigerate peanut butter mixture until firm enough to roll into balls, about 20 minutes.

3. Roll firmed peanut butter mixture into 120 bite-sized balls. Place on two parchment-lined baking sheets and refrigerate about 30 minutes.

4. Stir chocolate chips and coconut oil together in a small microwave-safe bowl. Microwave 1 minute. Cover and set aside 1 minute. Chocolate should be melted. Stir until well blended and smooth.

5. Use a fork to dip peanut butter balls in chocolate, tapping off excess chocolate. Lay chocolate-covered balls back on lined baking sheets. Refrigerate until chocolate coating is firm, about 20 minutes.

6. Store balls in a large airtight container in refrigerator up to 14 days, or in freezer up to 3 months. To serve, put out at room temperature, or eat cold.

PER SERVING (1 ball) Calories: 84 | Fat: 5.3 g | Protein: 1.5 g | Sodium: 12 mg | Fiber: 0.6 g | Carbohydrates: 7.8 g | Sugar: 6.4 g

Carrot Cake

Make this vegan Carrot Cake recipe and watch it disappear. It's moist, delicious, and topped with vegan cream cheese frosting!

INGREDIENTS | SERVES 14

For Cake

3 cups all-purpose flour
2 cups granulated sugar
1/3 cup vanilla soy protein powder
1 teaspoon salt
1 teaspoon ground cinnamon
1 teaspoon pumpkin pie spice
2 teaspoons baking soda
1½ cups whole walnuts, divided
2/3 cup vegetable oil
2 cups cold water
2 tablespoons apple cider vinegar
2 teaspoons vanilla extract
2 cups chopped peeled carrots

For Cream Cheese Frosting

1 (8-ounce) container vegan cream cheese
½ cup vegan butter
3 cups powdered sugar

1. Preheat oven to 350°F. Spray two 8" round cake pans with vegetable cooking spray.

2. **To make Cake:** in a large bowl combine flour, sugar, protein powder, salt, cinnamon, pumpkin pie spice, and baking soda. Set aside.

3. Place walnuts on an ungreased baking sheet and toast 5 minutes. Remove from oven and let cool about 5 minutes before chopping. Stir ½ chopped walnuts into flour mixture and set aside.

4. In a medium bowl combine vegetable oil, water, vinegar, and vanilla. Set aside.

5. Add chopped carrots to a food processor and pulse several times to shred. Pour shredded carrots into vegetable oil mixture. Stir to combine. Stir into flour mixture, then pour into prepared cake pans.

6. Bake 35 minutes until a toothpick inserted in center comes out clean. Remove from oven and allow cakes to cool 10 minutes before inverting onto a serving plate. Once inverted, allow cakes to cool completely, about 20 minutes.

7. **To make Cream Cheese Frosting:** combine vegan cream cheese and vegan butter in a medium mixing bowl until light and fluffy. Stir in powdered sugar ½ cup at a time.

8. Ice top of one cake with frosting. Top with ½ remaining chopped walnuts. Place second cake on top. Cover top and sides of cake with remaining frosting. Garnish with remaining chopped walnuts.

9. Store cake in a lidded cake container at room temperature up to 3 days, refrigerate up to 10 days, or freeze up to 3 months. To serve, allow slices to come to room temperature.

PER SERVING Calories: 551 | Fat: 23.8 g | Protein: 6.6 g | Sodium: 542 mg | Fiber: 2.1 g | Carbohydrates: 78.1 g | Sugar: 52.0 g

Pecan Pie

Everyone's favorite pie has been veganized. With simple ingredients and easy-to-follow instructions, you'll be enjoying this pie in no time!

INGREDIENTS | SERVES 8

For Pie Crust

2½ cups all-purpose flour, divided

1 teaspoon salt

2 tablespoons granulated sugar

1 (8-tablespoon) stick vegan butter, sliced

4 tablespoons vegetable shortening, cut into pieces

¼ cup cold vodka

¼ cup cold water

For Pie Filling

5 tablespoons vegan butter

1 cup packed light brown sugar

¾ cup corn syrup

4 tablespoons cornstarch

½ teaspoon salt

2 tablespoons light rum

1 teaspoon vanilla extract

1 cup silken tofu

2 cups whole pecans, toasted

1 container Reddi-wip Non-Dairy Almond whipped topping

1. Preheat oven to 350°F.

2. **To make Pie Crust:** pour 1½ cups flour, salt, and sugar into a food processor and pulse until combined, about 2 seconds. Add vegan butter and process until just combined. Add shortening and pulse until dough collects in clumps, about 15 seconds. Add remaining cup flour and pulse six times until mixture is evenly distributed. Empty mixture into a medium bowl.

3. Sprinkle cold vodka over dough and mix until combined. Add water, 1 tablespoon at a time, until dough is slightly tacky and sticks together.

4. Divide dough into 2 balls and flatten each into a 4" disk. Wrap each in plastic wrap and refrigerate at least 30 minutes, up to 5 days or freeze up to 1 month.

5. Roll 1 chilled crust to about ⅛" thickness and place in an ungreased 9" pie pan. Crimp edges of pie and use a fork to prick bottom of crust several times. Bake crust 20 minutes until golden brown. Remove from oven and set aside to cool during next step.

6. **To make Pie Filling:** in a medium saucepan combine vegan butter, brown sugar, corn syrup, and cornstarch. Cook over medium heat until comes to a boil, then reduce to a simmer over medium-low heat and cook 1 minute. Add salt, rum, and vanilla and stir to combine. Set aside.

7. In a food processor add silken tofu and pulse until smooth. Add corn syrup mixture and pulse again until combined. Add pecans (reserving 20) and stir. Pour mixture into pie dish and arrange reserved pecans on top.

8. Place a baking sheet on bottom rack of oven and place pie on sheet. Bake 1 hour until edges of pie are set. The center may still be a little jiggly. Remove from oven and let cool about 30 minutes.

9. Cover and store at room temperature up to 3 days, refrigerate up to 10 days, or cut slices and freeze up to 3 months. To serve, allow to come to room temperature and serve with whipped topping.

PER SERVING Calories: 731 | Fat: 34.3 g | Protein: 8.9 g | Sodium: 452 mg | Fiber: 3.5 g | Carbohydrates: 93.0 g | Sugar: 56.7 g

Southern Peach Cobbler

This easy vegan Southern Peach Cobbler is spiced with ginger and cinnamon on a buttery crust.

INGREDIENTS | SERVES 8

½ cup vegan butter
1½ cups granulated sugar, divided
1 tablespoon molasses
¼ teaspoon dried ginger
¼ teaspoon ground cinnamon
4 cups sliced peeled peaches
1 cup all-purpose flour
2 teaspoons baking powder
¼ teaspoon salt
1 cup plain soy milk
1 teaspoon apple cider vinegar

1. Preheat oven to 350°F.

2. Place vegan butter in a 13" × 9" baking dish. Place in heated oven 30 seconds until butter is melted. Remove from oven and set aside.

3. In a large bowl add ½ cup sugar, molasses, ginger, and cinnamon. Stir to combine. Add peaches and stir gently until peaches are coated. Set aside.

4. In a separate large bowl stir together flour, remaining 1 cup sugar, baking powder, and salt. Set aside.

5. In a small bowl combine soy milk and vinegar. Pour into flour mixture and stir until just combined. Pour batter over melted butter in dish. Spoon peaches over batter, being sure to distribute evenly across batter.

6. Bake 45 minutes until golden brown on top. Set aside to cool 20 minutes.

7. Cover and refrigerate up to 7 days. To serve, cook individual slices in a microwave in 30-second increments until heated through.

PER SERVING Calories: 297 | Fat: 5.4 g | Protein: 3.2 g | Sodium: 288 mg | Fiber: 1.8 g | Carbohydrates: 60.0 g | Sugar: 46.0 g

Oreo Cheesecake

*Get out your forks for this vegan Oreo Cheesecake with a cookie crust
and cookies throughout. Be prepared for awesome!*

INGREDIENTS | SERVES 12

For Pie Crust
25 Oreo Chocolate Sandwich Cookies
2 tablespoons coconut oil

For Cheesecake Filling
½ cup cashews
1 (15-ounce) can unsweetened coconut milk
2 (14-ounce) containers vegan cream cheese
1 (12-ounce) container firm silken tofu, pressed
1 cup granulated sugar
3 tablespoons cornstarch
½ cup vegan butter
1 tablespoon vanilla extract
¼ cup all-purpose flour
24 Oreo Chocolate Sandwich Cookies, roughly chopped, divided
2 cups water

1. **To make Pie Crust:** place cookies in a food processor and pulse until cookies resemble a crumbly flour. Add coconut oil and pulse another 2 seconds to combine. Press crust into an ungreased 8" springform pan. Set aside.

2. Preheat oven to 350°F.

3. **To make Cheesecake Filling:** place cashews and coconut milk in same food processor. Pulse 3 seconds to break down cashews. Push down any ingredients that might have risen to top of bowl. Pulse 1 minute until smooth and creamy. Add cream cheese and tofu and pulse again 1 minute until smooth and creamy.

4. Add sugar, cornstarch, vegan butter, vanilla, and flour. Pulse 1 minute until creamy. Add 12 chopped cookies and pulse to combine. Pour cheesecake filling into prepared crust and spread remaining chopped cookies over top. Wrap bottom of pan in foil.

5. Place cheesecake in a roasting pan and pour water into roasting pan. Place in oven and bake 1 hour. Then turn oven off and continue baking another 1 hour. Remove from oven.

6. Let cheesecake cool completely about 30 minutes, then cover and refrigerate up to 10 days or slice and freeze up to 3 months. To serve, allow to come to room temperature.

PER SERVING Calories: 681 | Fat: 42.2 g | Protein: 9.1 g | Sodium: 777 mg | Fiber: 1.7 g | Carbohydrates: 70.1 g | Sugar: 37.3 g

Chocolate Cheesecake with Raspberries

This vegan Chocolate Cheesecake with Raspberries may just be your new favorite dessert! Creamy layers of vanilla and chocolate cheesecake are topped with more chocolate.

INGREDIENTS | SERVES 12

For Pie Crust

25 Oreo Chocolate Sandwich Cookies

¼ cup coconut oil, softened

For Cheesecake Filling

2 (8-ounce) containers vegan cream cheese

½ cup cashews

1 (12-ounce) package silken tofu, pressed

1 cup granulated sugar

¼ cup all-purpose flour

⅓ cup cocoa powder

1½ teaspoons vanilla extract

2 cups water

For Chocolate Topping

1 cup dairy-free chocolate chips

¼ cup unsweetened almond milk

1 cup fresh raspberries

1. Preheat oven to 350°F.

2. **To make Pie Crust:** add cookies to a food processor. Pulse until crumbly. Add coconut oil and pulse again to combine. Press mixture into bottom of an ungreased 8" × 3" springform pan and refrigerate about 10 minutes.

3. **To make Cheesecake Filling:** add vegan cream cheese and cashews to food processor. Pulse about 1 minute until cashews are relatively smooth. Add tofu, sugar, flour, cocoa powder, and vanilla. Pulse again until combined and smooth, about 1 minute. Pour filling into prepared crust. Wrap bottom of pan in foil.

4. Place cheesecake in a roasting pan and pour water into roasting pan. Place in oven and bake 1 hour. Then turn oven off and continue baking another 1 hour. Remove from oven and let cool completely about 40 minutes.

5. **To make Chocolate Topping:** place chocolate chips in a small microwave-safe bowl with almond milk. Stir to coat all chips. Microwave 60 seconds, then stir. Drizzle over top of cooled cheesecake.

6. Top cheesecake with fresh raspberries, cover, and refrigerate at least 3 hours, up to 10 days. You can also freeze individual slices (without raspberries) up to 3 months once cake has been refrigerated 3 hours. To serve, allow slices to come to room temperature.

PER SERVING Calories: 491 | Fat: 28.3 g | Protein: 6.5 g | Sodium: 407 mg | Fiber: 3.6 g | Carbohydrates: 55.3 g | Sugar: 33.6 g

Two-Week Vegan Meal Plan

The following meal plans can be used as a starting point to help
you develop your own vegan meal plans in the future.

Week One

Day One
Breakfast: Peanut Butter Overnight Oats
(Chapter 3)
Lunch: Vegan Egg Salad Sandwiches (Chapter 9)
Dinner: Vegan Chick'n Taquitos (Chapter 9)

Day Two
Breakfast: Green Tea Banana Smoothie
(Chapter 5)
Lunch: Sweet Potato Black Bean Burgers
(Chapter 9)
Dinner: Pinto Bean Soup (Chapter 10)

Day Three
Breakfast: Leftover Peanut Butter Overnight Oats
(Chapter 3)
Lunch: Leftover Vegan Egg Salad Sandwiches
(Chapter 9)
Dinner: Vegan Taco Casserole (Chapter 17)

Day Four
Breakfast: Piña Colada Green Smoothie
(Chapter 5)
Lunch: Leftover Pinto Bean Soup (Chapter 10)
Dinner: Leftover Vegan Chick'n Taquitos (Chapter 9)

Day Five
Breakfast: Chocolate Peanut Butter Protein
Smoothie (Chapter 5)
Lunch: Leftover Vegan Taco Casserole
(Chapter 17)
Dinner: Basic Vegan Pepperoni Pizza (Chapter 13)

Day Six
Breakfast: Easy Vegan Biscuits and Gravy
(Chapter 3)
Lunch: Vegan Caesar Salad (Chapter 6)
Dinner: Ultimate Veggie Burgers (Chapter 9)

Day Seven
Breakfast: Banana Pancakes (Chapter 3)
Lunch: Leftover Basic Vegan Pepperoni Pizza
(Chapter 13)
Dinner: Leftover Vegan Taco Casserole
(Chapter 17)

Week Two

Day One
Breakfast: Easy Vegan Tofu Scramble
(Chapter 3)
Lunch: Vegan Tuna Salad Sandwiches
(Chapter 9)
Dinner: Vegan Cheeseburger Soup
(Chapter 10)

Day Two
Breakfast: Blueberry Overnight Oats
(Chapter 3)
Lunch: Freezer-Ready Vegan Club
Sandwiches (Chapter 9)
Dinner: Easy Vegan Lasagna (Chapter 13)

Day Three
Breakfast: Leftover Banana Pancakes
(Chapter 3)
Lunch: Leftover Vegan Cheeseburger Soup
(Chapter 10)
Dinner: Vegan Beef Stroganoff (Chapter 17)

Day Four
Breakfast: Blueberry Smoothie (Chapter 5)
Lunch: Leftover Easy Vegan Lasagna
(Chapter 13)
Dinner: Leftover Vegan Cheeseburger Soup
(Chapter 10)

Day Five
Breakfast: Basic Green Smoothie (Chapter 5)
Lunch: Leftover Freezer-Ready Vegan Club
Sandwiches (Chapter 9)
Dinner: Vegan Cobb Salad (Chapter 6)

Day Six
Breakfast: Whole-Wheat Vegan Waffles
(Chapter 3)
Lunch: One Pot Vegan Mac and Cheese
(Chapter 12)
Dinner: Crispy Orange Tofu (Chapter 17)

Day Seven
Breakfast: Chocolate Glazed Baked Donuts
(Chapter 3)
Lunch: Leftover Vegan Beef Stroganoff
(Chapter 17)
Dinner: Baked Nachos (Chapter 17)

APPENDIX B:

Vegan Shopping Guide

Accidentally Vegan Products

Life Cereal

Quaker Old Fashioned, Instant, and Steel Cut Oatmeal

Quaker Puffed Rice cereal

Guittard Semisweet Chocolate Baking Chips

Chick-O-Stick

Nabisco Oreo Cones

Airheads Bars Chewy Fruit Candy

Cracker Jack Original Caramel Coated Popcorn & Peanuts

Fritos Original Corn Chips

Lays Classic Potato Chips

Ritz Crackers Original

Wheat Thins Original

Hershey's Chocolate Syrup

Jell-O Cook & Serve Pudding & Pie Filling

Duncan Hines Classic Yellow Cake Mix

Duncan Hines Creamy Home-Style Frosting: Classic Chocolate, Vanilla, Caramel, Coconut Pecan, Dark Chocolate Fudge, Lemon Supreme, Strawberry Cream, and Homestyle Butter Cream

Smucker's Marshmallow Flavored Spoonable Ice Cream Topping

McCormick Bac'n Pieces Bacon Flavored Bits

Pillsbury Grands! Southern Homestyle Buttermilk Biscuits

Pillsbury Original Crescent Rolls

Pop-Tarts: Unfrosted Strawberry and Unfrosted Blueberry

Pepperidge Farm Puff Pastry Sheets

Nutter Butter Peanut Butter Sandwich Cookies

Nabisco Grahams Original

Teddy Grahams Chocolatey Chip

Sara Lee Cherry Pie

Standard US/Metric Measurement Conversions

VOLUME CONVERSIONS	
US Volume Measure	Metric Equivalent
⅛ teaspoon	0.5 milliliter
¼ teaspoon	1 milliliter
½ teaspoon	2 milliliters
1 teaspoon	5 milliliters
½ tablespoon	7 milliliters
1 tablespoon (3 teaspoons)	15 milliliters
2 tablespoons (1 fluid ounce)	30 milliliters
¼ cup (4 tablespoons)	60 milliliters
⅓ cup	80 milliliters
½ cup (4 fluid ounces)	125 milliliters
⅔ cup	160 milliliters
¾ cup (6 fluid ounces)	180 milliliters
1 cup (16 tablespoons)	250 milliliters
1 pint (2 cups)	500 milliliters
1 quart (4 cups)	1 liter (about)

WEIGHT CONVERSIONS	
US Weight Measure	Metric Equivalent
½ ounce	15 grams
1 ounce	30 grams
2 ounces	60 grams
3 ounces	85 grams
¼ pound (4 ounces)	115 grams
½ pound (8 ounces)	225 grams
¾ pound (12 ounces)	340 grams
1 pound (16 ounces)	454 grams

OVEN TEMPERATURE CONVERSIONS	
Degrees Fahrenheit	Degrees Celsius
200 degrees F	95 degrees C
250 degrees F	120 degrees C
275 degrees F	135 degrees C
300 degrees F	150 degrees C
325 degrees F	160 degrees C
350 degrees F	180 degrees C
375 degrees F	190 degrees C
400 degrees F	205 degrees C
425 degrees F	220 degrees C
450 degrees F	230 degrees C

BAKING PAN SIZES	
American	Metric
8 × 1½ inch round baking pan	20 × 4 cm cake tin
9 × 1½ inch round baking pan	23 × 3.5 cm cake tin
11 × 7 × 1½ inch baking pan	28 × 18 × 4 cm baking tin
13 × 9 × 2 inch baking pan	30 × 20 × 5 cm baking tin
2 quart rectangular baking dish	30 × 20 × 3 cm baking tin
15 × 10 × 2 inch baking pan	38 × 25 × 5 cm baking tin (Swiss roll tin)
9 inch pie plate	22 × 4 or 23 × 4 cm pie plate
7 or 8 inch springform pan	18 or 20 cm springform or loose bottom cake tin
9 × 5 × 3 inch loaf pan	23 × 13 × 7 cm or 2 lb narrow loaf or pâté tin
1½ quart casserole	1.5 liter casserole
2 quart casserole	2 liter casserole

Index

Note: Page numbers in **bold** indicate recipe category lists.

Vanilla Strawberry Lime Smoothie, 70
Vegan diet
    about: meal prep and, 6 (*See also*
        Meal prepping); overview of, 9–10
    accidental vegans and, 11
    benefits of, 11–14
    cancer risk reduction with, 13–14
    foods not eaten in, 10
    heart health and, 13
    "secular" vegans and, 10
    weight loss and, 12
Vegetables. *See also specific vegetables*
    about: buying frozen, 18; buying
        organic, 19–20; Dirty Dozen Plus,
        20
    Roasted Root Vegetables, 105
    Vegan Jambalaya, 180
    Vegan Pasta Primavera, 208
Veggie burgers. *See* Burgers,
    sandwiches, and wraps
Vodka, baking with, 252

Waffles, 34–35
Weekend gourmet meals, **279**–307
Weight loss, vegan diet and, 12, 24
Whole-wheat flours and breads, 34, 46
Wild Rice and Sweet Potato Skillet
    Dinner, 178

Yeast, working with, 49. *See also*
    Breads, biscuits, muffins, and pastries

Zucchini and zoodles. *See* Squash
    (including zucchini)

Meal Prep for Every Diet Need!

Pick Up or Download Your Copies Today!

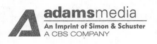
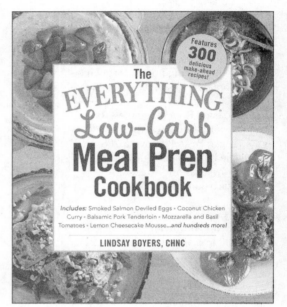

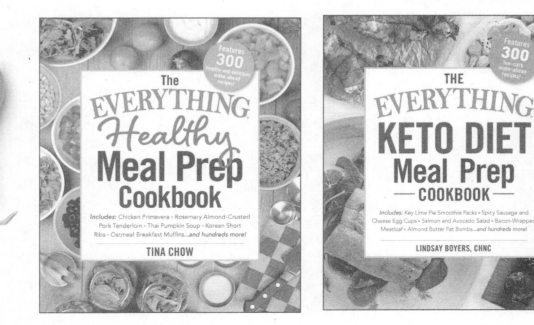